Chest Pain

Advanced assessment and management skills

Edited by

John W. Albarran and Jenny Tagney

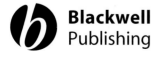

© 2007 by Blackwell Publishing

Blackwell Publishing editorial offices:
Blackwell Publishing Ltd, 9600 Garsington Road, Oxford OX4 2DQ, UK
Tel: +44 (0)1865 776868
Blackwell Publishing Inc., 350 Main Street, Malden, MA 02148-5020, USA
Tel: +1 781 388 8250
Blackwell Publishing Asia Pty Ltd, 550 Swanston Street, Carlton, Victoria 3053, Australia
Tel: +61 (0)3 8359 1011

The right of the Author to be identified as the Author of this Work has been asserted in
accordance with the Copyright, Designs and Patents Act 1988.

First published 2007 by Blackwell Publishing Ltd

ISBN: 978-1-4051-4422-3

Library of Congress Cataloging-in-Publication Data
Chest pain : advanced assessment and management skills / edited by
John W. Albarran and Jenny Tagney.
p. ; cm.
Includes bibliographical references and index.
ISBN: 978-1-4051-4422-3 (pbk. : alk. paper)
1. Chest pain.   2. Coronary heart disease–Diagnosis.   3. Diagnosis,
Differential.   I. Albarran, John W.   II. Tagney, Jenny.
[DNLM: 1. Chest Pain–diagnosis.   2. Chest Pain–therapy.
3. Medical History Taking–methods.   4. Physical Examination–methods.
WF 970 C5257 2007]
RC941.C444 2007
616.1′23075–dc22
2006024263

A catalogue record for this title is available from the British Library

Set in 10/12.5 pt Palatino
by SNP Best-set Typesetter Ltd., Hong Kong
Printed and bound in Singapore
by C.O.S. Printers Pte Ltd

The publisher's policy is to use permanent paper from mills that operate a sustainable forestry
policy, and which has been manufactured from pulp processed using acid-free and elementary
chlorine-free practices. Furthermore, the publisher ensures that the text paper and cover board
used have met acceptable environmental accreditation standards.

For further information on Blackwell Publishing, visit our website:
www.blackwellpublishing.com

We dedicate this book to the memory of
Lara Charmaine Albarran
(1984–2005)

She was, and still is, her parents' special princess

Contents

Foreword

I was delighted to be asked by John Albarran and Jenny Tagney to write the Foreword to this excellent book. Their knowledge and expertise within this field is well known and they have drawn together an excellent list of contributors right across the spectrum of cardiac care.

The treatment of patients presenting with chest pain has seen huge improvement over the past six years since the National Service Framework for Coronary Heart Disease was published in March 2000. This set a standard to treat people suffering from heart attack with thrombolytic drugs within an hour of them calling for professional help. The story is one of enormous change; before the NSF less than a quarter of patients suffering myocardial infarction received thrombolytic therapy within one hour of calling for expert help, today just over 60% do. This was achieved by the hard work and innovations in care delivered by NHS staff. These advances increased the demands on nurses and paramedics working with this group of patients; both have met the challenge.

Notable changes include expanded roles for nurses in the acute care setting; the role of 'chest pain or thrombolysis' specialist nurse is well established. A significant percentage of thrombolytic treatment is now given pre-hospital by paramedics, and rapid access chest pain clinics have been a great success with 98% of all patients now seen within 14 days of referral. Additionally primary angioplasty services for the treatment of myocardial infarction are now coming on stream and there is a project looking at the feasibility of delivering this across the country. These are all excellent examples of how services can be re-designed to speed up the patient journey and improve outcomes.

Jenny Tagney and John Albarran have produced a comprehensive guide to the diagnosis and treatment of the patient presenting with chest pain of medical or surgical origin. We know that speed to treatment is critical for saving lives and to quality of life for survivors, whether the cause is amenable to medical or surgical treatment.

This book will be of great use to nurses, cardiac physiologists, paramedics and other allied health professionals working with patients with chest pain. It will be a welcome addition and resource across both acute hospital, ambulance and primary care settings.

Maree Barnett RN MSc MBA
Deputy Branch Head Vascular programme / Nurse advisor
Department of Health

Acknowledgements

The editors would like to begin by thanking all our colleagues and friends for their time in proof-reading, making suggested editing changes and offering what was always helpful, constructive, detailed and wise advice.

We would like to particularly thank Jane Wathen, graphic designer, for her creative talents and advice in developing some of the images used in this textbook.

The editors would also like to extend their gratitude to the following:

- Blackwell Publishing for permission to reproduce images from *Physical Assessment for Nurses* (Cox 2004), *The ABC of Upper Gastrointestinal Tract* (Logan et al. 2002) and *Pocket Consultant: Gastroenterology* (Travis et al. 2005)
- BMJ publishing group for permission to reproduce a figure from the journal *Gut*

Contributors

John W. Albarran, MSc, PG Dip Ed (H/E), BSc (Hons), Dip N, RN, NFESC
Principal Lecturer in Critical Care Nursing, University of the West of England, Bristol

Jonathan R. Benger, MD, FRCS, DA, DCH, Dip IMC, FCEM
Consultant in Emergency Medicine, United Bristol Healthcare Trust, and Senior Research Fellow, University of the West of England, Bristol

Simon Binks, BMedSci, BM BS, MRCPCH, MCEM
Specialist Registrar in Emergency Medicine, Department of Accident and Emergency, Cheltenham General Hospital

Helen Cox, MA, BSc (Hons) RN
Senior Lecturer in Cardiac Nursing, University of the West of England, Bristol

Theresa M.D. Finlay, MSc, PG Dip Ed (H/E), BSc (Hons), RN
Senior Lecturer, Oxford Brookes University

Sarah Green, MSc, BSc (Hons), RN
Sister, Coronary Care Unit, Bristol Royal Infirmary, United Bristol Healthcare Trust

Rebecca Hoskins, MA, BSc (Hons), RN, FFEN
Nurse Consultant in Emergency Care, United Bristol Hospital Trust, and Senior Lecturer in Emergency Care, University of the West of England, Bristol

Jan Keenan, MSc, PG Dip Ed (H/E), RN
Nurse Consultant in Cardiac Medicine, Oxford Radcliffe Hospitals NHS Trust

Tom Quinn, MPhil, FESC, FRCN, RN
Professor of Cardiac Nursing and Consultant Cardiac Nurse, Coventry University

Jenny Tagney, MSc, BSc (Hons), RN, NFESC
Nurse Consultant in Cardiology, Bristol Royal Infirmary, United Bristol Healthcare Trust

Jackie Younker, MSN, PG Cert (H/E), RN
Senior Lecturer, University of the West of England, Bristol

Section 1
Principles of assessment and diagnosis

Chapter 1

Background to the assessment and management of patients with chest pain – using this book

John W. Albarran and Jenny Tagney

'Here I am dying of a hundred good symptoms'
Alexander Pope

Introduction

Chest pain is one of the most common reasons for people to seek healthcare advice within primary and secondary care settings in Europe and North America (Cayley 2005). However, skills and knowledge required to undertake thorough assessment and differentiation of the numerous alternative presentations of chest pain, particularly with regard to triaging potentially life-threatening conditions, remain elusive. A number of studies have reported that between 5 and 30% of patients are discharged with evidence of coronary heart disease (CHD) (Chan et al. 1998; Pope et al. 2000).

As far back as 1768, the physician Heberden produced a concise but influential account of angina pectoris based on observations of 100 patients. Heberden observed that many of these patients were often *'seized with a most disagreeable sensation in the breast while walking, which would seem to take their life away';* these symptoms would disappear with rest. Heberden also recorded that the majority of patients were generally overweight men, older than 50 years of age, and typically the victims of sudden death.

Today, CHD is the leading cause of morbidity and mortality among men and women in the United Kingdom (UK) and other developed nations. Due to the large numbers of patients affected and the burden on the National Health Service, a number of policy initiatives have been implemented to increase access to services and improve health outcomes. For example, many hospitals have introduced chest pain assessment units and rapid access chest pain clinics (RACPCs) and, subsequently, new posts have emerged to provide an efficient and cost-effective service that meets the needs of patients (Department of Health (DH) 2004; Goodacre et al. 2004; Pottle 2005). Fox (2005) adds that any successful strategy seeking to decrease the burden of resource misuse is inherently dependent on the effective assessment and management of patients. Without this

3

clinical expertise, demand for expensive investigations increases, resulting in a sizeable proportion of healthcare funds being unnecessarily consumed. Since many healthcare professionals, regardless of setting, have to deal with patients suffering from acute, discrete or chronic forms of chest pain, it is important that their physical assessment and diagnostic skills, as well as use of clinical interventions, are informed by a strong evidence base.

Challenges in accurately assessing chest pain

Central chest pain is the most common presenting symptom of coronary heart disease and it is characterised by radiation to the arms, shoulders, neck or jaw (Cooper et al. 2000; Fox 2005). Additional features may include feelings of tightness, constriction or heaviness across the chest that occur following exercise or during rest and that are relieved by sublingual nitrates. Complaints of chest pain represent between 20 and 30% of all medical admissions and, of these, only a third will be diagnosed as having an acute coronary syndrome (Capewell and Quinney 2001; Jowett and Thompson 2003). Likewise, of those who are seen in RACPCs, over two-thirds present without a cardiac cause (Fox 2005). In Pottle's (2005) study of 454 patients, 66.4% of those presenting at a RACPC had 'atypical' chest pain. Presentations of acute, undifferentiated chest pain are thus a common occurrence and a challenge for busy clinicians. However, the rapid identification of non-cardiac and non-life-threatening conditions may assist in ensuring that only those in need of hospital beds have immediate access. Establishing a diagnosis of CHD is not straightforward, as different conditions presenting with pain in the chest mimic cardiac ischaemia and other conditions. Reasons for inaccurate assessment are many and varied. For example, the distribution of nerve endings within the thorax often makes the interpretation of cardiac symptoms more difficult for the patient and examiner.

Hedges et al. (1995) identified a number of factors that are still relevant today, which illustrate the common problems in the evaluation of chest pain symptoms. These relate to:

- Age of patient: younger patients tend to have more missed diagnoses particularly in respect to myocardial infarction (MI), especially when their primary symptom is not chest pain but breathlessness (Pope et al. 2000).
- Presence of indigestion: in most cases the differences between cardiac and oesophageal pain can be discerned clinically although this is problematic in 20% of instances (Bennett 2001).
- Presence of sharp pain and chest wall tenderness: as many as 20% of patients with MI may present with sharp or pleuritic pain, which is often more characteristic of respiratory or pulmonary conditions. Moreover, Albarran et al. (2001) reported that patients with MI and those without MI use similar sensory and affective terms during their chest pain symptoms.
- Normal and non-specific electrocardiograms (ECGs): one of the difficulties is that the classic ECG features of MI may be missed due to the transient nature

of evolving ischaemia or absent in a proportion of patients (Adams et al. 1993). A small number of patients with either cardiac syndrome X or vasospastic angina may also have ECG features that can confuse the diagnosis and delay decision making (Chan et al. 1998).

- Gender differences: it is increasingly acknowledged that, with regard to CHD, women present with subtle and less specific symptoms than men with this disease (Albarran et al. 2002; McSweeney et al. 2005; Albarran et al. in press).
- Patient-orientated issues: some patients are poor at explaining their symptoms or may even trivialise the level of discomfort and others may deny they are unwell. In patients who do not speak English, the problems of obtaining a clear history are exacerbated and cultural differences in illness perceptions and pain tolerance may further confound information gathering.
- Interviewing skills: a lack of effective questioning techniques, listening skills and systematic clinical assessment framework can impact on the quality of data gained to contribute towards an informed diagnosis (Albarran 2002).

As misdiagnosis can occur in around 30% of all chest pain presentations, acute beds may be inappropriately occupied, leading to an overuse of expensive resources. The European Society of Cardiology (Erhardt et al. 2002) has produced international guidelines to support more effective diagnostic decision making in patients with chest pain.

Chest pain assessment units and emerging roles

Recent health service reforms are consistent in promoting the idea that all patients should receive care at the right time, in the right place by a suitably qualified person with the right skills (Thompson and Stewart 2002; Fox 2005). This may not always be a physician: indeed it may be a nurse, a physiotherapist or a registered paramedic. This shift in thinking is partly in response to the new Working Time Directives, the reduction in junior doctors' hours and increased patient demand to achieve NHS targets for patients presenting with chest pain. The process of responding to patient need is considered to begin when patients first come into contact with emergency services. Paramedics are expected to perform an initial assessment of symptoms en route to hospital. Role expansion in this area means that paramedics are now trained to recognise differential causes of chest pain, to accurately interpret the results of a 12-lead electrocardiograph (ECG), make a preliminary diagnosis on the available findings and treat the patient according to local protocols (Joint Royal Colleges Ambulance Liaison Committee 2004).

If an MI is not confirmed by the preliminary ECG, patients may be triaged within a hospital chest pain assessment unit. These units are equipped to undertake a rapid and accurate assessment of patients suspected of having acute coronary syndromes or other life-threatening illness, thus promoting outcomes of survival and recovery (Capewell and Quinney 2000; Goodacre et al. 2000, 2004).

Conversely, patients with milder symptoms may present to their General Practitioner (GP) or at a NHS walk-in centre and are then referred to a RACPC (Ryan et al. 2002; Pottle 2005). These services are often nurse-led, providing exercise testing facilities and access to other investigations that can be performed on the same day. Many senior nurses and some cardiac physiologists have become involved in establishing and running RACPCs, as have GPs developing a specialist interest in cardiology.

This concept of role redesign is seen as the way forward in facilitating expansion and development in healthcare (*New Ways of Working*, DH 2003). Accountability is an issue central to the expansion of new clinical roles, whether nurses, paramedics or cardiac physiologists. Practitioners must therefore be equipped with a blend of theory and skills to perform their responsibilities to the highest level of competency and safety. An ability to respond promptly and efficiently to symptom reports will greatly enhance their patients' chances of survival. This remit is likely to expand to other areas of hospital care as the traditional role of coronary care units is being re-evaluated (Quinn et al. 2005). This has been driven as a result of advances in pharma-cology, technology, workforce re-engineering and redefining of professional boundaries.

Competency

Nationally, there is increasing emphasis on the need for healthcare practitioners to broaden their skill base and expand areas of competency (DH 2000, 2005). Within the UK, documents such as *Liberating the Talents* (DH 2002) and *New Ways of Working* (DH 2003) aim to modernise the delivery of healthcare and achieve the targets of the NHS Plan. This is to be achieved by enabling the most appropriately equipped and trained healthcare professionals to provide the right care at the right time. Redesigning roles and organisational structures will give clinicians greater freedom in expanding their knowledge and skill base.

In response to the challenges presented by patients with chest pain associated with ischaemic heart disease, a *Coronary Heart Disease Competence Framework* (Skills for Health 2005) has also been launched. The focus is to enable healthcare professionals to develop competence in the areas of assessment, diagnosis and action planning in relation to CHD. It offers standards for benchmarking competency levels, courses and learning materials. The framework is structured around three workforce competencies that must be achieved:

- Contribute to assessing individuals with suspected CHD.
- Examine and assess individuals with suspected CHD and produce a diagnosis.
- Develop and agree a treatment plan with individuals diagnosed with CHD.

This textbook can be used to support this agenda and related objectives. It is directed at those health professionals who have to differentiate whether the presenting chest pain symptoms are life-threatening, regardless of whether they are in a home or community setting, hospital out-patient clinic, emergency department, GP practice or ward environment. The book is not intended as a step-by-step manual but as a reference text/resource to assist healthcare practitioners and students to expand their knowledge and skills, underpinned by an extensive evidence base.

Structure and aim of this book

In reviewing the conditions cited in this book, specialists would argue that some are often overlooked, misdiagnosed and mismanaged. Determining the cause of chest pain demands sleuthing skills as diagnoses do not arrive conveniently labelled. It is in connecting fragments of information and symptom cues that practitioners are able to establish underlying cause.

This book was conceived to enable practitioners to advance their practice by enhancing their intellectual and practical abilities. Specifically, the text aims to expand practitioners' knowledge and skills in order to enhance their competency in assessment, interpreting data, making a diagnosis, initiating treatment and managing the care of patients with undifferentiated chest pain conditions. Sparacino (1992) argues that these qualities are the hallmarks of advanced practice, which is achieved by incorporating a range of variables into the decision-making process, clinical judgements and actions.

In relation to the structure of the book, Section I comprises two distinct parts. Chapter 2 introduces current national policies relating to the strategic management of CHD. The other three chapters in this section form the foundation from which advanced knowledge and skill in assessment and management of patients with chest pain can develop in an integrated and logical manner. The focus is on learning how to perform a systematic clinical examination, taking a structured history, deciding on appropriate tests and investigations, and reviewing data obtained to reach a differential diagnosis in patients with chest pain. The underpinning principle is that treatment decisions depend very much on the quality of data gathered from the patient and whether it has been accurately interpreted. These chapters provide a structured format, which has been adopted throughout the book.

Section 2 deals with the advanced assessment and management of patients attending with specific conditions in which acute chest pain is a key feature. A number of cardiac and non-cardiac conditions are discussed and examined in detail. Each chapter has been constructed with key headings to guide the reader in a systematic fashion. These include:

- Background (incidence, trends in morbidity and mortality)
- Causative factors
- Pathophysiological factors
- Clinical presentation
- History taking
- Clinical examination
- Initial investigations
- Differential diagnosis

- Immediate management and interventions
- Further investigations
- Medium- to long-term management plan
- Key learning points
- References and websites for additional information

The contributors have drawn from their extensive clinical expertise and from current literature to produce a uniquely informative text.

Service demands continue to shape practice developments in both European and North American healthcare systems. It is important that healthcare practitioners equip themselves with appropriate skills and knowledge to be able to effectively respond to and, if appropriate, lead these developments. The evolution of new clinical roles raises countless professional issues, whilst offering tremendous opportunities to redefine roles, autonomy and, ultimately, status (Humphris and Masterson 2000; Albarran 2006). This book offers practitioners a means to advance the art and science of their practice, facilitate care delivery and improve the outcomes of patients presenting with chest pain.

References

Adams J, Trent R, Rowles J (1993) Earliest electrocardiographic evidence of myocardial infarction: implications for thrombolysis treatment. *British Medical Journal* **307**: 409–413.

Albarran JW (2002) The language of chest pain. *Nursing Times* **98**(4): 38–40.

Albarran JW (2006) New roles in critical care practice. In: Scholes, J. (ed.) *Developing Expertise in Critical Care*. Oxford, Blackwell Publishing.

Albarran JW, Chappel G, Durham B, Gowers J, Dwight J (2001) Are specific verbal descriptors useful in differentiating those with and without MI? Findings from a two-year study. *Infermería Intensiva* **12**(4): 164–174.

Albarran JW, Durham B, Gowers J, Dwight J, Chappel G (2002) Is the radiation of chest pain a useful indicator of myocardial infarction? A prospective study of 541 patients. *Accident and Emergency Nursing* **10**(1): 2–9.

Albarran JW, Clarke B, Crawford J (In press) 'It was not chest pain really, I can't explain it!' – an exploratory study on the nature of symptoms experienced by women during their myocardial infarction. *Journal of Clinical Nursing*.

Bennett J (2001) Oesophagus: atypical chest pain and motility disorder. *British Medical Journal* **323**: 791–794.

Capewell S, Quinney D (2001) What future for pain observation units? *Journal of Accident and Emergency Medicine* **18**: 3–4.

Cayley WE (2005) Diagnosing the cause of chest pain. *American Family Physician* **72**(10): 2012–2021.

Chan WK, Leung KF, Lee YE, Hung CS, Kung NS, Lau FL (1998) Undiagnosed acute myocardial infarction in the accident and emergency department: reasons and implications. *European Journal of Emergency Medicine* **5**: 219–224.

Cooper A, Hodgkinson D, Oliver R (2000) Chest pain in the emergency department. *Hospital Medicine* **61**(3): 178–183.

Department of Health (2000) *National Service Framework for Coronary Artery Disease*. London, The Stationery Office.

Department of Health (2002) *Liberating the Talents: Helping Primary Care Trusts to Deliver the NHS Plan.* London, The Stationery Office.

Department of Health (2003) *New Ways of Working.* London, The Stationery Office.

Department of Health (2004) *Winning the War on Heart Disease.* London, The Stationery Office.

Department of Health (2005) *Coronary Heart Disease Competence Framework (Skills for Health).* http://www.skillsforhealth.org.uk/chd/minor_area.php?area=60 (accessed 20th March 2006).

Erhardt L, Herlitz J, Bossart L, Halinen M, Keltai M, Koster R, Marcassa C, Quinn T, van Weert H (2002) Task force on the management of chest pain. *European Heart Journal* **23**: 1153–1176.

Fox K (2005) Investigation and management of chest pain. *Heart* **91**: 105–110.

Goodacre S (2000) Should we establish chest pain observation units in the UK? A systematic review and critical appraisal of the literature. *Journal of Accident and Emergency Medicine* **17**: 1–6.

Goodacre S, Nicholl J, Dixon S, Cross E, Angelini K et al. (2004) Randomised controlled trial and economic evaluation of a chest pain observation unit compared to routine care. *British Medical Journal* **328**: 254–260.

Hedges JR (1995) Pitfalls in accident and emergency chest pain evaluation. *Journal of the Royal Society of Medicine* **88**: 524–527.

Humphris D, Masterson A (2000) *Developing New Clinical Roles. A Guide for Healthcare Professionals.* London, Churchill Livingstone.

Joint Royal Colleges Ambulance Liaison Committee (2004) *Clinical Practice Guidelines: For Use in UK Ambulance Services.* http://www.asancep.org.uk/JRCALC/guidelines/ (accessed 26th April 2006).

Jowett N, Thompson DR (2003) *Comprehensive Coronary Care* (3rd Edition). London, Bailliere Tindall.

McSweeney JC, Lefler LL, Crowder BF (2005) What's wrong with me? Women's coronary heart disease diagnostic experiences. *Progress in Cardiovascular Nursing* **20**(2): 48–57.

Pope J, Aufderheide T, Ruthazer R, Woolard R, Feldman J, Beshanski J, Griffith J, Selker H (2000) Missed diagnoses of acute cardiac ischaemia in the emergency department. *New England Journal of Medicine* **342**: 1163–1170.

Pottle A (2005) A nurse-led rapid access chest pain clinic – experience from the first 3 years. *European Journal of Cardiovascular Nursing* **4**(3): 227–233.

Quinn T, Weston C, Birkhead J, Walker L, Norris R, on behalf of the MINAP Steering Group (2005) Redefining the coronary care unit: an observational study of patients admitted to hospital in England and Wales in 2003. *Quarterly Journal of Medicine* **98**: 979–982.

Ryan J, Heyworth J, Eslick G, Coulshed D (2002) Rapid assessment of chest pain. *British Medical Journal* **324**: 422.

Skills for Health Framework (2005) *Coronary Heart Disease.* http://www.skillsforhealth.org.uk/view_framework.php?id=60 (accessed 10th June 2006).

Sparacino P (1992) Advanced practice: the clinical nurse specialist. *Nursing Practice* **5**(4): 2–4.

Thompson DR, Stewart S (2002) Nurse directed services: how can they be more effective? *European Journal of Cardiovascular Nursing* **1**(1): 7–10.

Chapter 2

Coronary heart disease, healthcare policy and evolution of chest pain assessment and management in the UK

Tom Quinn

Introduction

The publication of the National Service Framework (NSF) for Coronary Heart Disease (CHD) (Department of Health (DH) 2000a) represented something of a watershed in health policy generally, and cardiovascular care in particular, within the National Health Service (NHS) in England. Similar initiatives have been launched in Scotland (Scottish Executive Health Department 2002) and Wales (National Assembly for Wales 2001). On the whole the broad thrust of the NSF, which applies solely to England, is similar to those in the devolved administrations of the United Kingdom in setting clear national standards, based on the best available evidence, alongside an infrastructure intended to support implementation. Northern Ireland does not have an 'NSF equivalent' at the time of writing. Some clinicians are uncomfortable with this consequence of political devolution (Brooks et al. 2005; Norell and Jennings 2006).

Aims

This chapter discusses the development and implementation of the NSF in the context of assessment and management of patients with chest pain, setting the context for other chapters in this book. Ongoing evolutionary change in health policy in England will also be discussed, in relation in particular to proposals strengthening the commissioning function and shift the focus of NHS provision away from the dominance of hospital care nearer to the patient's home.

Learning outcomes

On completion of this chapter, the reader should be able to:

- Describe the rationale for development of the National Service Framework for coronary heart disease and Rapid Access Chest Pain Clinics.
- Appreciate the burden of cardiovascular diseases (CVDs) and chest pain on National Health Service expenditure.
- Discuss changes in related NHS policies in England.

Burden of cardiovascular disease

Almost two fifths (238,000) of all UK deaths in 2002 were attributed to CVD, with CHD alone accounting for 117,000 deaths: one in five deaths in men and one in six in women (BHF 2004). CVD deaths as a whole have steadily declined since the 1970s, with a reported 27% reduction in mortality from heart disease, stroke and related diseases in people aged less than 75 years of age since 1996 (DH 2005a).

UK morbidity data suggest that CHD prevalence is increasing and this seems to be particularly marked in people aged 75 or more. A recent analysis by Majeed and Aylin (2005) suggests that, by 2031:

- The number of cases of CHD will rise by 44% (to 3,190,000), and hospital admissions related to CHD will increase by 32% to 265,000.
- The number of people with heart failure will rise by 54% (to 1,303,000), hospital admissions increasing by 55% to 124,000.
- The number of people with atrial fibrillation will rise by 46% (to 1,093,000), hospital admissions increasing by 39% to 85,000.

For a discussion of the public health implications of increased levels of obesity, the 'metabolic syndrome' (Alberti et al. 2005) and type 2 diabetes, refer to Chapter 6.

The burden of chest pain and stable angina

Typically, an early manifestation of CHD is discomfort across the chest, which may or may not radiate to the arms, shoulders, neck or jaw (Cooper et al. 2000). The individual may experience tightness or heaviness in the chest following exercise or during rest in more advanced cases. However, diagnosis is not straightforward (Albarran 2002) as the presentation may mimic other conditions, leading to misdiagnosis.

Chest pain is a major burden on patients and the NHS, resulting in an estimated 634,000 primary care consultations (Stewart et al. 2003) and 700,000 emergency department attendances annually in England and Wales (Goodacre et al. 2005). Stable angina pectoris is a common condition in the UK, with an estimated 341,500 people presenting as new cases each year (BHF 2005). Incidence rises with age and is higher in men. Fewer than 2 million people in the UK are estimated to be living with angina (BHF 2005), although these data may underestimate the true burden in an ageing population since many studies excluded people over 75 years of age. The cost of caring for angina patients has been estimated to consume 1% of the total NHS budget (Stewart et al. 2003).

National standards: the National Service Framework (NSF)

Before publication of the NSF, the state of cardiovascular prevention and care in England was considered by many to be below the standard of other comparable Western countries. The UK as a whole had higher mortality and morbidity from

CHD. Mortality was falling at a slower rate than elsewhere and there was clear evidence from published national and international studies that access to specialist care, including coronary revascularisation, was lower than in other countries. There was also evidence of inequalities in accessing services in a so-called 'postcode lottery' within the NHS, with, for example, much higher rates of revascularisation in some more prosperous parts of the country than in other, more deprived areas where disease was often more prevalent. In the United States, CHD mortality rates of 170 per 100,000 population compared very favourably to the 231 per 100,000 reported in England and Wales, as did rates of angioplasty (339 US versus 38 England, per 100,000), coronary bypass operations (203 versus 47) and the number of cardiologists (5.8 versus 0.9) (Ayanian and Quinn 2001). Moreover, while the evidence base for treatment of CHD in both emergency and primary care settings was substantial, there was important evidence that uptake of high quality care into routine clinical practice was suboptimal. For example, comparative audits of the management of patients with MI showed unexplained variation in the time taken to administer thrombolytic treatment once patients had reached hospital, and use of secondary prevention treatments such as aspirin, beta-blockers and statins to reduce the risk of a further acute event was patchy (Bowker et al. 1996; Birkhead 1999). A mere third of emergency departments across the UK provided thrombolytic treatment (Hood et al. 1998), resulting in additional delays in starting treatment while the patient was transferred to the cardiac care unit (CCU). Decades of underinvestment in infrastructure for coronary revascularisation meant that waiting times for surgery were long – a reported median 175 days for routine surgery in Manchester being but one example. With an estimated 500 deaths annually on the UK waiting list for coronary bypass surgery, waiting times were considered a 'significant but potentially treatable contribution' to overall CHD mortality (Bridgewater 1999).

Professional societies (de Bono and Hopkins 1994; Thompson et al. 1996; Wood et al. 1998) and governments had published guidelines and policies in previous years in an attempt to improve care, but these seemed to have little effect on clinical practice. A new concerted effort was required if lives were be saved and the overall burden of CHD reduced.

The election of the Blair government in May 1997 heralded enormous changes in the NHS (Stevens 2004). The publication of the White Paper *The New NHS* set out New Labour's vision of a service where long waiting times were abolished and quality was improved. The reforms introduced clinical governance, more systematic use of evidence and better monitoring of process and outcome through clinical audit and a national inspectorate of health service quality. The White Paper *Saving lives: our healthier nation* set a target for a 40% reduction, over a 10-year period, in CVD deaths in people aged less than 75 in line with the observed downward trend in mortality.

National standards were set for key conditions (selected on the basis of burden of disease, evidence base and perceived quality of care) such as cancer and mental health, with CHD chosen because it was common, possibly preventable, with a robust evidence base for the key interventions and, as previously discussed, with evidence of suboptimal care. Further evidence-based guidance and technology appraisals focusing on specific treatments are from time to time published by the National Institute for Clinical Excellence (NICE, subsequently re-formed as the National Institute for Health and Clinical Excellence to encompass public health interventions) on a range of cardiovascular-related topics including hypertension, implantable cardioverter defibrillators, intracoronary stents, dual chamber pacing, thrombolytic treatment for acute myocardial infarction, secondary prophylaxis following myocardial infarction, chronic heart failure, clopidogrel and glycoprotein IIb/IIIa inhibitors, use of myocardial perfusion scintigraphy, and statins. The list is not exhaustive, and further information on NICE and the Health Technology Assessment Programme (also published systematic reviews on topics such as assessment of chest pain in primary care, and the provision, uptake and cost of cardiac rehabilitation in under-represented groups) can be found at the relevant websites (www.nice.org.uk and www. ncchta.org). Delivery of the NSF standards, NICE guidance and other aspects of care provided by NHS organisations would be assessed by a newly established Commission for Health Improvement, later reinvented as the Healthcare Commission. For the first time, hospital in-patients with CHD benchmark England would be surveyed to help benchmark quality of care (Jenkinson et al. 2002).

The development of the NSF took over two years. An expert reference group was appointed to advise ministers, comprising heart patients and their carers, cardiologists, cardiac surgeons, a cardiac nurse, general practitioners, emergency physicians and an ambulance chief executive, together with public health doctors, epidemiologists, health economists, health service managers and civil servants. That this reflected a wider view of CHD than solely the preserve of the cardiological specialist, and that tackling CHD required a concerted effort on a number of fronts (including action on the wider determinants of health such as child poverty, maternal health, and helping individuals to remain healthy by increasing physical activity and improving diet), was perhaps an important step in achieving recognition of the concept of 'the community as the ultimate coronary care unit'.

Following the launch of the NSF on 6th March 2000 by Prime Minister Tony Blair and Secretary of State Alan Milburn, alongside cardiologist Dr Roger Boyle (newly appointed as national director for heart disease to provide clinical leadership for the implementation of the 10-year programme), CHD was firmly established as a priority area across government. The publication of the 10-year NHS Plan (DH 2000b) four months later reconfirmed key 'immediate priority' milestones for delivery of the NSF including the establishment of Rapid Access Chest Pain Clinics (RACPCs), increased revascularisation capacity and faster treatment including, where necessary, pre-hospital thrombolysis delivered by paramedics. Smoking cessation was given high priority as a 'key plank' of the wider public health programme; by 2004 at least a quarter of a million people had been helped to quit smoking for at least four weeks. A school fruit programme was instituted to ensure that around nine million children aged four to six years received at least one piece of fresh fruit every school day (Boyle 2004).

Among the host of reforms since 1997 one of the most significant underpinning the NSF was arguably the renegotiation of the general medical services contract for general practitioners (GPs), which introduced from April 2004 a system of financial reward for performance on key areas including CHD in primary care. A key component is the Quality and Outcomes Framework (QoF), rewarding GPs for improvements in patient care across four domains: clinical, organisational, 'additional services' and patient experience. CVD, with diabetes and hypertension, forms a major component of the 'points' attracting financial reward in the clinical domain. Use of disease registers in primary care, alongside improvements in clinical coding and protocols, also attract points under the organisational and patient experience domains (Capps 2004). The QoF data have also been useful in providing epidemiological insights into the relationship between CHD prevalence, quality of care and socio-economic deprivation (Strong et al. 2006).

Rapid Access Chest Pain Clinics (RACPCs)

The NSF set out plans to establish RACPCs across the English NHS so that patients with new onset chest pain, thought by the referring GP to be stable angina, could undergo timely specialist assessment (Department of Health 2000a). Observational studies published before the NSF helped to shape the policy, by demonstrating that this model of care enabled high-risk patients to be identified, and those without significant heart disease to be reassured and discharged back to their GP (Norell et al. 1992; Jain et al. 1997; Newby et al. 1998; Timmis 1999). The supporting evidence base, lacking a randomised controlled trial, has been subject to some criticism (Mant et al. 2004). Further research has been commissioned and preliminary findings suggest that the RACPC has provided an efficient and effective substitution for the traditional cardiology out-patient clinic model, subject to appropriate predefined referral criteria (Sekhri et al. 2006).

In England, the NSF has established RACPC services in most, if not all, general hospitals so that patients who are thought by their general practitioner to have new-onset stable angina can undergo specialist assessment within two weeks of referral: a considerable improvement on the lengthy waits for a general cardiology out-patient appointment in previous years.

Referral to an RACPC is facilitated by protocols agreed at the primary/secondary care interface supported by the local cardiac network. Standardised proformas are widely used to ensure appropriate use of the RACPC for its intended purpose (the RACPC is not appropriate for patients with suspected acute coronary syndromes or those with known CHD already under the care of the cardiology department) and to minimise delay. The proforma usually requires the referring GP to provide basic demographic information, describe symptom characteristics and duration, document CHD risk factors and ensure that the patient will be able to undertake exercise testing should it be required (for example, impaired mobility and aortic stenosis are contraindications to exercise testing). Specialist nurses or medical staff may 'screen' referrals to ensure that RACPC attendance is appropriate. Patients are provided with information by telephone or letter about appointment times and what to expect during clinic attendance, and are advised about medication (e.g. taking beta-blockers). Analysis of a patient's lipid profile, full blood count and other investigations are also commonly required to support early assessment. Some specialised cardiac centres provide RACPC 'slots' for symptomatic patients who have undergone interventional procedures.

The RACPC specialist nurse or doctor undertakes baseline history and clinical examination. A normal ECG does not rule out CHD (Norell et al. 1992) but provides a baseline and helps to exclude factors such as bundle branch block which would hamper analysis of an exercise test. If the clinical picture suggests new onset stable angina, an exercise tolerance test is usually performed. This test is extremely safe, with a mortality rate of 1 in 10,000 tests. Additional 'functional tests' (stress echocardiography, myocardial perfusion imaging or magnetic resonance imaging) may be required if the exercise test result is equivocal or the patient has been unable to perform the physical exertion required. In cases where these tests are negative, the risk of a major cardiac event in ensuing years is below 1% (Fox 2005).

Undifferentiated chest pain

Emergency care of the patient with chest pain is the subject of Chapter 6 on acute coronary syndromes (ACS). As discussed above, undifferentiated chest pain is a common reason for a patient seeking emergency medical help. One in 18 patients with acute chest pain calling 999 for an ambulance will have an ACS diagnosis (Deakin et al. 2006) and of the estimated 700,000 acute chest pain patients attending emergency departments in England and Wales each year (around 6% of adult attendances) approximately one-third of attendances and half of the admissions had a clinical diagnosis of ACS without clear ECG changes (Goodacre et al. 2005). It is possible that many such patients could be safely cared for in designated chest pain observation units (CPOUs): although widespread in the United States there is limited experience with such units in the UK (Goodacre and Dixon 2005).

Assessing the impact of the NSF

The impact of the NSF has been assessed in a number of ways. The Department of Health publishes annual reports setting out progress against the key standards (see Table 2.1). The Healthcare Commission undertook a formal evaluation of NSF implementation at the 'halfway stage' (Healthcare Commission 2005), reporting evidence of significant progress towards many of the national standards, particularly in relation to heart attack treatment, faster diagnosis of angina and reducing waits for revascularisation, underpinned by increased investment and targeted modernisation initiatives. The Commission report also recognised

Table 2.1 National Service Framework – progress against key standards. Reproduced with permission from Department of Health (2005a.) Crown copyright.

	Pre-NSF	Post-NSF
Adult smoking prevalence	28% (2000)	25% (2003)
Children receiving school fruit	0 (2000)	Over 2 million
Estimated lives saved by statins	2900 (2000)	9000 (2004)
Patients waiting over 12 months for heart surgery	1093 (March 2000)	Zero (Dec 2004)
Patients waiting over 9 months for heart surgery	2694 (March 2000)	Zero (March 2003)
Patients waiting over 6 months for heart surgery	2766 (April 2002)	Zero (Nov 2004)
Patients waiting over 3 months for heart surgery	—	Expected to be zero by end March 2005
% Door to needle less than 30 minutes	38% (2000)	84% (Dec 2004)
Consultant cardiologists	467 (1999)	694 (June 2004)
Heart surgeons	182 (1999)	240 (June 2004)

the significant advances made in development of primary care CHD registers, but highlighted further work needed to improve preventive work on a population basis and to provide better care for patients with heart failure or requiring cardiac rehabilitation. Key areas for attention identified by the Commission included action on health inequalities, concerted action in wider partnerships (e.g. local authorities) to tackle obesity, and improved information for, and communication with, patients. While the number of cardiologists has increased since the NSF, shortages of other key staff such as cardiac physiologists may hamper further service development, and the Commission report called for better integrated workforce planning at local level.

An unintended consequence of setting national standards for CHD alone, while resulting in welcome improvements for patients, may have been slower progress in developing services for patients with other cardiological conditions such as arrhythmias, valvular heart disease and adult congenital heart disease (Fifth Report 2002; Brooks et al. 2005; Tagney 2005). Arrhythmias have since been the subject of an additional NSF chapter (DH 2005b) and further policy development is under way for congenital heart disease. There is support for the setting of clear, unambiguous targets contained within regularly audited guidelines as a means of improving acute cardiac care (Graham et al. 2006). National comparative audit of the management of patients with acute coronary syndromes through the myocardial infarction national audit project (MINAP) has enabled reports of very significant changes (e.g. faster administration of thrombolytic treatment, and the changing role of the cardiac care unit as more patients with non-ST elevation MI are admitted) to be published both in peer-reviewed journals (Birkhead et al. 2004; Quinn et al. 2005) and in 'public' reports detailing performance of local hospitals and health systems (Royal College of Physicians 2005). Public disclosures of individual surgeons' results for some aspects of cardiothoracic surgery are gradually becoming a reality in the NHS (Keogh et al. 2004). NSF standards also form part of the wider assessment of hospital services (Healthcare Commission 2005).

Managed clinical networks for CHD are at an early stage in their development. These linked groups of health professionals and organisations spanning primary, secondary and tertiary care have been established to work across organisational boundaries in co-ordinating equitable provision of high quality, clinically effective care, with emphasis shifting from buildings and organisations towards services and patients (Baker and Lorimer 2000). At the time of writing, around 30 cardiac networks, intended to play a key role in, for example, informing local commissioning and workforce planning, have been established across England (NHS Modernisation Agency 2004).

Health Service reform in England

The NHS, since its inception in 1948, has provided universal coverage, free at the point of need, irrespective of ability to pay. It has done so, however, in the face of a rise in health technology (diagnostic, pharmaceutical and interventional) that has inevitably increased costs in a way that might possibly not have been predicted by the founding fathers of this 'cradle to grave' publicly funded service. As public expectations have risen, the NHS, once arguably the envy of the world, has suffered in comparison with other systems in comparable countries. According to the Organisation for Economic Co-operation and Development (OECD 2003) per capita health spending in the UK was $1813 compared with $2837 in France, $2580 in Canada, $2780 in Germany and $4540 in the United States. NHS buildings and equipment were seen as old and inadequate or even obsolete, and there were fewer health professionals relative to other countries (e.g. two doctors per 1000 population compared with 2.8 in the United States and 3.3 in France and Germany) (OECD 2003; Stevens 2004).

One of the key reforms instituted by the Blair administration was to commit to a 43% 'real terms' increase in health spending to meet comparisons with other wealthy European countries. Thus UK health spending is increasing from 6.8% of gross domestic product (1997) to over 9% in 2007–2008 (Stevens 2004). Investment in the NHS as a whole will have risen from £43.9 billion per annum at the time the NHS Plan was published in 2000 to £92.6 billion in 2008 (DH 2005c). Funding plans for following years have not yet been announced.

2005 onwards – the future NHS?

The current round of NHS reform in England is predicated on a desire to move from a 'politician led' NHS to one led by patients, recognising that the centralised setting of targets and a focus on performance management needs to be seen as only part of the mechanism for driving up standards of care. This is an ambitious – perhaps the most ambitious – set of reforms in the history of the NHS. There is an expectation that a more 'patient led' NHS will ensure that the process of improvement is continuous, with the service in perpetual response to patients' needs and expectations at a time when people want and indeed expect more from their tax-funded public services, and taking into account the impact of societal changes including access to information via the internet, rapid technological changes in pharmaceuticals, and so-called 'health tourism' where some people are happy to travel to obtain better care (DH 2005d). The current round of reforms is:

> '[R]ooted in the core values of the NHS: providing equal access to care that is available at the point of need regardless of ability to pay, personal to the individual patient and achieved within a taxpayer-funded system that must demonstrate value for money.' (DH 2005d: p. 2)

The complexity of the current round of NHS reforms has been described as 'incoherent and out of synch' by a former head of the DH's strategy unit (Harding 2005). The DH has described how the various reforms are intended to work together, to support NHS managers and health professionals in delivering the reforms, and to provide the 'necessary context' for developing NHS Foundation Trusts and changing strategic health authorities and primary care trusts as set out in *Creating a Patient-led NHS* (DH 2005c). The NHS is halfway through implementation of the NHS Plan reforms, informed by the Wanless Report (2002), both of which identified the need for sustained investment in and reform of the NHS to meet its core values, highlighting the importance of achieving consistently the best use of taxpayer-funded resources: value for money. These reports also stress the need for a greater focus on prevention of ill health through, for example, tackling inequalities of access and by empowering people to make choices to improve and protect their own health (DH 2005d).

The framework for reform of the NHS in England (DH 2005d) defines four related work streams:

- *Demand-side reforms* providing more choice and a much stronger patient voice; providing better information for the public about health and health services, especially to help those living with long-term conditions to manage their own health; and a new system of commissioning – practice based commissioning – to give primary care professionals the tools to innovate and to influence local service development (for patients, on behalf of the public and taxpayer), working closely with stronger primary care trusts (PCTs) and local partners, especially social services.
- *Supply-side reforms* giving NHS providers more freedom from central control (performance management) and greater local accountability through Foundation Trust status; introducing a wider range of providers from the private and voluntary sectors including new NHS social enterprises, to bring more capacity into the system alongside innovation and new ways of working in a so-called 'plurality of provision' that will include some services provided by PCTs. Workforce reform including flexible, productive working practices alongside the new contracts for almost all NHS staff (consultant and GP contracts, Agenda for Change) and a move from traditional occupational roles

towards defined competencies supported by new education, training, pay, workforce planning and regulation.

- *Transactional reforms* with 'money following the patient', rewarding the best providers and giving the rest clear incentives to improve through payment by results (PbR). Access to better information through the work of the National Programme for Information Technology (NpfIT or *Connecting for Health*) will help patients make better choices and enable providers to understand and respond to patients' needs, aligning service provision better with population need and enabling the tracking of quality and performance by practices, commissioners and regulators.
- *System management reforms* addressing governance, standards, licensing providers, setting rules for competition while protecting essential service provision and promoting co-operation, early identification and help for problems, and addressing serious clinical and financial failures, and setting prices by determining the level of NHS 'tariff'.

Implementation of the current round of reforms is expected to take three years and will be challenging for the NHS organisations and those working within them as organisational change. Transition will need to be achieved alongside maintenance of clinical and service standards and performance, and financial balance (DH 2005d).

A new direction for community services

At the time of writing a new health White Paper has been published by the Government. *Our health, our care, our say: a new direction for community services* (Secretary of State for Health 2006) sets out a vision for health and social care delivered outside hospitals, identifying five areas for change:

- Improved access and more funding following the patient ensuring personalised care, and expansion of walk-in (health) centres in the community.
- The shifting away of care from hospitals closer to people's homes, and investment in community hospitals and facilities.
- Improving working and information sharing between health and social care, and better co-ordination between the NHS and local councils.
- Budgets to increase choice by direct payment or care budget for people to pay for their own home help or care. PCTs required to act on findings of patient surveys.
- More action on prevention through introduction of the NHS 'life check' at key points in an individual's life, and linking the London 2012 Olympics to a 'Fitter Britain' campaign (Secretary of State for Health 2006).

The implications of these reforms for services for patients with chest pain are unclear, but it is possible that RACPC and similar 'ambulatory' services could be situated in diagnostic centres run by GPs or other practitioners with special interests, whether employed directly by the NHS or by independent providers commissioned locally.

Summary and conclusion

Cardiovascular diseases continue to exert a huge burden on patients, families, health services and society, both nationally and internationally. Chest pain alone forms a major part of that burden. Implementation of the NSF has been associated with improvements in care including faster access to care and uptake of evidence based treatments in both primary and secondary care settings. As the NHS undergoes significant reorganisation, it remains to be seen how the NSF, written for a very different health service structure, will continue to contribute to fighting the 'war against heart disease.'

References

Albarran JW (2002) The language of chest pain. *Nursing Times* **98**(4): 38–40.

Alberti KG, Zimmet P, Shaw J (2005) IDF epidemiology task force consensus group. The metabolic syndrome – a new worldwide definition. *Lancet* **366**: 1059–1062.

Ayanian JZ, Quinn TJ (2001) Quality of care for coronary heart disease in two countries. *Health Affairs* **20**: 55–67.

Baker CD, Lorimer AR (2000) Cardiology: the development of a managed clinical network. *British Medical Journal* **321**: 1152–1153.

Birkhead JS (1999) Trends in the provision of thrombolytic treatment between 1993 and 1997. Myocardial infarction audit group. *Heart* **82**: 438–442.

Birkhead JS, Walker L, Pearson M et al. (2004) Improving care for patients with acute coronary syndromes: initial results from the National Audit of Myocardial Infarction Project (MINAP). *Heart* **90**: 1004–1009.

Bowker TJ, Clayton TC, Ingham J, McLellan NR, Hobson HL, Pyke SD, Schofield B, Wood DA (1996) A British Cardiac Society survey of the potential for the secondary prevention of coronary disease; ASPIRE (Action on Secondary Prevention through Intervention to Reduce Events). *Heart* **75**: 334–342.

Boyle R (2004) Meeting the challenge of cardiovascular care in the new National Health Service. *Heart* **90**(Suppl. IV): iv3–iv5.

Bridgewater B (1999) Death on the waiting list for cardiac surgery. *Heart* **81**: 564.

British Heart Foundation (BHF) (2004) Coronary heart disease statistics database. www.heartstats.org.

British Heart Foundation (BHF) (2005) Coronary heart disease statistics database. www.heartstats.org.

Brooks N, Norell M, Hall J, Jennings K, Penny L, Khan M, Keogh B (2005) National variations in the provision of cardiac services in the United Kingdom. A report by a working group of the British Cardiac Society. *British Journal of Cardiology* **12**: 192–198.

Capps N (2004) Quality and outcomes framework of the new general medical services contract. Guest editorial. National Electronic Library for Health. Cardiovascular Diseases Specialist Library. http://libraries.nhs.uk/cardiovascular/default.asp?page=ED3.

Cooper A, Hodgkinson DW, Oliver RM (2000) Chest pain in the emergency department. *Hospital Medicine* **61**: 178–183.

Deakin CD, Sherwood DM, Smith A, Cassidy M (2006) Does telephone triage of emergency (999) calls using Advanced Medical Priority Dispatch (AMPDS) with Department of Health (DH) call prioritisation effectively identify patients with an acute coronary syndrome? An audit of 42,657 emergency calls to Hampshire Ambulance Service NHS Trust. *Emergency Medicine Journal* **23**: 232–235.

De Bono DP, Hopkins A (1994) The management of acute myocardial infarction: guidelines and audit standards. *Journal of the Royal College of Physicians of London* **28**: 312–317.

Department of Health (1999) *Saving Lives: Our Healthier Nation*. London, The Stationery Office.

Department of Health (2000a) *National Service Framework for Coronary Heart Disease*. London, The Stationery Office.

Department of Health (2000b) *The NHS Plan*. London, The Stationery Office.

Department of Health (2005a) *Leading the Way: the Coronary Heart Disease National Service Framework. Progress Report*. London, The Stationery Office.

Department of Health (2005b) Arrhythmias and Sudden Cardiac Death. *National Service Framework for Coronary Heart Disease*. London, The Stationery Office.

Department of Health (2005c) *Creating a Patient-led NHS: Delivering the NHS Improvement Plan*. London, DH.

Department of Health (2005d) *Health Reform in England: Update and Next Steps*. London, DH.

Fifth Report (2002) on the provision of services for patients with heart disease. *Heart* **88**(Suppl. 3): iii1–iii56.

Fox K (2005) Investigation and management of chest pain. *Heart* **91**: 105–110.

Goodacre S, Dixon S (2005) Is a chest pain observation unit likely to be cost effective at my hospital? Extrapolation of data from a randomised controlled trial. *Emergency Medicine Journal* **22**: 418–422.

Goodacre S, Cross E, Arnold J, Angelini K, Capewell S, Nicholl J (2005) The health care burden of acute chest pain. *Heart* **91**: 229–230.

Graham JJ, Timmis A, Cooper J, Ramdany S, Deaner A, Ranjadayalan K, Knight C (2006) Impact of the National Service Framework for Coronary Heart Disease on treatment and outcome of patients with acute coronary syndromes. *Heart* **92**: 301–306.

Harding M (2005) Ham hits out at 'policy incoherence'. *Health Service Journal* 15 December: 6.

Healthcare Commission (2005) Getting to the heart of it. Coronary heart disease in England: a review of progress towards national standards. London. Healthcare Commission. www.healthcarecommission.org.uk/assetRoot/04/01/05/85/04015185.pdf.

Hood S, Birnie D, Swan L et al. (1998) Questionnaire survey of thrombolytic treatment in accident and emergency departments in the United Kingdom. *British Medical Journal* **316**: 274.

Jain D, Fluck D, Sayer RW, Ray S, Paul EA, Timmis AD (1997) A one-stop chest pain clinic can identify high cardiac risk. *Journal of the Royal College of Physicians of London* **31**: 401–404.

Jenkinson C, Coulter A, Bruster S, Richards N (2002) The coronary heart disease in-patient experience questionnaire (I-PEQ (CHD)); results from the survey of National Health Service patients. *Quality of Life Research* **11**: 721–727.

Keogh B, Spiegelhalter D, Bailey A, Roxburgh J, Magee P, Hilton C (2004) The legacy of Bristol: public disclosure of individual surgeons' results. *British Medical Journal* **329**: 450–454.

Majeed A, Aylin P (2005) Dr Foster's case notes. The ageing population of the United Kingdom and cardiovascular disease. *British Medical Journal* **331**: 1362.

Mant J, McManus RJ, Oakes RA, Delaney BC, Barton PM, Deeks JJ, Hammersley L, Davies RC, Davies MK, Hobbs FD (2004) Systematic review and modelling of the investigation of acute and chronic chest pain presenting in primary care. *Health Technology Assessment* **8**(iii): 1–158.

National Assembly for Wales (2001) *Tackling CHD in Wales: Implementing Through Evidence.* Cardiff, Welsh Assembly Government.

Newby DE, Fox KAA, Flint LL, Boon NA (1998) A 'same day' direct access chest pain clinic: improved management and reduced hospitalisation. *Quarterly Journal of Medicine* **91**: 333–337.

NHS Modernisation Agency (2004) Establishing and developing cardiac networks. CHD Collaborative. www.modern.nhs.uk/serviceimprovement/1338/4668/21328/CHD_Network%20Guide.pdf.

Norell MS, Jennings KP (2006) National variations in cardiac service provision: how united is our kingdom? *Heart* **92**: 1–2.

Norell M, Lythall D, Coghlan G et al. (1992) Limited value of the resting electrocardiogram in assessing patients with recent onset chest pain: lessons from a chest pain clinic. *British Heart Journal* **67**: 53–56.

Organisation for Economic Co-operation and Development (2003) *OECD Health Data 2003*, 2nd edition. Paris, OECD.

Quinn T, Weston C, Birkhead JS et al. (2005) Redefining the coronary care unit: an observational study of patients admitted to hospital in England and Wales in 2003. *Quarterly Journal of Medicine* **98**: 797–802.

Royal College of Physicians (2005) How the NHS manages heart attacks. Fourth public report 2005. *Myocardial Infarction National Audit Project (MINAP).* www.rcplondon.ac.uk/pubs/books/minap05/HowHospitalsManageHeartAttacksJune2005.pdf.

Scottish Executive Health Department (2002) *Coronary Heart Disease and Stroke Strategy for Scotland.* Edinburgh, The Stationery Office.

Secretary of State for Health (2006) *Our Health, our Care, our Say: a New Direction for Community Services.* Command Paper 6737. London, The Stationery Office.

Sekhri N, Feder GS, Junghans C, Hemingway H, Timmis AD (2006) Rapid access chest pain clinics and the traditional cardiology outpatient clinic. *Quarterly Journal of Medicine* **99**(3): 135–141.

Stevens S (2004) Reform strategies for the English NHS. *Health Affairs* **23**: 37–44.

Stewart S, Murphy N, Walker A et al. (2003) The current cost of angina pectoris to the National Health Service in the UK. *Heart* **89**: 848–853.

Strong M, Maheswaran R, Radford J (2006) Socioeconomic deprivation, coronary heart disease prevalence and quality of care: a practice level analysis in Rotherham using data from the new UK general practitioner quality and outcomes framework. *Journal of Public Health (Oxford)* **28**(1): 39–42.

Tagney J (2005) Developing cardiac services for patients with arrhythmias: the next chapter (Editorial). *Nursing in Critical Care* **10**(5): 228–230.

Thompson DR, Bowman GS, Kitson AL, de Bono DP, Hopkins A (1996) Cardiac rehabilitation in the United Kingdom: guidelines and audit standards. National Institute for Nursing, the British Cardiac Society and the Royal College of Physicians of London. *Heart* **75**: 89–93.

Timmis AD (1999) Speeding up cardiac care. *Impact* **1**: 1–3.

Wanless D (2002) *Securing Our Future Health: Taking a Long Term View – Final Report.* London, HM Treasury.

Wood D, de Backer G, Faergeman O, Graham I, Mancia G, Pyorala K (1998) Prevention of coronary heart disease in clinical practice: recommendations of the Second Joint Task Force of European and other Societies on Coronary Prevention. *Atherosclerosis* **140**: 199–270.

Chapter 3

History taking

Jenny Tagney

'I told you I was ill'
Inscription on Spike Milligan's gravestone

Introduction

This chapter sets the scene in terms of history taking in the context of patients presenting with chest pain. It does not attempt to cover specific features of chest pain encountered in the various conditions described in the chapters of this book. Rather, it seeks to establish basic concepts and principles of history taking that the clinician can then expand with the specifics of each clinical scenario.

Aim

The aim of this chapter is to equip health practitioners with the general principles required in obtaining a clinical history through a systematic approach.

Learning outcomes

After reading this chapter and undertaking supervised practice the reader should be able to:

- Identify features of effective communication between practitioner and patient.
- Outline the approach required to obtain a meaningful clinical history.
- List the elements of a full health history.
- Discuss when a full or focused health history should be taken.

Background

Chest pain is one of the leading causes of emergency admission to hospital in Europe and North America and also accounts for one of the most common reasons to consult general practitioners (Cayley 2005). A number of conditions can give rise to chest pain and can be treated quite differently. In fact, recommended treatment for some conditions (e.g. thrombolysis in myocardial infarction) can be life-threatening in others (aortic dissection). It is therefore important to elicit relevant and specific information from the patient that will inform the differential diagnosis of their chest pain.

Eliciting an accurate clinical history from patients in combination with appropriate, targeted clinical examination will ensure that suitable management and treatment can be commenced promptly. The approach to both will vary according to the condition of the patient and whether they present as a life-threatening emergency or in more controlled circumstances. In either situation, the important elements of successfully obtaining an accurate clinical history include:

- Establishing effective communication with the patient (ensuring appropriate language, environment, understanding, etc.).
- Using a systematic approach.
- Eliciting the main features of the presenting complaint.
- Obtaining information regarding current symptoms and signs.
- Using targeted questions to obtain relevant past medical and medication history.
- Ascertaining the existence of any risk factors for development of particular disease processes (e.g. smoking, diabetes, family history).
- Using all available sources of information (e.g. any medications the patient may have with them, referral letters from GP/hospital, previous medical records if available, family, friends, bystanders as appropriate).

If the acute nature of the clinical presentation does not permit a full health history to be obtained during the initial consultation, this should be completed once the patient's condition is stabilised. Components of the full health history are identified in Table 3.1 and form the basis for structuring the chapter. However, there is no magic formula for conducting an effective consultation to obtain a health history, and the order of questioning will vary from situation to situation and patient to patient. Experienced clinicians are able to cover all areas in the order most appropriate for each individual patient and their current condition (Mallinson 2002; Tough 2004).

Practitioner–patient relationship

All healthcare practitioners need to recognise that they bring to any interaction with individual patients their own cultural beliefs and views of the world that are shaped by their own experiences. Obtaining a meaningful clinical history is not just about going through a list of questions with a patient but also about establishing a therapeutic relationship, ensuring that the patient feels listened to and understood (Seidel et al. 2003). It is therefore important for practitioners to acknowledge any potential bias or prejudice that may exist within themselves when interacting with patients. For example, smoking is a known risk factor in developing many disease processes, and clinicians have a responsibility to ensure that patients are equipped with health education regarding these risks. However, some clinicians may find it difficult to understand why a person with established disease continues to smoke. This should not influence their manner

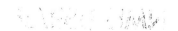

Table 3.1 Components of an adult health history. Adapted from Bickley (2006).

Identifying data	Age, gender, occupation, marital status, name and current address Source of this history – patient, friend, relative, through interpreter, referral letter, medical records Source of referral (in case summary report is needed on discharge)
Reliability	Varies according to patient's memory, mental status, trust, mood
Presenting complaint	One or more symptoms that caused the patient to seek care
History of current problem	Expands information regarding presenting complaint, describing how each symptom developed Includes patient's thoughts and feelings about the problem Pulls in relevant portions of 'review of systems' (see below) May include medications, allergies, habits of smoking, alcohol consumption, which are frequently related to development of the current problem
Past history	Lists previous illnesses with dates for any surgery or other hospital admissions, including obstetrics/gynae or psychiatric Includes health maintenance practices, e.g. exercise, diet, immunisations
Family history	Outlines or diagrams age and health or age and cause of death of siblings, parents and grandparents Documents presence of specific illnesses within the family, e.g. hypertension, diabetes, rheumatoid arthritis, asthma, etc.
Personal and social history	Describes educational level, family of origin, current household, personal interests, lifestyle
Review of systems	Documents presence or absence of common symptoms related to each major body system

with the patient. There should be no 'blame' apportioned and the clinician should not judge their patient, as it has been demonstrated that some patients will avoid seeking healthcare for fear of being criticised for risk-taking behaviours such as smoking (Richards et al. 2002).

Practitioners should also acknowledge their position of responsibility in being entrusted with information pertaining to each individual patient. It is important to establish the specific boundaries of the interaction and identify expectations from both practitioner and patient to avoid misunderstanding. Maintaining the patient's confidentiality is an obligation for all clinicians (Bickley 2006) but it is important to establish with the patient that diagnosing their symptoms may require information to be shared with other clinicians and formally documented.

Communication

Effective communication between clinicians and patients can improve health outcomes (Stewart 1995), whereas it has been demonstrated that patients are less

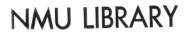

Table 3.2 Alternative questioning strategies – options for expanding and clarifying the patient's story. Adapted from Bickley (2006).

- Moving from open-ended to focused questions
- Using questioning that elicits a graded response
- Asking a series of questions, one at a time
- Offering multiple choices for answers (e.g. 'Which of these words might you use to describe your chest pain – sharp, dull, tight, a pressure, ache, stabbing, burning?')
- Clarifying what the patient means
- Offering continuers ('I see', 'Go on', nodding)
- Using echoing

likely to adhere to medical advice if they do not feel listened to, are interrupted during their explanations, are not comfortable asking questions or do not feel the clinician understands them (Mallinson 2002). Listening skills and effective questioning styles are therefore crucial in eliciting information from the patient that will help the clinician to understand what caused them to seek healthcare.

Questioning strategies are likely to change depending on the clinical condition of the patient plus the need to clarify or expand information given by the patient. Some alternative strategies are listed in Table 3.2.

Approaching the patient

Whether the patient has presented as an emergency or as a planned out-patient, it is likely that they feel at least a little apprehensive if not terrified at the prospect of their healthcare encounter. Clinicians should always bear this in mind when they first approach a patient as their initial behaviour may stem from this apprehension or fear. Putting patients at their ease is an often used expression but is really essential to develop any kind of meaningful interaction. First impressions are important, and a careful introduction including profession and title plus attention to cues, both verbal (tone of voice, language used – not too technical) and non-verbal (smile, open approach, eye contact, same level as patient – not 'looking down') will help to establish a rapport. Ensuring familiarity with any previously gathered information pertaining to this patient and the current presentation will help to avoid unnecessary repetition. Verifying some of this information can also be a helpful way of opening the interaction with the patient.

If patients have family and/or friends with them where the consultation is to take place, always check sensitively with the patient whether they are comfortable for these people to remain before commencing. Equally, it is important to be sensitive to cultural differences, such as the need for a chaperone with some women.

Additionally, if the patient has learning difficulties or their first language is not that of the clinician, it may be necessary to engage interpretation services or appropriate information support (e.g. pictures or diagrams for adults with learning difficulties).

Initial and identifying information

Date and time of presentation and consultation may seem obvious inclusions but are often missed. Without the initial date and time of presentation, many subsequent investigations and treatments may be jeopardised. It is always worth checking the patient's name, address and date of birth to ensure that any previously recorded details are updated.

Inviting the patient's story

Allowing the patient time to explain what caused them to seek healthcare is an important part of establishing an effective and therapeutic relationship, but in many cases, clinicians interrupt after only approximately 20 seconds (Mallinson 2002; Bickley 2006). If patients are allowed to tell their stories, most will finish within 2 minutes (Bickley 2006) and this should be facilitated if at all possible.

Even at this stage it is important to acknowledge that pain and discomfort are subjective experiences and patients' health expectations and cultural background may influence what is categorised as 'pain' (Sobralske and Katz 2005; Janzen et al. 2006).

Once the patient has explained what has been happening to them, the clinician can focus the interview or consultation towards eliciting specific factors that will assist in clarifying possible diagnoses. Careful use of open and closed questions utilising appropriate language will help to give structure to the process without discouraging patients. One suggested facilitative technique is to use the patient's own words once the clinician has clarified what the patient means by these.

Reliability

Relevant information should be documented such as 'vague historian' or 'appears confused' to indicate the circumstances in which any history was obtained (Bickley 2006). This may not become apparent until further into the history taking but should be highlighted early on within documentation.

The presenting or chief complaint

Patients should be encouraged to define as precisely as possible what caused them to seek healthcare at this time. This will include time of onset, any signs, symptoms, precipitating and relieving factors, previous episodes, frequency, increasing severity, deterioration, associated features or symptoms and subjective estimation of severity.

Chest pain may be described as the presenting complaint in a number of conditions, so it is important to gain an understanding as to the nature and severity of this symptom as soon as possible to inform differential diagnosis, initiate appropriate investigations and commence essential treatments.

Specific features of chest pain associated with particular conditions are discussed in the related chapters.

History of the current problem

This builds on information given regarding the presenting complaint so as to develop a more detailed clinical picture. If previous episodes have been experienced, it is important to ascertain whether these are increasing in severity and/or frequency and whether they are associated with any specific activities. This is relevant for several causes of chest pain including coronary heart disease (CHD) and oesophagastric diseases. The presence and development of any associated symptoms, such as breathlessness, lethargy or dizziness, are also useful indicators of symptom progression and possible measures of disease severity. Specific injuries acquired through contact sports or in the context of a road traffic collision should also be explored. Any elicited symptoms will also help to guide further questions and target the physical examination.

Past history

This pertains to anything that occurred prior to the current presentation and will include more general information regarding overall state of health, previous illnesses, hospitalisations (including those for obstetric or psychiatric reasons), operations and on-going treatments. In the context of chest pain, any known risk factor information such as raised cholesterol levels, hypertension, diabetes, thromboembolic disorders, and previous pulmonary, cardiac, gastro-oesophageal or thoracic musculoskeletal problems should be elicited. Depending on the circumstances, it may be relevant to review childhood illnesses, as some may impact on current health such as chicken-pox (re-activation of the varicella zoster virus in herpes zoster) or rheumatic fever (can affect heart valves). General enquiry regarding whether any recent coughs, colds or feelings of malaise have been experienced is also important to establish the circumstances of the current presentation. Vaccination history and any recent foreign travel or close association with anyone recently returned from foreign travel may be relevant, particularly if patients present with chest pain and a cough.

Information regarding current medications may also be taken at this stage plus lifestyle factors such as smoking, diet, exercise and alcohol consumption. Some of these may be considered sensitive areas and it may be difficult to obtain accurate information regarding quantities of cigarettes smoked and units of alcohol consumed. It may be worth returning to these areas once a clearer picture evolves.

Ask specifically about any alternative or supplementary medications the patient may be taking as these are often not mentioned and may be important. Terminology is important and, in this particular context, it might be worth asking a general, searching question such as 'The medications you've just told me about/brought with you – are these the only sort of tablets you take when you're at home?'

Family history

Here, information regarding any known inherited or familial problems should be elicited and documented as either text or diagram accordingly. Ascertaining if both parents are still alive and well, and, if not, how old they were when they died and whether any siblings died of similar causes can be a helpful start. Incidence of any gender-specific illness patterns should be identified. Establish whether there is a history of heart disease, cancer, diabetes, epilepsy, thyroid dysfunction, kidney disease, asthma or other allergic states (e.g. eczema, hay fever), rheumatoid arthritis, HIV-related illnesses and blood diseases (Bickley 2006). Knowledge of grandparents and what illnesses they may have suffered or what age they were when they died is often sketchy. Indeed, for some patients, family history is completely unknown because they were adopted.

Family history is particularly significant for cardiac conditions, especially if premature death (<60 years) is a feature. Additional information regarding cholesterol levels in families where such a history is identified may also reveal familial hypercholesterolaemia. Enquiries regarding the presence of cerebrovascular disease and hypertension in first-line blood relatives can also help to establish familial patterns.

Personal and social history

Asking questions regarding personal and home situations may require a sensitive approach. If, when clarifying identifying information, it was established that the patient is married, single or divorced, use this information to build upon. Do they have any children? Ascertaining whether the patient is in paid or unpaid employment and their enjoyment of their current position can give an indication of potential areas of stress or conflict. Occupation, level of education required to undertake this job, place of work and travel time can help to build a picture of a typical week and how their current condition has been interfering with these activities. Information regarding home life is also helpful such as number of people sharing accommodation, number of smokers (if any) in the house/flat, and if a flat whether there are stairs, is the patient self-caring or whether they have assistance with shopping/laundry/cleaning. If patients are younger, are they still in full-time higher education or training?

Review of systems

Depending on the urgency of the clinical situation and the condition of the patient, the practitioner systematically reviews all body systems through a series of questions. If the patient responds positively to any of the general questions, more specific and detailed questions are asked (Bickley 2006). If a more urgent assessment is required, a focused approach will be used, based on the presenting complaint and related systems.

These do not represent an exhaustive list of potential questions but give general areas for questioning and will also complement the physical examination.

- General constitutional symptoms such as fever, chills, general coughs, colds or feelings of tiredness, sleep patterns, night sweats, weight loss/gain.
- Diet: appetite, likes/dislikes, restrictions (vegetarian, religious, allergy, intolerance), use of vitamin and other supplements, use of caffeine containing drinks.
- Skin, hair and nails: rash or eruption, itching, pigmentation or texture change, excessive sweating, abnormal nail or hair growth.
- Musculoskeletal: joint stiffness, aches or pain in joints or muscles, restriction of movements, swelling, redness, heat, bony deformity.
- Head and neck: frequent or unusual headaches, their location, dizziness syncope, severe head injuries, moments of loss of consciousness.
  ○ Eyes: visual impairment – blurring, diplopia, photophobia, recent change in vision or appearance of the eyes, glaucoma, use of eye drops, recent trauma, family history of eye disease.
  ○ Ears: hearing impairment, pain, discharge, tinnitus (recent or chronic), vertigo.
  ○ Nose: sense of smell, frequent colds, obstruction, seasonal rhinitis (hay fever), epistaxis, sinus pain.
  ○ Throat and mouth: hoarseness or change in voice, frequent sore throats, bleeding or swelling of gums, recent tooth abcesses or extractions, soreness of tongue or buccal mucosa, ulcers, disturbance of taste.
- Endocrine and genital/reproductive: thyroid enlargement or tenderness, heat or cold intolerance, unexplained weight change, diabetes, polyuria, polydipsia, changes in distribution of body hair, skin striae.
  Males – puberty onset, erectile dysfunction, emissions, testicular pain, libido, infertility, contraception.
  Females – menstruation: onset, regularity, duration, dysmenorrhoea, last period, libido, sexual difficulties, infertility, contraception. Pregnancies – if any, deliveries, complications, abortions. Breasts – pain, swelling, palpable lumps, association with menstruation.
- Chest and lungs: pain related to respiration, dyspnoea, sputum (quantity and character), haemoptysis, exposure to TB.
- Heart and blood vessels: chest pain or distress, precipitating factors, timing and duration, relieving factors, palpitations, dyspnoea, orthopnoea, oedema, claudication, estimate of exercise tolerance, previous electrocardiogram or other cardiac tests.
- Haematologic: anaemia, bruise or bleed easily, thromboses, thrombophlebitis, known abnormality of blood cells, transfusions.
- Lymph nodes: enlargement, tenderness.

- Gastrointestinal: appetite, digestion, intolerance, dysphagia, heartburn, nausea, vomiting, haematemesis, bowels, constipation, diarrhoea, change in stool colour or content, flatulence, haemorrhoids, hepatitis, jaundice, dark urine, gallstones, polyps, tumour.
- Genitourinary: dysuria, loin or suprapubic pain, urgency, frequency, nocturia, haematuria, hesitancy, dribbling, oedema of the face, stress incontinence, hernias, sexually transmitted diseases.
- Neurologic: syncope, seizures, weakness or paralysis, abnormalities of sensation or coordination, tremors, loss of memory.
- Psychiatric: depression, mood changes, difficulty concentrating, nervousness, tension, suicidal thoughts, irritability, sleep disturbance.

Adapted from Seidel et al. (2003).

Concluding questions

At the end of obtaining the history, it can be helpful to ask the patient, 'Is there anything else that you think I should know?', to ensure nothing is missed. If several problems are elicited within the history, ascertain from the patient which problem bothers them most at present. It can also be helpful to explore with the patient what they perceive the cause of their current problems to be and the practitioner might begin to identify what the features presented in the history suggest. This is particularly important if, at the end of a thorough history, it seems likely that there is no biological or obvious psychiatric or psychological cause for the pain sensations experienced.

Unexplained chest pain

Despite the many potential physiological causes of chest pain discussed within this book, some patients suffer from unexplained chest pain (Janson Fagring et al. 2005). Compared with patients diagnosed with ischaemic heart disease, patients with unexplained chest pain tend to be younger and seek care more than once in six months. They may also experience more anxiety and pain and can be more preoccupied with bodily sensations than patients with cardiac disease (Esler and Bock 2004). One study proposed that patients with unexplained chest pain had a poor social support network and that being able to talk about their experience was therapeutic (Janson Fagring et al. 2005).

Next steps

The history will be used in conjunction with the physical examination to indicate which tests (if any) are most appropriate to confirm or exclude potential diagnoses. Where possible health practitioners should ensure that a shared understanding is reached with the patient regarding the meaning of all elicited signs and symptoms before continuing with further tests and investigations.

Key learning points

- Allow patients uninterrupted time to tell their story where at all possible.
- Remember that apprehension and fearfulness may alter their response to being questioned.
- Use a systematic approach.
- Be flexible in your questioning style to adapt to any given patient or clinical situation.
- Be mindful of the implications for patients of unexplained chest pain.

References

Bickley L (2006) *Bates' Guide to Physical Examination and History Taking*, 9th edition. Philadelphia, Lippincott Williams & Wilkins.

Cayley WE (2005) Diagnosing the cause of chest pain. *American Family Physician* **72**(10): 2012–2021.

Esler JL, Bock BC (2004) Psychological treatments for noncardiac chest pain. Recommendations for a new approach. *Journal of Psychosomatic Research* **56**: 263–269.

Janson Fagring A, Gaston-Johansson F, Danielson E (2005) Description of unexplained chest pain and its influence on daily life in men and women. *European Journal of Cardiovascular Nursing* **4**: 337–344.

Janzen JA, Silvus J, Jacobs S, Slaughter S, Dalziel W, Drummond N (2006) What is a health expectation? Developing a pragmatic conceptual model from psychological theory. *Health Expectations* **9**: 37–48.

Mallinson C (2002) Communication. In Kumar P, Clark M (Eds) *Clinical Medicine*, 5th edition, pp. 8–19. Oxford, WB Saunders.

Richards HM, Reid ME, Wyatt GC (2002) Socioeconomic variations in responses to chest pain: a qualitative study. *British Medical Journal* **324**: 1308–1312.

Seidel HM, Ball JW, Dains JE, William Benedict G (2003) *Mosby's Guide to Physical Examination*, 5th edition. St Louis, Mosby.

Sobralske M, Katz J (2005) Culturally competent care of patients with acute chest pain. *Journal of the American Academy of Nurse Practitioners* **17**(9): 342–349.

Stewart M (1995) Effective physician–patient communication and health outcomes: a review. *Canadian Medical Association Journal* **152**: 1423–1433.

Tough J (2004) Assessment and treatment of chest pain. *Nursing Standard* **18**(37): 45–53.

Chapter 4

Clinical examination skills for assessing the patient with chest pain

Jackie Younker

Introduction

Chest pain is a symptom most commonly associated with heart disease, but it may also be present in many different disease processes (Kumar and Clark 2005). A thorough history and clinical examination will help the practitioner make a correct diagnosis. The clinical examination is performed after taking a history from the patient. Subjective data obtained from the history will give insight into actual and potential problems and will provide a guide for the physical examination. Objective findings from the physical examination of the cardiovascular and peripheral vascular systems along with results of investigations support or refute each differential diagnosis for a patient who presents with chest pain. Chest pain may also be the result of a pulmonary or gastrointestinal problem, and findings from examining other systems (e.g. chest, thorax and abdomen) may impact judgements that will be made about the patient's presenting complaint. No system should be evaluated outside of the context of the full examination (Seidel et al. 2003).

Aims

This chapter provides an overview of clinical examination skills used for the patient presenting with chest pain. General techniques of inspection, palpation, percussion and auscultation are identified and used to describe examination of the cardiovascular, peripheral vascular, respiratory and abdominal systems.

Learning outcomes

At the end of this chapter the reader should be able to:

- Recognise life-threatening symptoms using a rapid ABCDE assessment approach.
- Describe the sequence used to examine the cardiovascular, peripheral vascular, respiratory and abdominal systems.
- Recognise normal and common abnormal findings.
- Document clinical examination findings.

The initial examination

The initial examination of the patient who presents with acute chest pain should be to determine if the symptoms are life threatening (Erhardt et al. 2002). Sudden cardiac arrest is commonly caused by ventricular fibrillation secondary to myocardial ischaemia or infarction. Recognising and responding to signs and symptoms of cardiac problems early may prevent cardiac arrest (ILCOR 2005). The critically ill patient will need a rapid assessment using an **A**irway, **B**reathing, **C**irculation, **D**isability and **E**xposure approach (Smith et al. 2002) in parallel with the history, investigations and full cardiovascular assessment. Use the following approach to quickly assess the patient (ILCOR 2005).

- **A**irway – Look for signs of airway obstruction and treat any airway obstruction as an emergency. Give oxygen as soon as possible at a high concentration.
- **B**reathing – Look, listen and feel for signs of respiratory distress. Count the respiratory rate while assessing depth and pattern of breathing. Treat any life-threatening conditions immediately (e.g. pneumothorax, acute severe asthma, pulmonary oedema). If breathing is inadequate or the patient has stopped breathing, it will be necessary to provide breaths with a pocket mask or bag-mask ventilation.
- **C**irculation – Perform a rapid assessment of the patient, noting colour of the hands and feet and temperature of the hands. Measure capillary refill time and assess the state of the veins. Measure the blood pressure and look for other signs of poor cardiac output such as a change in the level of consciousness. If the patient has primary chest pain and a suspected acute coronary syndrome, record a 12-lead ECG and treat initially with oxygen, aspirin, nitroglycerine and morphine.
- **D**isability – A rapid initial assessment of the patient's conscious level is made using the AVPU method: **A**lert, responds to **V**ocal stimuli, responds to **P**ainful stimuli or **U**nresponsive. Common causes of unconsciousness are hypoxia, hypercapnia, and cerebral hypoperfusion due to low blood pressure.
- **E**xposure – Full exposure of the body is necessary to examine the patient properly.

Patients presenting with chest pain who are having an ST elevation myocardial infarction will need reperfusion therapy quickly (e.g. thrombolytic therapy or percutaneous coronary intervention). There may not be time to do a full clinical examination until the patient has been stabilised.

The following sections in this chapter will provide more detailed examination techniques for the stable patient.

Preparing for the examination

Before beginning the physical examination, take time to prepare yourself and the patient. Examining the chest, thorax and abdomen requires the patient to be undressed. It is important to provide a suitable environment giving consideration to temperature, privacy and dignity, and lighting. Handwashing is essential before touching the patient. Prepare the equipment prior to starting the examination and be certain it is immediately available.

Examination of the chest, thorax and abdomen should ideally be done with the examiner at the patient's right side. This position has a few advantages: jugular venous pressure is better estimated from the right side, palpation of the apical impulse is more comfortable, and abdominal organs are more easily palpated (Bickley and Szilagyi 2003). Depending on the nature of the examination, the patient may need to be at 30–45°, sitting upright, or supine. Some patients have difficulty sitting up or standing and the examiner may consider positioning the patient supine to examine the anterior chest, and then have the patient roll on to the left side to examine the posterior chest.

The cardiovascular examination

Examination of the cardiovascular system includes assessing heart function and arterial and venous circulation. The cardiovascular examination must be performed in a systematic way that is comfortable for the examiner and includes inspection, palpation and auscultation. The patient should be supine with the head of the bed elevated to 30–45° for most of the examination. The patient may also need to turn on the left side and sit upright (Seidel et al. 2003).

General examination

- Eyes, mouth and face
  - Colour, expression, sweating, pallor
  - Conjunctivae for anaemia
  - Around eyes for xanthelasma (irregularly shaped, yellow-tinted lipid deposits on periorbital tissue suggestive of hyperlipidaemia)
  - Periphery of the cornea for arcus (precipitation of cholesterol crystals)
  - Around mouth, lips and tongue for pallor, or blue or grey colour (indicating central cyanosis and poor perfusion)
  - Signs of thyroid disease (hypothyroidism – dry, thin, coarse hair; hyperthyroidism – exophthalmos)

- Upper extremities
  - Fingernail clubbing (suggests cyanotic heart disease or respiratory disease)
  - Splinter haemorrhages under the nails (may represent microembolism in endocarditis or other vascular conditions)
  - Colour of hands and fingers (blue, pale or mottled suggests poor perfusion)
  - Temperature of extremities (offers clues about peripheral perfusion)
  - Capillary refill time (a prolonged CRT > 2 seconds may indicate poor peripheral perfusion)

- Lower extremities
  - Colour, temperature (blue, pale or mottled suggests poor arterial and/or venous circulation)

  ○ Hair distribution (hair loss occurs with arterial insufficiency)
  ○ Size, symmetry, oedema
  ○ Venous pattern (signs of varicose veins)

- Signs of shortness of breath or distress, general symmetry of chest, use of accessory muscles.

- Palpate radial pulses for rate, rhythm, quality and equality. An electrocardiogram is used to confirm findings.
  ○ Tachycardia > 100 beats/minute
  ○ Bradycardia < 50 beats/minute
  ○ Regular rhythm or normal variation on breathing = sinus rhythm
  ○ Regularly irregular = type 1 – second-degree heart block, or coupled extrasystoles (pulsus bigeminus)
  ○ Irregularly irregular = atrial fibrillation, ventricular ectopic beats
  ○ Bounding = exercise, anxiety, fever/sepsis
  ○ Weak, difficult to palpate = low cardiac output
  ○ Inequality between left and right = impaired circulation

- Measure blood pressure in both arms – readings may normally vary by as much as 10 mmHg and a variable pulse from atrial fibrillation may make a precise reading difficult. A difference of >20 mmHg systolic between arms suggests arterial occlusion (Cox 2004).

- Inspect jugular venous pressure (see Figures 4.1 and 4.2)
  ○ Position the patient supine to fill the jugular veins
  ○ Gradually raise the head of the bed to approximately 45°. Shining a torch at an angle across the neck, look for jugular venous pulsations between the angle of the jaw and clavicle.
  ○ Measure vertical height in centimetres about the manubriosternal angle, using the pulsating external jugular vein or upper limit of internal jugular pulsation. It may be helpful to place a ruler on the patient's chest and draw an imaginary line from the jugular pulsation to the ruler to estimate pressure.

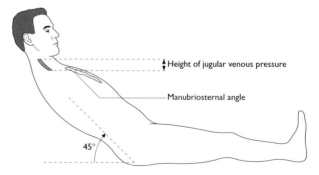

Height of jugular venous pressure

Manubriosternal angle

45°

Figure 4.1 Assessing vertical height of jugular venous pressure. Reproduced with permission from Cox (2004).

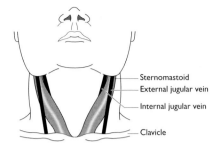

Figure 4.2 External jugular vein. Reproduced with permission from Cox (2004).

- ○ Normal JVP is approximately 1–9 cm
- ○ Some conditions make this exam difficult:
  - ■ Severe right heart failure, tricuspid insufficiency, constrictive pericarditis and cardiac tamponade may cause extreme elevation of JVP
  - ■ Hypovolaemia makes it difficult to detect JVP
  - ■ Obesity makes it difficult to see the jugular vein pulsations

Inspection

- ● Inspect the precordium
  - ○ Look for deformities of the chest wall (e.g. pectus excavatum or kyphoscoliosis)
  - ○ The apical impulse should be visible at approximately the midclavicular line, 5th intercostal space, and is best observed when the patient is sitting up and the heart is closer to the chest wall (see Figure 4.3)
  - ○ Inspection of the apical impulse is easily obscured by obesity, large breasts, or a muscular chest and doesn't necessarily present an abnormal finding
  - ○ A readily visible and bounding apical impulse suggests a large left ventricle

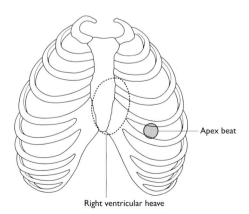

Figure 4.3 Location of apical impulse. Reproduced with permission from Cox (2004).

○ Right ventricular hypertrophy or atrial enlargement may cause a heave over the left parasternal area

Palpation

- Use the proximal halves of four fingers or the whole hand to palpate the apex, left sternal border and base of the heart. Use a gentle touch, because sensation will decrease as you increase pressure.
- It is also helpful to palpate the precordium with the patient supine and sitting upright.
- Feel for the apical beat or point of maximal impulse (PMI). This is usually at 5th intercostal space, midclavicular line in adults. It may shift slightly to the 6th intercostal space, just left of the midclavicular line in older adults – its radius is usually no more than 1 cm (see Figure 4.3).
- Ask the patient to lean forward or lie on the left side if the PMI is difficult to find. Apical impulses may be difficult to feel due to thickness of the chest wall.
- Assess the character of the impulse
  - ○ More vigorous than expected is described as a *heave* or *lift*
  - ○ Forceful or widely distributed – may indicate increased cardiac output or ventricular hypertrophy
  - ○ Thrusting displaced apical beat – suggests volume overload, possibly from mitral or aortic valve incompetence, left-to-right shunt, or cardiomyopathy
  - ○ Tapping apex beat – occurs in mitral stenosis
- Palpate the left sternal border and the base.
- Feel for thrills (a palpable murmur that feels like a fine, rushing vibration).
- Describe sensations in terms of intercostal space, and relationship to midsternal, midclavicular and axillary lines.

Auscultation

Palpation of the precordium may have provided some clues about the heart that can be considered during auscultation. A forceful left ventricular beat may be because of aortic or mitral valve disease so listening carefully for a murmur is important. The key is to use a systematic approach listening and describing what is heard in each area. There are five main areas and it is useful to listen over each with the bell and diaphragm of the stethoscope. The diaphragm transmits louder, harsh sounds, while the bell transmits softer sounds. Listen with the patient supine and sitting up, leaning slightly forward. Take time to listen carefully for each heart sound, isolating each component of the cardiac cycle. Avoid jumping from one area to the next. Concentrate on heart sounds, noting systole and diastole. It can be helpful to palpate an arterial pulse to assist in determining systole and diastole, particularly when an irregular rhythm such as atrial fibrillation is present. Note any added sounds, then listen for murmurs (Bickley and Szilagyi 2003).

- Five key areas to listen (these areas represent sounds transmitted in the direction of blood flow as it passes through valves, not surface markings of the valves (Figure 4.4))
    - Aortic valve area – 2nd right intercostal space, right sternal border
    - Pulmonary valve area – 2nd left intercostal space, left sternal border
    - Second pulmonic area (Erb's point) – 3rd left intercostal space, left sternal border
    - Tricuspid area – 4th left intercostal space, lower left sternal border
    - Mitral (apical) area – apex of the heart, 5th left intercostal space, midclavicular line

- Heart sounds are described by pitch, intensity, duration, and timing in the cardiac cycle. Sounds produced are generally low pitched. S_1 and S_2 result from valve closure and are the most distinct sounds and provide useful clues about heart function (Figure 4.5).

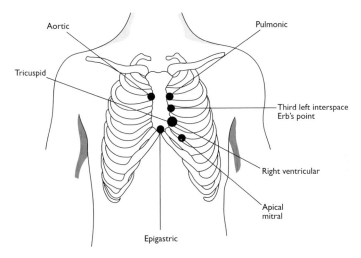

Figure 4.4 Auscultation site landmarks. Reproduced with permission from Cox (2004).

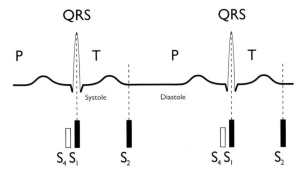

Figure 4.5 Relationship of heart sounds to electrocardiogram. Reproduced with permission from Cox (2004).

○ S_1 – closure of mitral and tricuspid (AV) valves; indicates the beginning of systole, best heard towards the apex.

○ S_2 – closure of aortic and pulmonic (semilunar) valves; indicates the end of systole, best heard in aortic and pulmonic areas.

○ S_2 is higher pitched and shorter in duration than S_1.

○ **Splitting of S_2** – S_2 is made up of two sounds that merge during expiration. Aortic valve closure (A_2) contributes most of the S_2 sound when heard in the aortic and pulmonic areas and tends to override the sound from pulmonic valve closure (P_2). During inspiration, P_2 occurs a little later and gives S_2 two phases or a split S_2. Listening while asking the patient to take in a deep breath may reveal a split S_2. It is easier to hear in younger patients. In older adults a delayed closure of P_2 may be associated with right ventricular hypertrophy or pulmonary hypertension. It will be very difficult to assess splitting if the patient is breathless and unable to hold his breath in or out.

○ S_3 – First phase of rapid ventricular filling in early diastole – increased with exercise, fast heart rate, elevation of legs, and increased venous return. Often described as a ventricular gallop.

○ S_4 – Second phase of ventricular filling – atrial contraction causing ventricular filling towards the end of diastole – physiological S_4 may be heard in middle-aged adults, particularly after exercise. In older adults suspect hypertensive disease, coronary artery disease, myocardial ischaemia, infarction, congestive heart failure. Often described as an atrial gallop.

- Extra heart sounds – heart valves usually open without making a noise unless thickened or roughened. *Ejection clicks* are heard when abnormal aortic and pulmonic valves open. This sound is heard early in systole. *Opening snaps* are associated with an abnormal mitral or tricuspid valve and are best heard in diastole. A *pericardial friction rub* may be heard when inflammation of the pericardial sac causes the parietal and visceral surfaces to become rough. This produces a rubbing or grating sound heard with the stethoscope. Pericardial friction rub is often heard loudest at the apex and usually covers systole and diastole (Seidel et al. 2003). A prosthetic mitral valve will produce a distinct click early in diastole.

- Murmurs – murmurs are generally caused by some disruption in blood flow into, through, or out of the heart. Diseased valves that do not open or do not close normally are the most common causes of murmurs. Other reasons for murmurs may include high output states (thyrotoxicosis, pregnancy), structural defects, altered blood flow in major vessels near the heart, obstructive disease in cervical arteries, and vigorous left ventricular ejection (Seidel et al. 2003). A full examination as well as other diagnostic testing is useful in accurate diagnosis of a murmur. Murmurs are classified according to timing (systole or diastole), pitch, intensity, pattern, quality, location, radiation and relationship to respiration (see Tables 4.1 and 4.2).

Table 4.1 Gradation of murmurs. Adapted from Bickley and Szilagyi (2004).

Grade 1	Very faint, may be barely audible with a stethoscope in a quiet room
Grade 2	Quiet, but heard when the stethoscope is placed over the heart
Grade 3	Moderately loud
Grade 4	Loud, with palpable thrill
Grade 5	Very loud, thrill palpated easily
Grade 6	Audible when stethoscope not in contact with chest wall, thrill palpated easily

Table 4.2 Timing of murmurs. Adapted from Kumar and Clark (2005).

Timing	Likely causes
Midsystolic S_1 S_2	Innocent murmurs (no CV abnormality) Physiologic murmur (pregnancy, sepsis, anaemia) Aortic stenosis or aortic sclerosis Pulmonic stenosis Hypertrophic cardiomyopathy
Pansystolic S_1 S_2	Mitral regurgitation Tricuspid regurgitation Ventricular septal defect
Late systolic S_1 S_2	Mitral valve prolapse Hypertrophic cardiomyopathy Coarctation of aorta
Early diastolic S_1 S_2 S_1	Aortic regurgitation Pulmonary regurgitation
Mid–late diastolic S_1 S_2 S_1	Mitral stenosis Tricuspid stenosis

Peripheral arteries and veins

Palpation of radial pulses, measurement of blood pressure, and examination of jugular venous pressure were included in general examination. It is important to complete a full examination of the vascular system even if there were no obvious initial signs to gain a clear picture of the state of the cardiovascular system (Munro and Campbell 2003). This part of the examination should be performed in a systematic way that is comfortable for the examiner.

- Peripheral pulses – palpate pulses and compare with opposite side (Figure 4.6)
  - Carotid – medial to and below angle of the jaw – do *not* palpate both sides simultaneously
  - Brachial – medial to biceps tendon
  - Radial – medial and ventral side of the wrist

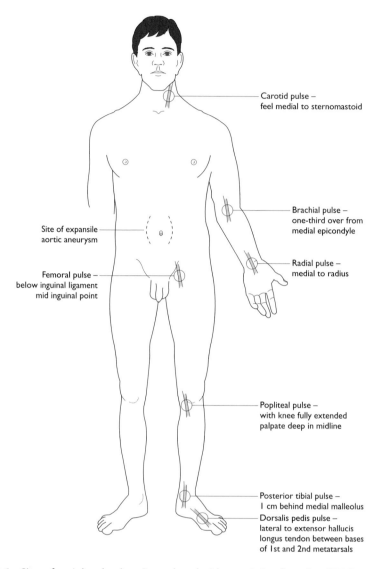

Carotid pulse –
feel medial to sternomastoid

Brachial pulse –
one-third over from
medial epicondyle

Site of expansile
aortic aneurysm

Radial pulse –
medial to radius

Femoral pulse –
below inguinal ligament
mid inguinal point

Popliteal pulse –
with knee fully extended
palpate deep in midline

Posterior tibial pulse –
1 cm behind medial malleolus

Dorsalis pedis pulse –
lateral to extensor hallucis
longus tendon between bases
of 1st and 2nd metatarsals

Figure 4.6　Sites of peripheral pulses. Reproduced with permission from Cox (2004).

○ Femoral – may be difficult to palpate in obese patients but helpful to identify any potential problems if this route is to be used for access in coronary angiography
○ Popliteal – popliteal fossa – helpful if the patient is prone with knee flexed
○ Dorsalis pedis – medial side of the dorsum of the foot with foot slightly dorsiflexed
○ Posterior tibial – behind and just inferior to medial malleolus of the ankle

○ Abdominal aorta – this may be included as part of the abdominal exam and is done by pressing on both sides of the aorta, feeling for any lateral pulsation suggestive of an aneurysm
- Auscultation – using the stethoscope to listen over arteries for a bruit. Bruits are caused by turbulent blood flow due to constriction or altered flow. Sites to auscultate include:
  ○ Carotid – if clinical signs of carotid stenosis, older adults; ask the patient to hold a breath for a few seconds
  ○ Abdominal aorta – if clinical signs of aortic aneurysm
  ○ Femoral arteries – if signs of peripheral arterial disease in lower limb

The respiratory examination

Examination of the respiratory system is an important element when assessing the patient with chest pain. The function of the respiratory system is to work closely with the cardiac and peripheral vascular systems to enable exchange of oxygen and carbon dioxide in the lungs and tissues and achieve regulation of acid–base balance. Differential diagnoses for chest pain such as bronchitis or pleuritic pain must be considered (Kumar and Clark 2005). Inspection, palpation, percussion and auscultation are used to examine the chest and thorax. The patient should ideally be sitting upright during examination of the posterior thorax, and supine during examination of the anterior chest and thorax (Bickley and Szilagyi 2003).

General examination

- Note general appearance, mental alertness, agitation, anxiety, facial expressions
- Activity tolerance – note the patient's breathing at rest and with activity (e.g. while walking, transferring to the bed or exam table, dressing/undressing)
- Respiratory rate – count for one minute (10–12 breaths per minute is average in healthy adults)
- Signs of respiratory distress
  ○ Tachypnoea (increased respiratory rate)
  ○ Dyspnoea (breathlessness)
  ○ Nasal flaring
  ○ Use of accessory muscles
  ○ Signs of cyanosis (can be central – seen in tongue and lips, or only peripheral – nails and skin of extremities)

- Evidence of respiratory failure – it is useful to learn from the history if the patient has chronic hypoxia or hypercapnia
  ○ Hypoxia (central cyanosis, change in level of consciousness)
  ○ Hypercapnia (change in level of consciousness, confusion, coarse tremor/ flap of hands)
  ○ Clubbing (see below)

- Pattern of respiration
  - Orthopnea – shortness of breath that occurs when patient is supine, associated with heart failure, severe asthma, chronic obstructive pulmonary disease, mitral valve disease
  - Tachypnoea – persistent increased breath rate (>24 breaths/minute), rapid, shallow breathing pattern
  - Bradypnoea – persistent decreased breath rate (<8–10 breaths/minute) may indicate neurologic or electrolyte disturbance, response to protect from pleuritic chest pain
  - Kussmaul breathing or hyperventilation – increase in depth and rate of breathing, Kussmaul is associated with metabolic acidosis
  - Cheyne-Stokes – alternating hyperventilation with intervals of apnoea usually caused by severe increased intracranial pressure, drug-related respiratory compromise, high altitude, left ventricular failure
  - Air trapping – results with prolonged, inefficient expiratory effort, respiratory rate increases and breathing becomes shallow to compensate
  - Biot respiration (ataxic breathing) – unpredictable, erratic pattern of irregular respirations varying in depth and interrupted by periods of apnoea, associated with neurologic disease/disorders
  - Obstructive airway disease – pattern of pursed lip breathing and use of accessory muscles
  - Wheezing – caused by airway constriction, may be associated with bronchospasm, asthma, anaphylaxis and heart failure
  - Stridor – partial obstruction of the upper airways, retractions of sternum and intercostal spaces may also occur as interpleural pressure becomes increasingly negative and the muscular structures pull back to try to overcome the blockage (Seidel et al. 2003). Immediate treatment must be used to relieve airway obstruction

- Peripheral examination
  - Finger clubbing (seen in patients with intrathoracic tumours, chronic obstructive pulmonary disease, chronic hepatic fibrosis, congenital heart defects; may also be congenital and present with no underlying disease process)
  - Nicotine staining on fingers
  - Colour of extremities (peripheral cyanosis)

Inspection

- Inspect the chest with the patient sitting upright and undressed to the waist if possible. Look at the shape and symmetry of the chest from the front and back, comparing hemithoraces. The anterior–posterior (AP) diameter is normally less than the transverse diameter. Note colour, contour and condition of skin, noting any bruises, lesions or scars. The prominence of the ribs and presence of underlying fat will offer some clues about nutritional status (Seidel et al. 2003).

- Changes to chest wall
  - Asymmetry – decreased size of one side or the other associated with flail chest, lung collapse, or fibrosis
  - Barrel chest – increased AP diameter associated with compromised respiration and commonly seen in chronic asthma, emphysema, or cystic fibrosis; moderate changes may also be normal in older adults
  - Kyphosis or scoliosis – deviation of the spine either posteriorly (kyphosis) or laterally (scoliosis)
  - Pectus carinatum (pigeon chest) – prominent sternal protrusion
  - Pectus excavatum (funnel chest) – indentation of lower sternum

Palpation

Palpation of the chest may be integrated with the cardiac examination. Feel for general condition of the thorax, including ribs, clavicles, sternum and scapulae, noting any areas of crepitus (air in subcutaneous tissue), pain or tenderness (Cox 2004).

- Tracheal position
  - Inspect the position of the trachea to assess position: it should be midline (Figure 4.7). Tracheal deviation may be caused by tension pneumothorax, tumour or node enlargement on the opposite side. Moderate displacement may be present with atelectasis, thyroid enlargement or pleural effusion (Seidel et al. 2003)
  - Move the trachea gently side to side with the index finger in the suprasternal notch to assess position

- Respiratory excursion (thoracic expansion)
  - Place thumbs on both sides of the spinal processes at about the 10th rib; wrap the hands gently around the chest wall. Ask the patient to take a deep breath and note if there is symmetrical movement of the thumbs

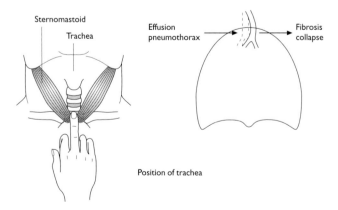

Figure 4.7 Position of trachea. Reproduced with permission from Cox (2004).

○ Repeat this anteriorly by placing thumbs along the costal margin and xiphisternum, noting symmetrical movement of the thumbs when the patient takes a deep breath

○ Asymmetrical movement may indicate pathology such as pneumonia, pleural effusion (>500 ml), pneumothorax, or collapse of bronchus (Kumar and Clark 2005)

- Tactile fremitus – palpable vibration of the chest wall that results from speech, useful assessment tool when pathology (emphysema, pleural effusion, pulmonary oedema, or bronchial obstruction) is present
  ○ Use the palmar surfaces or ulnar surfaces of the hand and apply firm touch to patient's back between the spinal processes and scapulae. Ask the patient to repeat a few numbers or words (e.g. 'Ninety-nine') and note vibrations on both sides. Fremitus is best felt at the 2nd intercostal space, the level of bifurcation of the bronchus.

Percussion

Percussion is done by using the finger of one hand as a hammer and a finger of the other hand is placed against the chest and used as a striking surface. Good technique should produce a sound wave or percussion tone. The degree of the percussion tone is determined by the tissues that are below the area being percussed (see Table 4.3).

- Percuss anterior and posterior aspects of the chest at the top, middle, and lower segments (Figure 4.8). Make comparisons side to side rather than percussing from top to bottom fully on each side. If a dull area is present, map it out by percussing from a resonant area to a dull area (e.g. liver borders).
- Anterior and lateral percussion
  ○ It is helpful to ask the patient to raise the arms overhead
  ○ Percuss over intercostal spaces rather than on top of ribs

Table 4.3 Classification of percussion tones. Adapted from Bickley and Szilagyi (2003).

Sound	Description	Example where heard
Flatness	Soft intensity, high pitch, short duration, very dull sound	Over muscle
Dullness	Moderate intensity, moderate pitch, moderate duration, thud-like sound	Over liver, other organs, and solid masses
Resonant	Loud intensity, low pitch, long duration, hollow sound	Healthy lung tissue
Hyper-resonant	Very loud intensity, low pitch, long duration, boom-like sound	Emphysema, pneumothorax
Tympanic	Loud intensity, high pitch, moderate duration, drum-like sound	Air in stomach and intestines (predominant sound in abdominal examination)

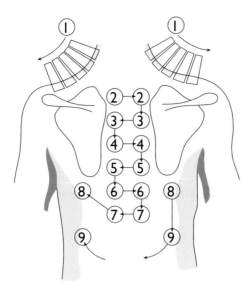

Figure 4.8 Percussion sequence of the chest. Reproduced with permission from Cox (2004).

- Posterior percussion
  - ○ Ask the patient to bend the head forward and cross arms in front. This moves the scapulae laterally and exposes the lung
  - ○ Percuss over intercostal spaces
- Increased resonance (hyper-resonance) indicates hyperinflation and may occur in pneumothorax and emphysema
- Decreased resonance (dullness or flatness) over lung fields suggests alveolar collapse (atelectasis), pleural effusion, or neoplasm

Auscultation

Listening to breathing with a stethoscope may provide important clues about the condition of the lungs and pleura. The patient should sit upright and breathe deeply through the mouth. Be aware this somewhat exaggerated breathing may be difficult for some patients and it is useful to listen to lung bases before the patient becomes fatigued. The diaphragm of the stethoscope is generally used because it transmits higher-pitched sounds. The stethoscope must be over bare skin. The examiner should use a systematic approach listening anteriorly, posteriorly and laterally, and making comparisons from side to side (Figure 4.9). Listen carefully to inspiration and expiration at each point (Munro and Campbell 2003).

- Normal breath sounds are characterised by pitch, intensity, quality and relative duration during inspiration and expiration
  - ○ Tracheal/bronchial (tubular) – heard over the upper and lower aspect of the trachea with expiration longer than inspiration and a characteristic, high-pitched, loud, harsh sound

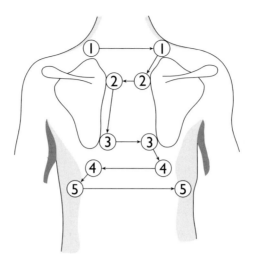

Figure 4.9 Sequence for auscultation. Reproduced with permission from Cox (2004).

- ○ Bronchovesicular – heard over the main bronchus and large upper airways with inspiration and expiration about equal and a medium pitch and intensity
- ○ Vesicular – heard over most of lung fields with inspiration longer than expiration and low pitch and soft intensity
- ● Adventitious (added or abnormal) breath sounds – sounds may be continuous and heard throughout the respiratory cycle (rhonchi, wheezes) or discontinuous and heard during part of the respiratory cycle (crackles) (see Table 4.4)
  - ○ Crackles (other terms include rales, crepitations and creps) – caused by alveoli popping open with inspiration or fluid in the lungs and usually described as fine, medium or coarse
  - ○ Wheezes (other terms include sibilant rale, musical rale, or rhonchus) – caused by high velocity airflow through a constricted area that produces a whistling-type sound and may be heard on inspiration or expiration
  - ○ Rhonchi (other terms include sonorous wheezes) – caused by passage of air through a large airway partially obstructed with mucus or secretions
  - ○ Bronchial – used to describe harsh, loud breath sounds heard in an area of the lungs other than the upper or lower trachea and caused by consolidation
  - ○ Diminished – caused by either lack of air movement or air or fluid obstructing sound conduction (e.g. bronchial obstruction, effusion, pneumothorax). If the patient is critically unwell, this requires immediate intervention
  - ○ Pleural friction rub – caused by inflammation of the pleura (pleurisy); produces a dry, crackly, grating, low-pitched sound

Table 4.4 Description of adventitious breath sounds. Adapted from Munro and Campbell (2003).

Sound	Characteristic and possible causes
Crackles (discontinuous)	Fine – high pitched, soft, crackling sound; heart failure, alveolitis Medium – lower, more moist sound, not cleared by cough; infection or fluid in alveoli Coarse – loud bubbling noise heard throughout inspiration, not cleared by cough; bronchiectasis or pulmonary oedema
Wheezes (continuous)	Musical or whistling sound during inspiration and expiration, may be louder on expiration; asthma, bronchitis, pulmonary oedema, congestive heart failure
Rhonchi (continuous)	Loud, low, coarse, may sound like a snore, heard during inspiration and expiration and may be cleared with coughing; mucous secretions, pulmonary oedema, ineffective cough effort
Bronchial	Loud, harsh sound heard in the lung fields; consolidation from pneumonia (most common), neoplasm, fibrosis, or abcess
Pleural friction rub	Dry, rubbing or grating sound, like rubbing pieces of leather together, heard during inspiration or expiration; inflammation of pleural surfaces

The abdominal examination

Elements of an abdominal examination may help to exclude some differential diagnoses for chest pain. Gastrointestinal diseases such as hiatus hernia, reflux oesophagitis, cholecystitis, peptic ulcer disease and pancreatitis may all be possible causes for chest pain. Aortic dissection is another possible cause (Kumar and Clark 2005). Before beginning the examination, take a history from the patient and note any statements that would lead to more thorough assessment of the abdomen. Clues from the history may include:

● History of indigestion
● Vague onset of pain or discomfort
● Related to eating or drinking (note if before or after meals)
● Lasts for several hours; unrelated to effort
● Patient does not need to stop activity
● Relief from antacids
● Onset of pain may happen at any time
● Left upper quadrant pain
● Back or flank pain
● History of increased alcohol intake
● Recent weight loss

Inspection

A good abdominal examination requires adequate lighting, a relaxed patient and full exposure of the abdomen (Figure 4.10). The patient should be positioned supine with a pillow under the head and perhaps under the knees, and the arms should be resting comfortably at the sides. Begin the examination by looking at

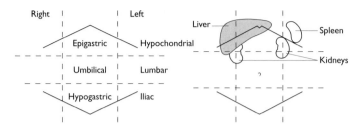

Figure 4.10 Abdominal of quadrants for examination. Reproduced with permission from Cox (2004).

the patient's mouth and throat. This provides clues about the alimentary system as well as giving an indication of cyanosis (Kumar and Clark 2005).

- Inspect surface characteristics and contour of the abdomen. The colour and surface of the skin on the abdomen should be the same as the rest of the body. Cyanosis (blue) or jaundice (yellow) is an unexpected finding and offers clues about other problems
- The contour of the abdomen may be flat, rounded, or scaphoid and there should be overall symmetry
- Aortic pulsation may be visible in the upper midline in thin adults. A marked or very strong pulsation may indicate increased pulse pressure or abdominal aortic aneurysm (Seidel et al. 2003)

Auscultation

Auscultation primarily provides information about bowel motility. It may be done before palpation and percussion to avoid altering the frequency of bowel sounds (Cox 2004).

- Listen over four quadrants. Clicks and gurgles are normally heard and range from 5 to 35 per minute.
- Auscultate for at least 3 minutes before deciding bowel sounds are absent.
- It is useful to listen over the abdominal aorta in the epigastric region for a systolic bruit, indicating an abdominal aortic aneurysm. The bell of the stethoscope may also be used to listen for bruits over renal, iliac and femoral arteries (Seidel et al. 2003).

Palpation

Light and deep palpation is generally used to assess the organs in the abdominal cavity. It will also help to detect muscle spasm, fluid, and areas of tenderness. The patient should be supine with a pillow under the knees and arms alongside the body to help relax the abdomen. It is important to look at the patient's facial expressions for any grimace indicating discomfort. It is also important to ask the patient to report any discomfort or tenderness during the examination (Bickley and Szilagyi 2003). The examination is performed from the patient's right side.

- Begin with light palpation of four quadrants using the palmar surface of the hand and depressing the abdominal wall approximately 1 cm. Use a smooth and even motion and avoid jabbing, short, quick movements.
- The abdomen normally feels smooth with consistent softness. Generalised muscular resistance is usually due to the patient's difficulty in relaxing. Discomfort or tenderness is usually related to an affected organ or generalised inflammation.
- Deep palpation is used to map out abdominal organs and detect the presence of any masses. It should also be done with the palmar surface of the hand in a smooth, even way. The use of the fingertips should be avoided.
- The liver, spleen and kidneys are specific structures that may be felt with deep palpation in some normal people, but this is not common (Kumar and Clark 2005). Further information about organ palpation can be found in clinical examination textbooks (Bickley 2003; Munro and Campbell 2003; Seidel et al. 2003).

Percussion

Percussion is generally used to determine the presence of fluid, air, or solid masses. It may also be used to assess the size and density of organs.

- Using the same technique described in the respiratory examination section, percuss over four abdominal quadrants. Table 4.3 provides a description of normal percussion tones.
- Tympany is the predominant sound heard over the stomach and intestines. Dullness will be heard over the liver, an enlarged spleen, or solid mass. Further information about techniques for liver and spleen percussion is found in clinical examination textbooks (Bickley 2003; Munro and Campbell 2003; Seidel et al. 2003).

Conclusion

Chest pain is a common symptom of heart disease. It may, however, also be present with other disease processes. The practitioner must take a thorough history and perform a clinical examination to make the correct diagnosis. This chapter has outlined techniques used to rapidly examine a patient with acute chest pain. A systematic approach to examination of the cardiovascular, peripheral vascular, respiratory, and abdominal systems has also been outlined. Further details about clinical examination techniques are available in a range of clinical examination textbooks.

Example

The following is an example of documentation for clinical examination of a 55-year-old male presenting with a two-day history of recurring stable angina.

Patient sitting on examination table. No chest pain at present.
Pulse 72, regular, BP 130/76 left arm, 132/78 right arm
CV:
Capillary refill < 2 seconds
JVP +3 cm, normal character, no oedema
Apical impulse barely palpable at 5th ICS, 4 cm from midsternal line – no heaves, lifts, or thrills
Heart sounds I + II, no extra sounds or murmur
Peripheral pulses:

	Radial	Brachial	Carotid	Femoral	Dorsalis pedis	Posterial tibial
R	+	+	+	+	+	+
L	+	+	+	+	+	+

Lower extremities warm, pink with symmetric hair distribution; superficial varicosities in lower extremities (L > R)

RESP
No pallor, cyanosis, or clubbing
Trachea central
AP diameter < lateral with 1:2 ratio; respiratory effort symmetric; no use of accessory muscles
Expansion reduced, but symmetrical
Resonant percussion throughout
Vesicular breath sounds throughout; no adventitious sounds

ABDO
Normal oral mucosa
Abdomen soft, rounded, faded small scar around umbilicus (previous laporoscopy)
Aorta midline with no visible pulsation
Bowel sounds present in 4 quadrants; no aortic bruit
Tympanic percussion tones over 4 quadrants
No pain or tenderness to light or deep palpation
Liver, spleen, kidneys not palpable

References

Bickley L, Szilagyi P (2003) *Bates' Guide to Physical Examination and History Taking.* Philadelphia, Lippincott Williams and Wilkins.

Cox C (2004) *Physical Assessment for Nurses.* Blackwell, Oxford.

Erhardt L, Herlitz J, Bossaert L, Halinen M, Keltai M, Koster R, Marcassa C, Quinn T, van Weert H (2002) Task force report on the management of chest pain. *European Heart Journal* **23**: 1153–1176.

International Liaison Committee on Resuscitation (ILCOR) (2005) Part 4. Advanced Life Support 2005 International Consensus on Cardiovascular Resuscitation and Emergency Cardiovascular Care Science and Treatment Recommendations. *Resuscitation* **67**: 213–247.

Kumar P, Clark M (2005) *Clinical Medicine.* Oxford, Elsevier Saunders.

Munro J, Campbell I (2003) *Macleod's Clinical Examination.* London, Churchill Livingstone.

Seidel H, Ball J, Dains J, Benedict GW (2003) *Mosby's Guide to Clinical Examination.* St. Louis, Mosby.

Smith G, Osgood V, Crane S (2002) ALERT – a multiprofessional training course in the care of the acutely ill adult patient. *Resuscitation* **52**: 281–286.

Useful websites

Heart Sounds Tutorial: http://www.blaufuss.org/

Rale Repository of Lung Sounds: http://www.rale.ca/

Yale University School of Medicine – Cardiothoracic Imaging: http://info.med.yale.edu/intmed/cardio/imaging/contents.html

Chapter 5

Assessment and differential diagnoses in the patient with chest pain

Jonathan R. Benger

Introduction

Chest pain is a common presenting complaint in both primary and secondary care. In the United Kingdom it is estimated that 20–30% of emergency medical admissions are due to chest pain (Kendrick et al. 1997), and the underlying diagnosis can range from the trivial to the immediately life threatening. Careful assessment of the chest pain patient is therefore mandatory. A strategy of caution is often adopted, with many of the patients who are admitted to hospital for further assessment being subsequently shown to be free of serious disease (Goodacre et al. 2004).

Traditional patient assessment follows a well defined process of:

(1) Taking a detailed history (Chapter 3)
(2) Performing a thorough clinical examination (Chapter 4)
(3) Requesting those investigations that will assist in diagnosis

Chest pain is no exception, but it is true to say that the majority of the diagnosis is based on the patient's history, and that clinical examination is often unhelpful. Inexperienced clinicians tend to seek a battery of test results to reassure them that their clinical impression is correct. However, many tests add nothing to the diagnosis, may generate confusing false positive or false negative results, sometimes cause patient harm and are expensive. Investigations should therefore be targeted to address specific questions and only performed when they will alter patient management.

Aims

This chapter aims to guide the reader through the principles of assessment and accurate diagnosis in the patient with chest pain, paying particular attention to those conditions which represent the greatest risk to the patient, and which need to be 'ruled out' in order to provide a safe management plan (see Table 5.1). This chapter aims to help the reader build on the principles described previously (Chapters 3 and 4), by following the layout of history, examination and investigation, concentrating on the key differentials. The various theories that help to inform sound clinical reasoning and successful diagnosis are then explored to

Table 5.1 Key differential diagnoses in the patient with chest pain.

- Acute coronary syndrome, including myocardial infarction and unstable angina
- Aortic rupture or dissection
- Pericarditis and/or myocarditis
- Pulmonary embolism
- Pneumonia
- Oeophageal rupture
- Pneumothorax (tension or simple)
- Major chest trauma, including haemothorax, open pneumothorax, flail segment

assist the reader in understanding where 'pattern recognition' is appropriate, where other cognitive process should be utilised and how to recognise their own biases.

Learning outcomes

On completion of the chapter, the reader will be able to:

- Describe the process of assessment in a patient with chest pain.
- Understand the diagnostic processes in a patient with chest pain.
- List key differential diagnoses and understand the available strategies for further investigation in a patient with chest pain.
- Describe common approaches to diagnostic reasoning and the potential pitfalls that may occur.

History taking

Because history is the most important part of chest pain assessment, it is essential to listen carefully to everything the patient has to say, and seek collateral information (e.g. from relatives, friends, the ambulance service) whenever possible. Patients asked to recount the problem in their own words usually do so in less than two minutes (Langewitz et al. 2002), so there is often no need to cut short this part of the consultation, which can then be followed by more detailed and specific questioning. It is important to bear in mind that cardiac pain may be described in various vague terms by some people: 'pressure', 'ache' and 'tightness' should all be considered significant, even if the patient is keen to downplay their symptoms. This can be a particular problem in people who are worried that their symptoms may indicate heart disease: they may have been brought unwillingly by a spouse or friend to the consultation, and be keen to reassure the clinician and themselves that all is well. Similarly, a patient with suspected cardiac disease whose pain has now reduced to 'mild ache' still has significant symptoms that require further assessment and treatment. The key questions relating to a history of chest pain are summarised in Table 5.2 and the following sections.

Table 5.2 Key questions when taking a history from the patient with chest pain.

- Is there a history of chest injury?
- How long has the pain been present?
- How did the pain begin?
- What is the character of the pain?
- Does the pain go anywhere else (radiate)?
- Are there any associated symptoms?
- Does the pain come and go, or is it there all the time?
- Does anything make the pain better or worse?
- Has pain like this been experienced previously?
- What risk factors does the patient have?

Is there a history of chest injury?

This key question directs the clinician down one of two routes: traumatic versus non-traumatic chest pain. Diagnosis in traumatic chest pain is often straightforward, with a greater challenge lying in the assessment of non-traumatic pain. Usually the answer to this question is obvious, but problems can arise when patients or clinicians attribute non-traumatic pain to recent activity (such as digging the garden) or a minor injury that is actually unrelated. Patients may be keen to find a trivial cause for chest pain that is worrying them, and it is essential that the clinician does not get drawn into the same trap. Even the presence of chest wall tenderness is unhelpful, since this has been described in both acute coronary syndrome and pulmonary embolism. Therefore, where uncertainty exists, it is sensible to assume that the chest pain is non-traumatic in origin.

How long has the pain been present?

Severe pain of short duration is often more significant than longer-standing symptoms. Pain that has been present for years is more likely to be attributable to musculoskeletal or psychological causes.

How did the pain begin?

Pain from the organs within the chest (mainly the heart and lungs) is mediated by the autonomic nervous system and tends to build up (and decline) over minutes, rather than being instantaneous in onset and offset. It is often taught that *pleuritic* chest pain (worse on breathing in, coughing and sneezing) is of sudden onset in pulmonary embolism, but this actually has no predictive value (Rodger and Wells 2001). Whilst it is true that a pulmonary embolism occurs suddenly, the associated pain is due to inflammation of the *parietal pleura* (the external lining of the lungs) that follows lung ischaemia, and is therefore more gradual in onset. In a larger pulmonary embolism, shortness of breath may occur very suddenly but pain follows later or sometimes not at all. In a smaller pulmonary embolism there may be no shortness of breath, just a gradual onset of pleuritic chest pain, which may vary over days or weeks. Chest pain of very sudden onset may be musculoskeletal in origin, or less commonly due to a perforation of the upper gastrointestinal tract (oesophagus or stomach) or dissection of the thoracic aorta. Chest pain that rapidly comes and goes, and lasts for less than a minute, is very rarely due to any serious disease.

What is the character of the pain?

It is worth taking some time to understand the character of the patient's pain. Cardiac pain may be severe but is rarely felt as 'sharp': the patient will frequently describe a sensation of pressure as if there is a heavy weight on their chest. Pleuritic chest pain is often due to inflammation of the pleura and may be caused by pneumonia, less specific infection (e.g. viral pleurisy), pulmonary embolism, or chest wall pain due to trauma or localised inflammation. Severe, sharp or tearing pain of sudden onset suggests dissecting thoracic aneurysm (Klompas 2002), though it is worth noting that in this condition the pain is slightly more likely to be in the anterior chest than in the classically described location of the back (Hagan et al. 2000). Pain reproduced by specific movements may have a musculoskeletal cause such as a muscle injury or nerve root irritation, but, as discussed above, chest wall tenderness is generally unhelpful and can even be misleading.

Does the pain go anywhere else (radiate)?

Pain that *radiates* into the neck, jaw, one arm or both arms often suggests a cardiac cause (Panju et al. 1998). In some patients, particularly the elderly or diabetic patient where autonomic function is impaired, chest pain or discomfort may be entirely absent and jaw or arm pain may be the only symptom of significant cardiac ischaemia (see Chapter 7). Pain radiating into the back suggests aortic dissection, but is not uncommon in acute coronary syndrome. Pleuritic pain rarely radiates, but some nerve entrapment syndromes may cause a shooting 'electric' pain to or from the shoulder or spine. Oesophageal pain sometimes radiates to the shoulder or jaw, whilst diaphragmatic irritation secondary to intra-abdominal pathology (such as bowel perforation or ruptured ectopic pregnancy) may be felt as pain in the shoulder tip. This is a form of *referred pain* because the spinal nerve roots that supply the diaphragm (C3, C4 and C5) also supply the shoulder.

Are there any associated symptoms?

Cardiac chest pain is traditionally associated with autonomic symptoms such as nausea, vomiting, sweating and pallor. Transient neurological disturbance, or the loss of pulses in the limbs, suggests aortic dissection. Shortness of breath (*dyspnoea*) is commonly associated with chest pain, and it is useful to distinguish dyspnoea that simply occurs in association with chest pain from pleuritic pain that is triggered or increased by inspiration. The latter suggests pathology in the pleura or chest wall, and often gives a subjective impression of dyspnoea;

however, the two problems may co-exist in some conditions, such as pneumonia. Patients with an increased respiratory rate or effort may develop musculoskeletal chest pain over time, and persistent coughing can have a similar effect, even to the point of causing a 'cough fracture' of one or more ribs. This phenomenon is more common in the elderly, or those with pre-existing osteoporosis. Sudden onset of shortness of breath occurs in larger pulmonary embolisms, and may be associated with *haemoptysis* (coughing up blood). However, haemoptysis also occurs in respiratory infections, when the patient's cough may also produce purulent sputum. Oesophageal reflux can produce an unpleasant taste in the mouth, and a sore throat or cough, particularly when the patient lies down and at night. It may also be associated with upper abdominal pain, but this is not exclusive to gastrointestinal pathology, and abdominal pain can also occur in inferior myocardial infarction and lower lobe pneumonias (Ravichandran and Burge 1996; Pope et al. 2000).

Does the pain come and go, or is it there all the time?

Pleuritic pain tends to be relatively constant, whereas the pain of cardiac ischaemia may come and go over time and increase with exertion. Similarly, gastro-oesophageal pain may be variable in its intensity. Constant pain is usually more troublesome at night when the patient is trying to sleep: at this time there are few distractions and ample opportunity to concentrate on the pain, thereby increasing its intensity and significance.

Does anything make the pain better or worse?

Angina tends to be precipitated by exercise, such as climbing a flight of stairs, and relieved by rest. Musculoskeletal pain may be reproduced by certain movements, or in certain positions. Chest pain due to reflux of stomach contents into the oesophagus is often made worse by lying flat, and the pain's intensity may be related to periods of eating and starvation. Psychogenic chest pain may be precipitated by life stressors, but these may also precipitate acute coronary syndrome in susceptible individuals (Bass and Mayou 2002).

Has pain like this been experienced previously?

A recurrence of previously experienced pain may provide an indication of the cause. However, whilst symptoms identical to previous ischaemic cardiac pain are obviously worrying, it is important to note that patients experiencing a second myocardial infarction often have very different symptoms from those of their first episode, which can lead to delayed presentation (Dracup et al. 1997). Therefore symptoms that are different from previous ischaemic cardiac pain should not be regarded as particularly reassuring. Patients experiencing a repeat pulmonary embolism are often certain of the diagnosis before they see a clinician, and this question can be particularly useful in identifying patients with recurrent psychogenic chest pain.

What risk factors does the patient have?

Risk factors for cardiac and venous thromboembolic disease should be established in all patients presenting with chest pain (see Chapter 6). The more major risk factors that are present, the more likely that disease becomes. Risk factors for cardiac disease are listed in Table 5.3 (see also Chapters 6 and 7), and for venous thromboembolism in Table 5.4 (see also Chapter 10).

Table 5.3   Risk factors for cardiac disease.

Major risk factors
- Personal history of ischaemic heart disease
- Family history of ischaemic heart disease
- Smoking
- Diabetes
- Hypertension
- Hypercholesterolaemia

Minor risk factors
- Male sex
- Obesity
- Physical inactivity
- Heavy alcohol use
- Psychological stress
- Cocaine use

Table 5.4   Risk factors for venous thromboembolism.

Major risk factors
- Personal history of venous thromboembolism
- Family history of venous thromboembolism
- Active cancer
- Immobility
- Recent major surgery
- Recent trauma
- Pregnancy and postpartum
- Smoking

Minor risk factors
- Older age
- Intravenous drug use
- Obesity
- Oestrogen
- Long-distance travel
- Inflammatory bowel disease

Clinical examination

Patient examination should be careful and thorough: this provides the best opportunity to identify abnormal findings, and is crucial in reassuring the patient. Key stages in the examination of a chest pain patient are listed in Table 5.5 and described in detail in Chapter 4. Additional examination of legs, ankles and associated arterial pulses

Table 5.5 Stages in the examination of a patient with chest pain.

● General impression	● Chest percussion
● Hands and pulse	● Chest auscultation
● Face and neck	● Abdominal examination
● Chest inspection	● Vital signs
● Chest palpation	

may be indicated depending on the history obtained (e.g. if the patient describes *claudication* (calf pain) when walking, or is suffering from chest pain and breathlessness following swelling in one leg, this suggests deep venous thrombosis and pulmonary embolism).

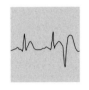

Clinical investigations

For a proportion of patients with chest pain a clear diagnosis is readily reached and no investigations are required. However, a handful of investigations may be indicated in reaching a diagnosis and forming a subsequent management plan. Although sublingual nitroglycerin and oral antacids are frequently administered during the assessment of non-traumatic chest pain in adults, neither are of any value in distinguishing cardiac pain from other causes, and should not be used for this purpose (Simpson et al. 1984; Diercks et al. 2005).

The electrocardiogram

The 12-lead electrocardiogram (ECG) is increasingly used in primary and community care as well as in hospital practice. The ECG may be abnormal in acute coronary syndrome, pulmonary embolism, pericarditis or aortic dissection, but a normal ECG can also occur in all of these conditions (see other related chapters). This means that the 12-lead ECG has high specificity but low sensitivity. However, it is such a cheap, non-invasive and rapid investigation that it is widely employed in adults with non-traumatic chest pain. Under certain circumstances additional leads may be recorded, or continuous ECG monitoring undertaken during provocative testing, such as exercise on a treadmill (see Chapters 6 and 7 for more detail).

Chest x-ray

Chest x-rays are commonly taken in acute chest pain of both traumatic and non-traumatic origin, particularly in patients presenting to hospital. In significant chest trauma an early x-ray is mandatory since major injuries may not be apparent on initial clinical examination. These may include fractures to the ribs, clavicles or spine, lung contusions, haemothorax, pneumothorax, pericardial effusion, mediastinal injury or diaphragmatic rupture (see Chapter 11). In non-traumatic chest pain, chest x-ray may reveal a small spontaneous pneumothorax that cannot be detected clinically, pneumonia, or underlying cardiac disease.

Laboratory tests

Whilst blood testing is frequently carried out in the hospital evaluation of adults with chest pain, the results rarely alter immediate clinical management. However, the following exceptions are generally recognised:

- In chest trauma, haemoglobin measurement assists in the detection of significant haemorrhage. Blood should also be cross-matched in preparation for transfusion where appropriate.
- In patients with chest pain of possible ischaemic cardiac origin, serum cardiac *troponin* is an excellent tool for risk stratification (see Chapters 6 and 7 for further discussion). However, its practical value is limited by the fact that troponin levels are only reliable 8–12 hours after the onset of the patient's worst pain, introducing delays that may inconvenience the patient and sometimes necessitate hospital admission. Where troponin is measured correctly, and found to lie within the normal range, the risk of a significant cardiac event during the next 30 days is substantially less than 1%, permitting further investigation and management on an outpatient basis (Hamm et al. 1997). On the other hand, an elevated troponin level is associated with a much poorer prognosis and usually mandates hospital admission. It is worth noting that troponin is also elevated in significant pulmonary embolism, cardiac contusion and some other conditions that do not normally cause chest pain, such as renal failure (Ammann et al. 2004).
- In patients who are judged to be at low clinical risk of pulmonary embolism, a normal *D-dimer* assay (see Chapter 10) reduces the risk of pulmonary embolism to less than 1%, at which point most clinicians would consider the disease to be 'ruled out'. Clinical risk assessment can be undertaken using the '*Wells Criteria*' (Wells et al. 2000), which are reproduced in Table 5.6. It is worth noting that D-dimers are raised in a wide variety of diseases, including significant infection and aortic dissection (Jolobe 2006).

Table 5.6   Criteria for assessment of pre-test probability for pulmonary embolism.

Criteria	Points
Suspected DVT	3.0
An alternative diagnosis is less likely than PE	3.0
Heart rate >100 beats per minute	1.5
Immobilisation or surgery in the previous 4 weeks	1.5
Previous DVT or PE	1.5
Haemoptysis	1.0
Malignancy (on treatment, treated in the past 6 months or palliative)	1.0

Score range	Mean probability of PE, %	% with this score	Interpretation of risk
<2 points	3.6	40	Low
2 to 6 points	20.5	53	Moderate
>6 points	66.7	7	High

DVT = deep venous thrombosis; PE = pulmonary embolism.

- In patients with suspected pulmonary pathology, such as pneumonia, chest trauma or pulmonary embolism, arterial blood gas analysis is useful in assessing disease severity and guiding therapy.

Inexperienced clinicians often use blood testing to supplement their clinical judgement, in the mistaken belief that laboratory tests have greater utility than is really the case. For example, *C-reactive protein* (CRP) is not useful in the diagnosis of lower respiratory tract infection (van der Meer et al. 2005). It is essential to consider to what extent the results of an investigation will alter patient management, and to avoid the temptation to arrange unnecessary tests which run the risk of generating both false negative and false positive results, as well as wasting valuable healthcare resources.

Other investigations

More specialised investigations, such as computerised tomography (CT) scanning or echocardiography, are indicated in certain circumstances, and are considered in more detail in the relevant chapters of this book.

Putting it all together – making a diagnosis

Diagnostic decision making in adult patients with chest pain is notoriously treacherous (Swap and Nagurney 2005). This is because mild chest discomfort may be the only evidence of life-threatening illness, and examination is often unrewarding. As a result, many clinicians opt for a policy of safety, which may involve a period of hospital observation and a series of investigations designed to exclude serious pathology. This is, however, taxing on healthcare resources, and various strategies have been used to improve the process of care whilst containing costs. These include the adoption of point-of-care testing and the establishment of low risk chest pain assessment or observation units (see Chapter 2).

In its purest form, diagnosis requires the identification and causal explanation of an abnormal health state. The traditional structure outlined above, following a logical sequence of history, examination and investigations, is a useful guide in reaching a diagnosis, but may need to be modified according to the patient's immediate clinical needs (e.g. resuscitation) and personal circumstances. Novice clinicians tend to take an *exhaustive* approach, collecting as many facts as possible during their initial assessment, and then endeavouring to make subsequent sense of these. This is inevitably inefficient and tiring, and tends to be superseded by a more focused approach, asking questions to support or refute possible causes of chest pain (the *hypothetico-deductive* method), before undertaking a targeted examination and any specific investigations that may be indicated to gather additional relevant information.

Traumatic chest pain

In reaching a diagnosis it is helpful to divide patients with chest pain into those with traumatic and non-traumatic causes, though with the caveat previously described that some patients with non-traumatic pain may ascribe their symptoms to possible, or unrelated, trauma. Where the pain can be confidently identified as arising from trauma, then the diagnostic process becomes a logical search for possible injuries. The likelihood, and severity, of injury is determined by:

- The mechanism of injury
- Underlying susceptibility in the patient (such as older age and osteoporosis)
- The degree of injury already known to exist

A common error in trauma diagnosis is to stop searching for further problems once a single injury has been found (*search satisfying*). This occurs because searching in everyday life differs from searching in clinical diagnosis: in everyday life, once the lost item has been found, further searching becomes pointless. Conversely, when searching in trauma every injury found increases the likelihood of further injury being present. Therefore the identification of an injury in the context of chest trauma should prompt additional efforts to seek other injuries (e.g. a small pneumothorax accompanying a fractured rib), rather than an abandonment of the diagnostic process. An understanding and adoption of the need for this approach (known as a *cognitive forcing strategy*) reduces the likelihood of common diagnostic errors (Croskerry 2003).

Non-traumatic chest pain

In patients with non-traumatic chest pain, however, different diagnostic strategies are required. Most clinicians with a reasonable degree of previous experience appear to rely on a process of *'pattern recognition'* for much of the time. In this diagnostic approach patients are fitted to 'prototypes' of disease that are developed and held in the clinician's mind, and which are subject to modification in the light of experience and learning. Pattern recognition, which is closely related to the use of *heuristics* ('rules of thumb' or tacit knowledge, developed by a clinician as a result of experience), allows diagnoses to be made rapidly and with minimal cognitive effort. It follows that more experienced clinicians will be more successful in this approach since they have a greater range of better developed prototypes on which to draw (for example, pattern recognition will fail when the clinician first encounters a rare disease of which they were previously unaware).

Pattern recognition is usually successful, but can also have disastrous consequences in the context of an atypical patient presentation, which may be ascribed to the wrong prototype. This can be compounded by the problem of *anchoring*, in which the clinician refuses to revise their diagnosis in the light of new information, and in some circumstances only seeks or accepts information that supports the diagnosis they have already made (*confirmation bias*). When diagnostic errors occur, it is often possible to identify instances where contradictory information has been ignored or explained away, rather than triggering a reconsideration of the original diagnosis, and this is supported by the consistent

observation of *order effects*, in which information presented early in the consultation is given greater weight than that presented later.

Bayes' theorem

Many researchers believe that humans tend to favour the relative ease of pattern
recognition, and move only reluctantly to higher order cognition in response to
difficult or unusual problems (Reason 1990). *Bayes' theorem*, which indicates that
the probability of each diagnostic possibility can be mathematically revised
according to the pre-test probability of that disease and the properties of any
test applied, is often cited as a diagnostic paragon but is rarely used explicitly
in practice. However, when the word 'test' is expanded to include the answer to
each question in the history and each finding on examination, it then becomes
apparent that most clinicians do use *Bayesian reasoning*, in a non-mathematical
way, to guide their assessment and estimate the likelihood of various diagnostic
possibilities. Thus, the more cardiac risk factors that are elicited by the clinician,
the more likely a cardiac diagnosis becomes in their mind. The main weakness
in this approach is the lack of a mathematical context, in that most clinicians
have little idea of the pre-test probability of key diseases, or of the properties of
the 'tests' they are using. This leads to relatively imprecise thinking, in which
disease probabilities are arbitrarily divided into 'high' and 'low' categories on
the basis of clinical impression and previous experience, rather than objective
criteria.

Whilst Bayesian reasoning has proved invaluable in some areas of chest pain
diagnosis (it underpins the use of D-dimer to 'rule out' pulmonary embolism in
low risk patients), it is also susceptible to various cognitive biases. Probability
revisions are seldom linear, and estimates of pre-test probability are clearly
influenced by recent experience or received wisdom. Clinicians are prone to
overestimate the probability of easily recalled events (such as those associated
with negative outcomes), or may place undue emphasis on life-threatening
disease. For example, patients with severe chest pain radiating to the back are
often immediately investigated for dissecting thoracic aneurysm, even though
they are far more likely to have an acute coronary syndrome (ACS). This is
because ACS is 100 times more common than dissection, even when the patient's
symptoms are atypical.

Rule out all serious things

In response to the risks associated with non-traumatic chest pain diagnosis in
adults, clinicians may assemble a list of the life-threatening possibilities, and
then attempt to 'rule out' each one in turn using clinical assessment and targeted
investigations. This may be described as a strategy of 'ROAST' ('Rule Out All
Serious Things'). The principle of 'rule out' and 'rule in' is again encompassed
by Bayesian reasoning, in that, if the probability of a disease falls below a certain
threshold (conventionally 1%), that possibility is discarded. Conversely, if the
probability rises to an arbitrary treatment threshold (conventionally 80–90%),

then no further testing occurs, the diagnosis is considered made and treatment begins. In this situation it is particularly difficult to revise the diagnosis in the light of new information unless a conscious effort is made to avoid anchoring bias. 'ROASTing' patients with chest pain may reduce risks for the patient and clinician but also tends to lead to an absence of diagnosis, rather than a clear explanation of symptoms and a treatment plan, which many patients find unsatisfactory.

Expert reasoning

Expert diagnosticians appear to move easily from one form of thinking to another, relying on pattern recognition and heuristics for straightforward cases, but shifting readily to more complex cognitive processes when the situation demands this. The use of *metacognition* (thinking about one's own thought processes) and the adoption of explicit cognitive forcing strategies may also help to reduce diagnostic error. Nevertheless, the study of expertise remains very challenging, and it is unclear how experts decide which form of thinking to use and when to change approach.

Any clinician undertaking diagnosis in chest pain patients is inevitably accepting an element of risk, which must be managed and minimised but cannot be eradicated. Very cautious clinicians, who simply refer all patients for a battery of diagnostic tests, have abdicated their responsibilities and risk inflicting unnecessary harm and inconvenience. On the other hand, those who choose to develop their clinical acumen and diagnostic skills on the basis of a simple bedside assessment will gain the approval of their patients, but cannot expect to be right every time.

Key learning points

- In the patient with chest pain, successful diagnosis is founded on the process of taking a careful history, performing a thorough clinical examination and requesting those investigations that will genuinely influence subsequent management.
- It is useful to distinguish between traumatic and non-traumatic chest pain, though even this is not always entirely reliable.
- Life-threatening disease may present with minimal symptoms.
- Listen carefully to the patient, but do not be unduly influenced by any desire they may have to downplay their symptoms.
- Making a diagnosis inevitably involves an element of risk. Logical thinking and an understanding of common cognitive biases helps to minimise this.

References

Ammann A, Pfisterer M, Fehr T, Rickli H (2004) Raised cardiac troponins. *British Medical Journal* **328**: 1028–1029.

Bass C, Mayou R (2002) The ABC of psychological medicine: chest pain. *British Medical Journal* **325**: 588–591.

Croskerry P (2003) Cognitive forcing strategies in clinical decision making. *Annals of Emergency Medicine* **41**: 121–122.

Diercks DB, Boghos E, Guzman H, Amsterdam EA, Kirk JD (2005) Changes in the numeric descriptive scale for pain after sublingual nitroglycerin do not predict cardiac etiology of chest pain. *Annals of Emergency Medicine* **45**: 581–585.

Dracup K, Alonzo AA, Atkins JM, Bennett NM, Braslow A, Clark LT, Eisenberg M, Ferdinand KC, Frye R, Green L, Hill MN, Kennedy JW, Kline-Rogers E, Moser DK, Ornato JP, Pitt B, Scott JD, Selker HP, Silva SJ, Thies W, Weaver WD, Wenger NK, White SK (1997) The physician's role in minimizing prehospital delay in patients at high risk for acute myocardial infarction: recommendations from the National Heart Attack Alert Program. *Annals of Internal Medicine* **126**: 645–651.

Goodacre S, Nicholl J, Dixon S, Cross E, Angelini K, Arnold J, Revill S, Locker T, Capewell SJ, Quinney D, Campbell S, Morris F (2004) Randomised controlled trial and economic evaluation of a chest pain observation unit versus routine care. *British Medical Journal* **328**: 254–257.

Hagan PG, Nienaber CA, Isselbacher EM, Bruckman D, Karavite DJ, Russman PL, Evangelista A, Fattori R, Suzuki T, Oh JK, Moore AG, Malouf JF, Pape LA, Gaca C, Sechtem U, Lenferink S, Deutsch HJ, Diedrichs H, Marcos y Robles J, Llovet A, Gilon D, Das SK, Armstrong WF, Deeb GM, Eagle KA (2000) The International Registry of Acute Aortic Dissection (IRAD): new insights into an old disease. *Journal of the American Medical Association* **283**: 897–903.

Hamm C, Goldman B, Heeschen MD, Kreymann G, Berger J, Meinertz T (1997) Emergency room triage of patients with acute chest pain by means of rapid testing for cardiac troponin T or troponin I. *New England Journal of Medicine* **337**: 1648–1653.

Jolobe OM (2006) Venous thromboembolism: potentially dangerous pitfalls arise from diagnostic tests. *British Medical Journal* **332**: 364.

Kendrick S, Frame S, Povey C (1997) Beds occupied by emergency patients: long term trends in patterns of short term fluctuations in Scotland. *Health Bulletin (Edinburgh)* **55**: 167–175.

Klompas M (2002) Does this patient have an acute thoracic aortic dissection? *Journal of the American Medical Association* **287**: 2262–2272.

Langewitz W, Denz M, Keller A, Kiss A, Rüttimann S, Wössmer B (2002) Spontaneous talking time at start of consultation in outpatient clinic: cohort study. *British Medical Journal* **325**: 682–683.

Panju AA, Hemmelgarn BR, Guyatt GH, Simel DL (1998) Is this patient having a myocardial infarction? *Journal of the American Medical Association* **280**: 1256–1263.

Pope JH, Aufderheide TP, Ruthazer R, Woolard RH, Feldman JA, Beshansky JR, Griffith JL, Selker HP (2000) Missed diagnosis of acute cardiac ischemia in the emergency department. *New England Journal of Medicine* **342**: 1163–1170.

Ravichandran D, Burge DM (1996) Pneumonia presenting with acute abdominal pain in children. *British Journal of Surgery* **83**: 1707–1708.

Reason J (1990) *Human Error*. Cambridge, Cambridge University Press.

Rodger M, Wells PS (2001) Diagnosis of pulmonary embolism. *Thrombosis Research* **103**: V225–238.

Simpson FG, Kay J, Aber CP (1984) Chest pain – indigestion or impending heart attack. *Postgraduate Medical Journal* **60**: 338–340.

Swap CJ, Nagurney JT (2005) Value and limitations of chest pain history in the evaluation of patients with suspected acute coronary syndromes. *Journal of the American Medical Association* **294**: 2623–2629.

van der Meer V, Neven AK, van den Broek PJ, Assendelft WJJ (2005) Diagnostic value of C reactive protein in infections of the lower respiratory tract: systematic review. *British Medical Journal* **331**: 26.

Wells PS, Anderson DR, Rodger M, Ginsberg JS, Kearon C, Gent M, Turpie AG, Bormanis J, Weitz J, Chamberlain M, Bowie D, Barnes D, Hirsh J (2000) Derivation of a simple clinical model to categorize patients' probability of pulmonary embolism: increasing the model's utility with the SimpliRED D-dimer. *Thrombosis and Haemostasis* **83**: 416–420.

Useful websites

The 'BestBETs' Best Evidence Topics for emergency medicine, available at: http://www.bestbets.org.

The 'Cardiac' section of the Bandolier website for evidence-based care, available at: http://www.jr2.ox.ac.uk/bandolier/booth/booths/cardiac.html.

The 'Clinical Evidence' website of the *British Medical Journal*, available at: http://www.clinicalevidence.com.

Section 2

Advanced assessment and
management of patients
presenting with chest pain

Chapter 6

Assessing and managing the patient with chest pain due to an acute coronary syndrome

Sarah Green and Jenny Tagney

Aims

The overall aim of this chapter is to develop the reader's understanding of chest pain in the context of the spectrum of acute coronary syndromes. Despite being a major cause of morbidity and mortality throughout the developed world, acute coronary syndromes are often misdiagnosed and misunderstood. This chapter endeavours to address the confusion that surrounds acute coronary syndromes and explore ways in which rapid diagnosis and risk stratification may be facilitated to enable rapid commencement of appropriate treatments.

There are significant guidelines published by the European Society of Cardiology (ESC) and the American College of Cardiology/American Heart Association (ACC/AHA), which the reader should refer to in addition to reading this chapter.

Learning outcomes

At the end of the chapter, following pertinent background reading and appropriate supervised practice the reader will be able to

- Discuss the pathophysiology of acute coronary syndromes.
- Identify the clinical presentation of acute coronary syndromes and consider it in relation to the differential diagnosis of chest pain.
- Perform an assessment of a patient and identify characteristics that are highly suggestive or negate a potential diagnosis of an acute coronary syndrome.
- Request and correctly interpret appropriate diagnostic tests for acute coronary syndromes.
- Discuss the management of the whole spectrum of acute coronary syndromes.
- Undertake the process of risk stratification in a patient with an acute coronary syndrome and identify appropriate treatment strategies according to individual risk.

Background

Cardiovascular disease remains the main cause of death in the United Kingdom today, with half of these deaths resulting from coronary heart disease (CHD). Despite a significant reduction in mortality rates for CHD over the last 25 years and the introduction of the National Service Framework (NSF) for CHD in 2000, the British Heart Foundation (BHF 2005) statistics show that CHD continues to account for 113,895 deaths per year in the UK. This is compared with 33,420 deaths a year from lung cancer, 16,142 deaths from colo-rectal cancer and 12,625 deaths from breast cancer (BHF 2005). Most deaths from CHD are the consequence of an acute myocardial infarction, of which 260,000 occur each year. Acute coronary syndromes (ACS) are usually, but not always, caused by atherosclerotic CHD and are associated with increased risk of cardiac death and myocardial infarction (Braunwald et al. 2002).

ACS refers to a clinical spectrum of the same disease process resulting in reduced coronary arterial blood flow causing acute myocardial ischaemia, which leads to unstable angina, ST segment elevation myocardial infarction (STEMI) or a non-ST segment elevation myocardial infarction (N-STEMI). When a complete occlusion occurs, ST segment elevation or a bundle branch block pattern appears on the 12-lead electrocardiogram (ECG) as myocardial necrosis progresses from the subendocardium to the subepicardial layers. This is termed an ST segment elevation myocardial infarction (STEMI).

If thrombus creates a partial or incomplete occlusion of the coronary artery, damage may not extend to the full thickness of the myocardium. Instead, unstable angina or N-STEMI may develop. The difference between unstable angina and N-STEMI is determined by the cardiac marker serum troponin, which is released during myocardial cell damage. The pathological and clinical outcomes depend on whether the thrombus partially or completely occludes the coronary artery and on the degree of myocardial damage (Edwards et al. 2005).

Whilst incidence and mortality rates remain a cause for concern, evidence suggests that the severity of acute coronary events has lessened (Dauerman et al. 2000; Goff et al. 2000; Hellermann et al. 2002) and mortality rates are decreasing (Abildstrom et al. 2003). There has also been a significant change in the pattern of ACS within the last few years, with a larger proportion of patients with myocardial infarction having N-STEMI and fewer experiencing STEMI (Rogers et al. 2000). Of patients who survive and reach hospital, approximately 12% will present with STEMI and 13% with N-STEMI. Of those diagnosed with unstable angina, 8% will die within 6 months of their presentation (Fox 2004).

Causes

Angiographic evidence demonstrates that the disruption of a vulnerable atherosclerotic plaque and subsequent thrombus formation account for over 90% of ACS with ST segment elevation (Braunwald et al. 2002), some occurring in mild to moderate coronary artery stenoses (Bertrand et al. 2002). However, thrombus in the coronary artery is responsible for clinical changes in 35–75% of cases of

ACS without ST segment elevation (N-STEMI and unstable angina) (Braunwald et al. 2002). Braunwald et al. (2002) identify a further four possible explanations for non-ST elevation ACS that are also characterised by a myocardial oxygen supply and demand mismatch. These are:

- Dynamic obstruction
- Severe narrowing without spasm or thrombus
- Arterial inflammation
- Secondary unstable angina

Dynamic obstruction

A dynamic obstruction to blood flow may be caused by transient and focal coronary artery spasm, sometimes known as Prinzmetal/variant angina, in which ST elevation is produced on the 12-lead ECG that usually does not, but may, progress to myocardial infarction. This vasospasm is caused by hypercontractility of the vessel wall and may also be induced by cocaine use (see also Chapter 15).

Severe narrowing without spasm or thrombus

Severe narrowing of the coronary arteries without vasospasm is described by Braunwald et al. (2002) as occurring in some patients with 'progressive atherosclerosis' or with restenosis after percutaneous coronary intervention.

Arterial inflammation

The inflammatory process in general has been shown (in studies measuring high sensitivity C-reactive protein levels) to have an impact upon plaque destabilisation (Burke et al. 2002; Sano et al. 2003; James et al. 2005). In particular, arterial inflammation, perhaps related to infection, has been a factor that Braunwald et al. (2002) believe has an impact upon plaque destabilisation and subsequent rupture.

Secondary unstable angina

This can occur in conditions such as:

- Fever, tachycardia and thyrotoxicosis, which increase myocardial oxygen demand
- Anaemia and hypoxia, which reduce oxygen delivery to the myocardium
- Hypotension, which reduces coronary perfusion

When these conditions occur in those with underlying atherosclerotic CHD, an ACS may be precipitated.

The Framingham Heart Study 1963 (Fox et al. 2004) made a significant contribution to our understanding of the risk factors for CHD, and the findings are reflected in the Joint British Societies' Guidelines on prevention of cardiovascular disease (Wood et al. 2005). The guidelines essentially focus on the following risk factors:

- Tobacco smoking
- Blood pressure and hypertension
- Blood lipids and dyslipidaemia
- Glycaemia and diabetes mellitus
- Physical inactivity
- Obesity and body fat distribution
- Positive family history of CHD, which is defined as the development of CHD in a first degree male relative <55 years of age and a female first degree relative <65 years

Whilst one cannot change a positive family history, health professionals can work with 'at risk' individuals to ensure that modifiable risk factors are identified early and controlled. Studies have consistently demonstrated that modifiable risk factors such as hypercholesterolaemia, hypertension, smoking and a sedentary lifestyle independently and significantly increase the risk of an acute coronary event (Wood et al. 2005). The presence of an individual risk factor doubles the risk of developing ACS, and when two or more of the major modifiable risk factors are present, relative risk is multiplied rather than added (Jamrozik 2002).

- Tobacco smokers are known to have poorer endothelial function and an increase in migration of lipoproteins into the vessel wall from the bloodstream. Smoking creates 'sticky' platelets and high levels of fibrinogen, which significantly increase the chances of an atherothrombotic event (Neunteufl et al. 2002; Ambrose and Barua 2004). Findings in Himbert et al. (2005) and Rosengren et al. (2005) suggest that smoking is strongly associated with STEMI.
- Hypertension is prevalent in those patients with ST elevation and non-ST elevation ACS but particularly in the latter group (Khot et al. 2003; Rosengren et al. 2005). The role of hypertension in advancing atherogenesis is well documented but remains less clear in acute coronary events, though it is suggested that elevated blood pressure may promote growth of, rather than instability of, existing plaques.
- The risks associated with CHD increase as concentrations of total blood cholesterol rise (Wood et al. 2005). Cardiovascular risk is essentially determined by concentrations of LDL and HDL cholesterol (inversely) and the preferred target for treatment strategies is LDL (Wood et al. 2005). Those with familial hypercholesterolaemia have a CHD mortality risk 10 times greater than the general population (Wood et al. 2005).
- Although a risk factor for all acute coronary events, obesity according to Rosengren et al. (2005) is seen more frequently in patients who present with ACS without ST elevation and is strongly associated with other factors such as diabetes mellitus, hypertension and dyslipidaemia, which are related to the development of CHD.

- Glycaemia has a continuous relationship with cardiovascular risk. In comparison with those demonstrating a normal glucose tolerance, those with impaired glucose tolerance have a 1.5 times relative risk of developing CHD and those with established diabetes have a two- to four-fold risk of developing CHD (Wood et al. 2005). The particular role of diabetes in atherosclerotic plaque development and plaque rupture is unclear; however, the high rate of MI in patients with diabetes suggests that diabetes creates susceptibility to plaque rupture. Additionally, diabetic patients have more diffuse and distal disease, and experience increased frequency of cardiac complications, higher morbidity and mortality rates with acute coronary events (Grundy et al. 2004).

Metabolic syndrome

The new diagnostic label of metabolic syndrome is based upon a number of interrelated cardiovascular risk factors (see Tables 6.1a and 6.1b). The presence of these factors together is associated with higher rates of CHD, increased levels of fibrinogen and thus a prothrombotic situation (Grundy et al. 2004; Birhanyilmez et al. 2005).

Incidence of atherosclerosis is also known to be age dependent. This and a family history of early onset of CHD are associated with increased risk of an ACS. The absolute risk for the development of CHD rises with age in both men and women, the majority of first events of CHD occurring over the age of 65. This is particularly true for women in whom the onset of CHD is around 10 years later than in their male counterparts (Chandra et al. 1998; BHF 2005; see also Chapter 7).

Table 6.1 Definition of metabolic syndrome.

(a) National Cholesterol and Education Program (NCEP 2001) guidelines (cited in Wood et al. 2005)
Clinical diagnosis of metabolic syndrome is made if three of the following criteria are met

- Central obesity, waist circumference in Caucasians >102 cm (males) and >88 cm (females)
- Fasting glucose 6.1 mmol/l
- Blood pressure 130 / 85 mmHg
- Serum triglycerides 1.7 mmol/l
- HDL cholesterol <1.0 mmol/l (males) and <1.3 mmol/l (females)

(b) International Diabetes Federation (2005)
Central obesity (according to ethnic specification – see below) plus any two of the following:

- Triglyceride levels >1.7 mmol/l or specific treatment for elevated triglyceride levels
- Reduced HDL cholesterol levels <1.03 mmol/l in men and <1.29 mmol/l in women, or specific treatment for reduced HDL cholesterol
- Blood pressure ≥130/85 mmHg or previously diagnosed hypertension
- Fasting plasma glucose ≥5.6 mmol/l or previously diagnosed with type 2 diabetes

Waist circumference by ethnicity

Europids	Male >94 cm	Female >80 cm
South Asians and Chinese	Male >90 cm	Female >80 cm
Japanese	Male >85 cm	Female >90 cm

Pathophysiology

The coronary circulation perfuses the myocardium, which in turn is responsible for producing adequate output and blood flow to perfuse all of the body's organs, including the heart itself. Compromised coronary perfusion attenuates the pumping function of the heart, which in turn further compromises coronary blood flow. The heart is dependent upon a rich oxygen supply with the myocardium of the left ventricle withdrawing around 75% of the oxygen supplied by the coronary arteries at rest (Fiegl and Schaper 2002), thus the myocardium has very little anaerobic capacity. Any increase in oxygen consumption must be quickly balanced by an increase in oxygen delivery via the coronary arterial blood flow, which is usually achieved by a local intrinsic mechanism (Fiegl and Schaper 2002).

Atherosclerosis is a disease of the large and medium-sized arteries, and is characterised by a loss of elasticity and thickening of the vascular wall. The disease process occurs in the intimal layer of the artery wall where lipoprotein-derived lipid cells and inflammatory cells permeate and form intimal plaques and create fibrosis to various degrees in a focal or multifocal rather than a uniform manner. The plaques or atheromas may be described as raised fibro-fatty lesions and consist of a largely cholesterol lipid core covered by a fibrous cap. Atherosclerotic lesions not only reduce the lumen size of the coronary artery but also produce turbulent blood flow around the stenotic lesion, which reduces the speed, energy and pressure of the blood flow distal to the lesion (Fiegl and Schaper 2002). The reduction in pressure may lead to inadequate perfusion within the distal microvascular bed, particularly during periods when myocardial oxygen demand is higher such as during exercise, i.e. in stable angina or during conditions such as fever, tachycardia or thyrotoxicosis (secondary unstable angina – see causes and risk factors section).

Symptoms and clinical conditions that are associated with ACS are generally related to the deterioration of the plaque rather than its maturation (Hansson and Nilsson 2002). Certain factors (see Table 6.2) are proposed that may reduce the tensile strength of the fibrous cap.

The plaque may concede to the pressure from the pulsating blood flow through the coronary artery, creating either small fissures through the endothelium down into the plaque, or areas of endothelial desquamation increasing the plaque's vulnerability to sudden rupture or thrombus formation (Hansson and Nilsson 2002). The sudden rupture of the atherosclerotic plaque leads to the

Table 6.2 Characteristics of a vulnerable plaque.

Large lipid core
Greater density of inflammatory cells
Thin fibrous cap which is depleted of collagen and smooth muscle cells
Large numbers of macrophages increase enzyme levels which
● Inhibit collagen formation
● Stimulate apoptosis of endothelial and smooth muscle cells
Inflammatory activity impairs the process of repair of the fibrous cap

formation of an occlusive or subocclusive thrombus, referred to as the culprit lesion(s). In the presence of an occlusive thrombus and poor collateral blood supply, myocardial ischaemia leads to myocyte necrosis within 15–20 minutes and spreads from subendocardium to subepicardium (Braunwald et al. 2002). The time taken to restore adequate blood flow within the artery dictates the size of the myocardial infarction. In non-ST elevation ACS, the thrombotic response is often associated with vasospasm. This causes intermittent obstruction to blood flow during which fragments of the thrombus can break off and flow down the artery, lodging in smaller vessels. These distal emboli can cause small areas of infarction without a complete occlusion of an epicardial vessel (Bertrand et al. 2002). Like vulnerable plaque, several areas of thrombus formation may be seen simultaneously, either within the same coronary artery or in different ones (Chew and White 2004).

Clinical presentation

Clinical presentation and outcomes are dependent upon the location of the culprit lesion(s) plus the severity and duration of the myocardial ischaemia. Patients may present with a cardiac arrest, with ventricular fibrillation (VF) being the commonest fatal arrhythmia in the first 24 hours of acute MI (Channer and Morris 2003). Inferior infarction/ischaemia may be accompanied by transient or prolonged bradyarrhythmias. The artery that supplies the sinoatrial (SA) and atrioventricular (AV) node is usually a branch of the right coronary artery (RCA). In patients with an inferior infarction where the RCA is occluded, the reduced blood supply to the SA and AV nodes may result in a variety of arrhythmias and transient degrees of heart block, the most commonly occurring of which are complete heart block (CHB, also known as third degree AV block) and Wenkebach or Möbitz type 1 second degree AV block. CHB may also be seen in the presence of an anterior MI but is not usually transient and indicates an extensive infarct and thus generally a poor prognosis. As a consequence of a poorly functioning left ventricle in the presence of ischaemia/infarction, patients may also present with acute left ventricular failure.

Central chest discomfort or pain remains the prominent clinical indicator of the whole spectrum of ACS. Classically, the discomfort is reported to be retrosternal, radiating to the neck, jaw and left shoulder or arm (Bertrand et al. 2002; Braunwald et al. 2002; Van de Werf et al. 2003; Antman et al. 2004). In reality, symptoms are often ill defined and the patient may describe a heavy feeling, tightness or a dull ache rather than 'chest pain' (Horne et al. 2000; Albarran 2002). Chest discomfort resulting in an ACS may also be confused with indigestion, or described as a numb or tingling feeling, and often radiates down the right or both arms into the fingers. Chest pain associated with ACS may occur at rest, may be precipitated by exercise or may have been associated with increased frequency and severity over a short period of time (e.g. crescendo angina). Other factors such as stress are also relevant, whilst many, particularly women, also report recent fatigue and weakness (Ryan et al. 2005; see also Chapter 7 for more detailed review of presenting symptoms in women with CHD).

Significant numbers of patients present with minimal symptoms or without any chest pain or discomfort at all. Consequently, many STEMIs or N-STEMIs may remain unrecognised by the patient and are classified as clinically 'silent' events (Canto et al. 2000; Horne et al. 2000). Associated symptoms frequently include shortness of breath, nausea, diaphoresis (severe perspiration) and sometimes light-headedness. Silent and atypical symptom presentations are acknowledged as important features of an acute coronary event, with studies linking these to unfavourable outcomes (Brieger et al. 2004). Unusual presentations may impede diagnosis, leading to delays in establishing initial treatment plans and ensuing hospital management, which is often suboptimal as a result (Canto et al. 2000; Brieger et al. 2004).

The large numbers of patients that present with various causes of chest pain create a challenge for healthcare professionals. Skilled assessment and expertise are required to identify those with ACS, which often comprise a relatively small number. It is particularly difficult to accurately differentiate between ACS patients without myocardial injury (as in those with unstable angina) and those that have moderate myocardial injury on initial presentation.

History taking

Because chest pain is associated with a number of other clinical conditions, it is vital to clearly establish the character of the symptoms in order to differentiate between myocardial ischaemia and non-ischaemic or non-cardiac chest pain. Braunwald et al. (2002) describe five important factors, ranked in order of importance, to assist in distinguishing patients with ACS:

- The nature of the chest pain
- Prior history of CHD
- Gender
- Age
- The number of traditional risk factors present

General assessment of the patient's chest pain history should focus upon eliciting information regarding site, radiation, character, severity, duration, aggravating factors and relieving factors as well as any associated symptoms such as breathlessness, nausea and diaphoresis (Macleod et al. 1995).

As previously mentioned, symptoms of ACS are varied and may consist of a deep and poorly localised chest pain, tightness or discomfort and/or arm, jaw, neck, ear or epigastric discomfort. The chest discomfort may also be described as a 'pressure', 'squeezing' or 'crushing sensation' or even a sensation of 'fullness'; it is often severe and prolonged, lasting more than 20 minutes. Many patients also present solely with arm, neck or jaw discomfort (Wallentin et al. 2002). In those who present without chest pain, new onset or worsening, unexplained, exertional dyspnoea is the most commonly experienced symptom. Patients presenting with atypical symptoms are more likely to be older in age, female, hypertensive and diabetic and to have a history of heart failure (Brieger et al. 2004). Although typical features are known to increase the likelihood that chest pain occurs as a result of CHD, Braunwald et al. (2002) acknowledge that stabbing, pleuritic pain and pain reproduced by palpation, do not necessarily exclude ACS. Larger numbers of males have ACS than females, and the likelihood of CHD increases with age. Traditional risk factors are less significant in the predictive process of ACS compared with clinical history and 12-lead ECG findings. However, they are an important part of assessment and risk stratification processes because of their significant contribution to CHD and their association with adverse outcomes.

Recent cocaine ingestion is a significant contributory factor to the development of ACS. Thus it is important to establish evidence of illicit drug use in patients presenting to hospital with chest pain (see Chapter 15 for more detailed information).

Clinical examination

On initial assessment the patient may report chest discomfort and appear pale, cool and clammy with an elevated respiratory rate, blood pressure and pulse rate in response to the pain and other symptoms. In both STEMI and N-STEMI, diaphoresis is a common feature and hypertension is often identified in the early stages, which may be associated with the level of pain and anxiety that the patient is experiencing. The patient may also feel nauseous and vomit. Some patients, however, particularly women, may be pain-free but present with shortness of breath as their primary symptom for seeking medical treatment.

Those presenting with an inferior infarction with right ventricular involvement may have hypotension and an elevated jugular venous pressure. If confirmed this is treated with fluids to increase filling pressures. In contrast, persistent hypotension with an extensive infarct in and consequent hypoperfusion in the presence of high filling pressures is indicative of cardiogenic shock, and is associated with mortality rates of over 60% (Braunwald et al. 2002). In some patients with ACS, initial examination may be unremarkable.

Heart sounds may remain entirely normal on auscultation but the following may be present:

- A third (S3) or fourth heart sound (S4) may be heard indicating decreased ventricular compliance as a result of ischaemia.
- The presence of a pansystolic murmur heard best at the apex suggests mitral regurgitation as a result of ischaemia-induced diastolic dysfunction, or papillary muscle dysfunction. If a pansystolic murmur is heard at the left sternal edge, a ventricular septal defect is a possibility. In either case an urgent transthoracic echocardiogram is indicated.

On pulmonary auscultation, crackles may be heard at the bases to mid zones of the lungs, indicating the presence of pulmonary oedema as a result of left ventricular dysfunction.

As with clinical history, assessment for evidence of peripheral vascular disease is a vital component in identifying those with ACS. Findings may consist of absence or diminution of peripheral pulses, particularly in the lower limbs, and the presence of carotid or femoral bruits.

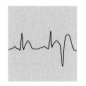

Initial investigations

The 12-lead ECG and biochemical cardiac markers have important parts to play in confirming the diagnosis of ACS, calculating risk and identifying appropriate treatment strategies. In those patients with good clinical histories of ACS but with an equivocal or borderline ECG and biochemical markers, echocardiogram and/or myocardial stress tests may be indicated.

Electrocardiogram

The 12-lead ECG is central to decisions regarding treatment strategies for ACS patients, but must be used as an adjunct to clinical history and physical examination due to the many variations in 'normal' ECG presentation that can mimic ACS patterns (e.g. ST elevation in precordial leads of young black males, Newby et al. 2005).

Extensive evidence identifies that ACS patients with ST segment elevation benefit greatly from early reperfusion therapy (Van de Werf et al. 2003; Antman et al. 2004), whereas ACS patients without ST segment elevation benefit from early access to an aggressive and interventional strategy, including anti-platelet therapy and percutaneous coronary intervention (PCI) (Bertrand et al. 2002; Braunwald et al. 2002).

Within the early stages of ACS, the 12-lead ECG may be normal (Morris et al. 2003). Around 10% of patients diagnosed with a myocardial infarction on the basis of clinical history and biochemical markers failed to develop ST segment changes (Morris et al. 2003). However, in most patients with ACS, serial 12-lead ECG recordings tend to show evolving changes that generally follow recognised patterns.

ACS with ST segment elevation

A third of patients with ST segment elevation die within 24 hours of the onset of ischaemia (Antman et al. 2004). Overall mortality rates are highest in those with left bundle branch block and anterior ST segment elevation (Antman et al. 2004), thus rapid and accurate diagnosis of STEMI is vital as rapid reperfusion improves prognosis.

The very early evidence of STEMI on the 12-lead ECG includes:

- Increased T wave amplitude in the affected area
- Hyperacute T wave changes (T waves become more prominent and peaked)

These changes are subtle and often only present for around 5–30 minutes prior to the development of ST segment elevation (Morris et al. 2003). As the STEMI evolves, the ST segment elevation develops, the T wave becomes broad and the ST segment loses its normal concavity and often becomes more convex (Morris et al. 2003). It reaches its maximum height in around an hour after the onset of infarction (Jaffe and Davidenko 2002).

12-lead ECG criteria for reperfusion therapy* (Morris et al. 2003)

- ST elevation ≥1mm in two contiguous limb leads (see Figure 6.1 inferior STEMI), or
- ST elevation ≥2mm in two contiguous chest leads (see Figure 6.2 antero-lateral STEMI), or
- New left bundle branch block, or
- Isolated ST segment depression V1–V3 indicating a posterior infarct

(*Individual health service protocols may vary slightly. It is vital that you check the protocol in your specific area.)

Other characteristics that may be identified on a 12-lead ECG indicating STEMI may be reciprocal ST segment depression in opposing leads (see Figure 6.2 of an antero-lateral STEMI with reciprocal inferior ST depression) and pathological Q waves (please refer to Morris et al. 2003).

ACS without ST elevation

The 12-lead ECG recorded at rest when the patient first presents is critical not only to identify or rule out STEMI but also to gather information to support suspicions of CHD. Transient ST segment depression ≥0.5mm, which develops during chest pain and resolves when the patient becomes asymptomatic, is strongly suggestive of acute ischaemia (Braunwald et al. 2002). Non-ST elevation ACS may be identified on the ECG in a variety of ways. These include:

- Horizontal ST segment depression
- T wave inversion
- ST deviation of less than 0.5mm
- Biphasic T waves (especially in the anterior leads, which suggest a lesion in the left anterior descending artery)
- A normal ECG (1–6%, Braunwald et al. 2002)

Patients with any of the above changes are initially considered to have non-ST elevation ACS and may later be diagnosed with N-STEMI or unstable angina according to analysis of biochemical markers, which identify myocardial necrosis in the bloodstream. The findings on a 12-lead ECG in patients with non-ST elevation ACS indicate the appropriate treatment besides providing independent prognostic information (Braunwald et al. 2002). ST deviation ≥0.5mm associated with chest pain at rest strongly suggests severe CHD and is associated with high mortality and re-event rates (Braunwald et al. 2002), particularly in those with a larger magnitude of ST segment depression (Chew and White 2004).

Laboratory investigations

Serum cardiac markers are laboratory tests that play a significant part in the diagnostic and risk stratification processes in ACS. Damage to the cell membrane

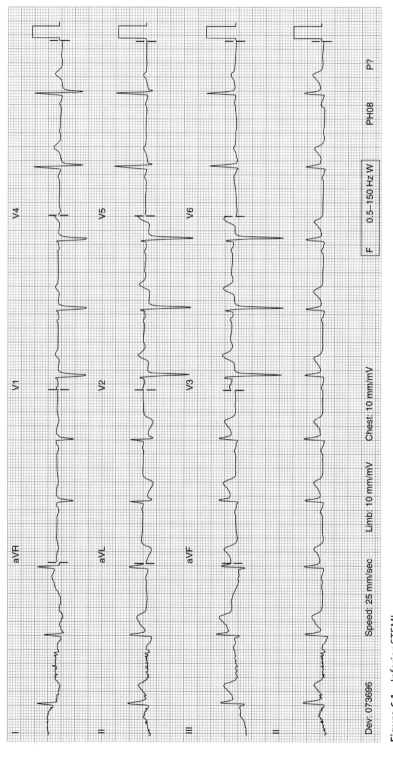

Figure 6.1 Inferior STEMI.

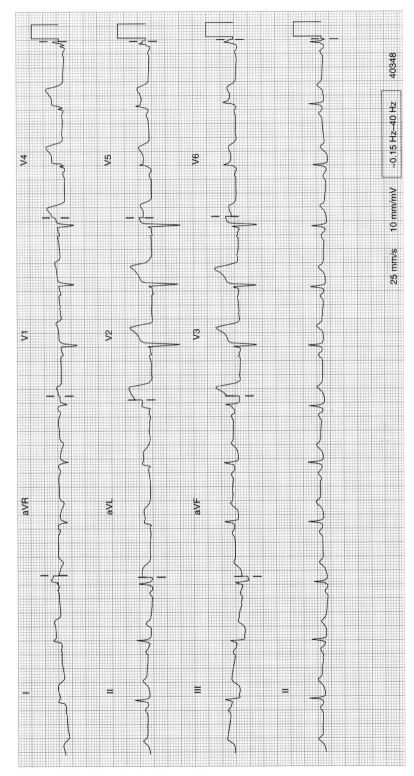

Figure 6.2 Antero-lateral STEMI with reciprocal inferior changes.

during necrosis causes cellular contents to leak into cardiac interstitium, lymphatics and cardiac vasculature and finally into the peripheral circulation where they can be detected via a venous blood sample (Van de Werf et al. 2003).

Whilst other traditional markers such as creatine kinase (CK), CK-MB (an isoenzyme of CK) and myoglobin may have some advantages, cardiac troponins (I and T) in conjunction with clinical history and the 12-lead ECG have emerged as the most appropriate markers of ACS (Bertrand et al. 2002; Braunwald et al. 2002; James et al. 2005). Cardiac troponins are found solely within the myocardial cells, are detectable within the bloodstream within 4 hours of ischaemic injury and remain elevated for up to 2 weeks (James et al. 2005). Elevation of troponin I (TnI) and troponin T (TnT) are useful not only for diagnostic purposes but also in predicting adverse outcomes (James et al. 2005). Elevated TnI or TnT levels identify those who are at much higher risk of death and recurrent myocardial infarction, both in the short and long term (Lindahl et al. 2000). There is a direct proportional relationship to the risk of mortality (Antman et al. 2004), i.e. as the level of troponin rises, so does the risk of death and re-infarction. Thus, cardiac troponin has a significant role in risk stratification of those with N-STEMI and unstable angina, aiding identification of patients who will most benefit from treatment strategies such as glycoprotein IIb/IIIa inhibition and early percutaneous coronary intervention as opposed to more conservative strategies and routine coronary angiography. Other biochemical markers such as C-reactive protein (CRP), brain natriuretic peptide (BNP) and renal dysfunction have also been documented as potential markers for risk stratification of ACS patients. For further discussion or information please refer to James et al. (2005).

Cardiac troponins are accurate in identifying myocardial necrosis. However, such necrosis may be due not to an ACS but to hypoxia, pulmonary embolus or heart failure or in the presence of renal failure. Consequently, the use of cardiac troponins and their role in risk stratification for acute coronary syndrome is limited to those who present with a clinical history and/or ECG criteria consistent with ACS.

Radiography

Chest x-ray findings are generally normal in ACS. However, potential abnormal findings may include pulmonary oedema and/or increased cardiac ratio as a result of left ventricular dilatation. Essentially, the value of a chest x-ray in ACS is in excluding other potential causes of chest pain rather than providing specific information for the early diagnosis of ACS. Thus, performing a chest x-ray should not delay the initiation of treatment such as thrombolysis, unless a contraindication, for example aortic dissection, is suspected (Antman et al. 2004).

Echocardiography

An echocardiogram (ECHO) can identify regional wall abnormalities that occur in myocardial ischaemia and necrosis (Van de Werf et al. 2003). Consequently it may be useful in identifying ACS in patients who present with chest pain and non-specific ECG patterns (Antman et al. 2004). However, wall abnormalities are not specific to acute ischaemia and may be as a result of an old infarct (Van de Werf et al. 2003), and thus the role of ECHO in an acute situation is limited. However it has been suggested that ECHO may be useful in the diagnostic process of other causes of chest pain such as aortic dissection and pulmonary embolus (Van de Werf et al. 2003).

Myocardial stress testing

Patients who initially present with a *suspected* ACS who *do not have*:

- Further chest pain during the period of observation
- ST segment depression or ST elevation
- Elevated cardiac biochemical markers on initial and repeat bloods (performed between 6 and 12 hours)

are considered to be at low risk for developing adverse events such as myocardial infarction or death (Bertrand et al. 2002). In these cases a stress test, usually an exercise tolerance test (ETT), is indicated to establish whether the underlying cause is CHD. This management strategy has been used successfully within the chest pain assessment unit environment to assist 'rule-out' criteria and thus avoid hospital admission (Goodacre et al. 2004). For further information on ETT please refer to Hill and Timmis (2003). For additional strategies to aid diagnosis in women, please refer to Chapter 7.

Differential diagnosis

The main priority in the assessment of a patient with chest pain is the identification of a potentially life-threatening condition which needs particular attention and fast track to treatment (Erhardt et al. 2002). ACS is among these high risk conditions.

ACS shares symptoms and clinical features with other conditions, which may lead to misdiagnosis (see Table 6.3). Epigastric conditions such as peptic ulcer disease are often mistaken for ACS and vice versa (Ghuran et al. 2003). Patients suffering from such conditions may present with chest/epigastric pain which may be associated with nausea and diaphoresis; however, ECG tracings are likely to be normal. Aortic dissection is often a sudden-onset tearing pain that radiates to the

Table 6.3   Differential diagnosis in ACS.

Pericarditis	Peptic ulcer disease
Myocarditis	Tension pneumothorax
Hypertrophic cardiomyopathy	Muscular skeletal chest wall pain
Aortic dissection	Pleurisy
Pulmonary embolus	Biliary or pancreatic pain
Gastro-oesophageal reflux and oesophageal spasm	Cervical disc or neuropathic pain
Psychogenic pain disorder	Costochondritis

back and frequently lasts for a significant period of time (Antman et al. 2004). Physical assessment findings may reveal absent peripheral pulses and abnormal heart sounds (an aortic regurgitant murmur may also be heard). Evidence of a dissection may also be identified on a chest x-ray and an ECHO. Acute pericarditis is often mistaken with STEMI as it shares similar features of ST segment elevation on a 12-lead ECG. In pericarditis, however, the ST segments tend to be saddle shaped; such changes tend to be more widespread and the PR segment may be depressed. Pericarditic chest pain is often constant and pleuritic in nature and relieved by sitting forward (see Chapter 8). A careful clinical history and physical examination help to distinguish between the many differential diagnoses.

Immediate management and interventions

Treatment goals for all patients with ACS are to provide:

- Adequate pain relief – with opiate analgesia and/or nitrates
- Adequate arterial oxygen concentration – with supplemental oxygen
- Continuous cardiac monitoring to identify and be able to rapidly act upon potential cardiac arrhythmias or ongoing ischaemia (if 12-lead monitoring available)
- Venous access – for rapid drug administration
- Aspirin 300 mg chewed
- Serial 12-lead ECGs

For further clinical management in the acute phase, treatment strategies to relieve ischaemia are separated into management of ST segment elevation ACS and management of non-ST elevation acute coronary syndromes. The different treatment regimes and their effectiveness for STEMI, N-STEMI and unstable angina are based on current knowledge of the different underlying pathology and disease processes (Edwards et al. 2005).

ST elevation ACS

The current European Society of Cardiology (Van der Werf et al. 2003) and American College of Cardiology/American Heart Association (Antman et al. 2004) guidelines recommend early pharmacological or mechanical reperfusion therapy for those who present with persistent ST segment elevation or new left bundle branch block. Both ESC and AHA/ACC guidelines state that patients with STEMI in the absence of contraindications (see Table 6.4) should receive reperfusion by either thrombolysis within 30 minutes of presentation to hospital or primary percutaneous coronary intervention (PCI) performed within 90 minutes of medical contact. The sooner reperfusion is achieved, the greater the chance of salvaging myocardium. It is clear that fibrinolysis in STEMI (in the absence of contraindications) improves outcomes when administered within 12 hours of symptom onset (Menozzi et al. 2005). Maximal efficacy in terms of survival occurs within the first 2–3 hours and significant benefits decrease as the thrombus 'ages' (refer to the Boersma curve, Boersma et al. 1996). Limitations

Table 6.4 Absolute contraindications to thrombolysis.

- Recent CVA
- Recent gastrointestinal bleed
- Surgery within the last month (Including abdominal, neurological and eye surgery; liver biopsy and dental extraction are also considerations)
- Lumbar puncture within the last month
- Pregnancy or post-partum
- Trauma
- Aortic dissection
- Aortic aneurysm
- Prolonged CPR
- Systemic hypertension

Absolute and relative contraindications for thrombolysis exist; relative contraindications vary from area to area; consult the protocols in your clinical area.

of pharmacological reperfusion include its relative and absolute contraindications, increased risk of bleeding, haemorrhagic stroke, and restoration of TIMI-3 flow in the affected vessel of less than half of the patients who receive fibrinolysis (Menozzi et al. 2005). In cases where thrombolyisis is unsuccessful (<50% reduction in ST segments 90 minutes post-thrombolysis), there is evidence to show that rescue PCI is beneficial (Silber et al. 2005).

In comparison, primary percutaneous coronary intervention (P-PCI) achieves TIMI-3 flow rates in >90% of treated patients (Menozzi et al. 2005) and the reocclusion rate is <5% (Keeley et al. 2003). Higher risk patients with STEMI such as those with cardiogenic shock have the greatest survival benefits in P-PCI (Hochman et al. 1999). However, highly skilled and experienced teams who are able to offer the service without significant delay must perform P-PCI in order to achieve such impressive results. P-PCI is also time dependent: if the difference between door to needle and door to balloon inflation time is >90 minutes, the advantages of the latter are likely to be lost (De Luca et al. 2004). Delays in either treatment strategy lead to poorer outcomes (Antman et al. 2004). However, the choice of reperfusion therapy is not merely a clinical treatment decision but is affected by organisational, resource and clinical restrictions such as:

- Availability of suitably skilled teams to perform P-PCI over 24 hours, 7 days per week
- Distance to P-PCI centres in some rural areas
- National strategies to focus on early thrombolysis leading to resources being directed to paramedic-led thrombolysis

Thus reperfusion therapy for patients with STEMI must be based upon evaluation of clinical and organisational resources, ensuring that clear protocols are available to guide clinicians.

Non-ST elevation ACS

Where the risks of adverse events of ST segment elevation are highest within the first few hours, these risks continue over time for those with non-ST elevation

ACS. Biochemical markers (preferably TnI or TnT) should be measured both at time of presentation and at 6–12 hours after onset of symptoms. It is the presence of a characteristic rise and fall of troponin levels which provides a diagnosis of myocardial infarction and thus separates N-STEMI from unstable angina (Fox 2004).

The current ESC (Bertrand et al. 2002; Silber et al. 2005) and AHA/ACC (Braunwald et al. 2002) guidelines recommend that all non-ST segment ACS patients be risk stratified into high or low risk groups (see Table 6.5 for high-risk characteristics). The risk of death and recurrent infarction varies among those who present with ACS (Fox 2004) and the process of risk stratification in patients with non-ST elevation ACS helps to appropriately target the sort and intensity of medical therapies and interventions. Both the ESC and the AHA/ACC guidelines state that high-risk patients benefit from more aggressive treatment regimes, and those at low risk may be able to be discharged early and safely from hospital.

In both low- and high-risk patients, five initial therapies are recommended (Bertrand et al. 2002; Braunwald et al. 2002): aspirin, clopidogrel and low molecular weight heparin, with the addition of beta-blockers and nitrates in those with ongoing ischaemia. Two further treatments should be aimed at high-risk individuals: glycoprotein IIb/IIIa inhibitors and early coronary angiography to provide information regarding the coronary vessels and the extent of any atherosclerotic obstruction, and the suitability of revascularisation (invasive strategy). A small group of patients may require a coronary angiogram within the first hour (Bertrand et al. 2002). This includes those who experience evidence of significant ongoing ischaemia or cardiac arrhythmias and who are haemodynamically unstable.

Further investigations and treatments

Treatment strategies are determined according to individual risk in all ACS patients. Patients who are haemodynamically unstable, have on-going ischaemia

Table 6.5 High risk characteristics in patients with non-ST elevation ACS. (Braunwald et al. 2002; Silber et al. 2005).

Prolonged chest pain at rest (>20 min)
Recurrent pain at rest
Evidence of left ventricular dysfunction – pulmonary oedema, gallop rhythm, tachycardia
New or worsening mitral regurgitation
Ventricular arrhythmias
Dynamic ST segment changes >1 mm
Elevated troponin 1, troponin T or CK-MB levels
Hypotension
Bradycardia
Aged >75 years
Increased tempo of chest pain within 48 hours of presentation
Early post-infarction unstable angina
Diabetes mellitus

or experience cardiac arrhythmias as a result of any ACS require urgent invasive investigation (Bertrand et al. 2002). Haemodynamic support in the form of an intra-aortic balloon pump and/or inotropes may also be initiated in the presence of cardiogenic shock, and temporary pacing may be required for bradyarrhythmias in those with ischaemia affecting the conduction pathway.

In patients receiving successful thrombolytic treatment, current ESC guidelines recommend angiography and any further revascularisation within 24 hours (Berrtand et al. 2002).

In patients with atherosclerotic lesions suitable for myocardial revascularisation, an evaluation is made as to the most suitable method: either percutaneous or surgical revascularisation. If, as in some cases, angiography demonstrates no viable option for revascularisation as a result of severe, diffuse coronary artery disease, or in those who have mild to moderate plaques, patients will be managed by maximising their medical therapies.

Glucose levels are a strong independent predictor of long-term mortality of patients with diabetes, thus effective control of glucose levels is a vital part of the treatment during the acute phase and long-term management of diabetic patients with ACS (Malmberg et al. 2005).

Patients with low risk characteristics should be managed with antiplatelet regimes such as aspirin, clopidogrel and beta-blockers. A full stress test such as an exercise tolerance test is recommended to determine the need for further invasive strategies in the low-risk group (Bertrand et al. 2002).

Medium- to long-term management plan

The broad aims of care during this phase should generally focus upon preparing the patient to return to normal activities, using the acute event to evaluate lifestyle and risk factors. Continued medical therapies (unless contraindicated) include aspirin, a beta-blocker, ACE inhibitor and statin, plus nitrates if there is evidence of on-going ischaemia (DH 2000; NICE 2001 – revised version expected 2007). Clopidogrel is recommended for at least 9–12 months in non-ST elevation ACS (NICE 2004). Increased understanding of major risk factors and significant actions taken to modify transmutable risk factors may account for an alteration in the pattern and prevalence of the traditional risk factors and thus changes in both the clinical presentation and impact of ACS. However, if this trend is to continue, lifestyle and risk factor interventions or modifications according to current guidelines must be maintained.

Availability of cardiac rehabilitation programmes varies across Europe and North America. In England, cardiac rehabilitation should be offered to all those who have experienced myocardial infarction or revascularisation (percutaneous coronary intervention or coronary artery bypass grafting) (DH 2000). It is also recommended for other patients such as those who are newly diagnosed with angina or who have been hospitalised due to unstable angina (SIGN 2002). There are many issues around availability and accessibility of appropriate programmes that are beyond the scope of this chapter to address. However, aggressive risk factor management is essentially the mainstay of secondary prevention treatment in patients with CHD, to reduce the risk of further non-fatal or fatal events and to improve both length and quality of life. Interventions should focus upon smoking cessation, normalisation of hypertension and hyperlipidaemia, control of diabetes, obesity management and promotion of regular exercise. Tailoring support to enable individuals to achieve a reduction in their cardiovascular risk will remain a challenge for healthcare professionals.

Key learning points

- Acute coronary syndromes encompass ST segment elevation myocardial infarction, non-ST segment elevation myocardial infarction and unstable angina.
- Collate all available data: include current and past clinical history, physical examination, ECG results and biochemical markers (if applicable) and base treatment strategies on the individual patient's calculated risk.
- First phase of management for all ACS consists of IV access, opiate analgesia (+/- nitrates), aspirin, oxygen, 12-lead ECG and continuous cardiac monitoring.
- The second phase of management is based upon the presence or absence of ST elevation.
- In the presence of STEMI, urgent reperfusion therapy is indicated (primary PCI or thrombolysis).
- Risk stratification is paramount in those with non-ST elevation ACS.
- Target non-ST elevation ACS patients who have high risk features with aggressive antithrombotic therapies and an early invasive strategy.
- All ACS patients require aggressive risk factor management to prolong life and improve its quality.

References

Abildstrom SZ, Rasmussen S, Rosén M, Madsen M (2003) Trends in the incidence and case fatality rates of acute myocardial infarction in Denmark and Sweden. *Heart* **89**(5): 507–511.

Albarran JW (2002) The language of chest pain. *Nursing Times* **98**(4): 38–40.

Ambrose JA, Barua RS (2004) The pathophysiology of cigarette smoking and cardiovascular disease: an update. *Journal of American Cardiology* **43**(10): 1731–1737.

Antman EM, Anbe DT, Armstrong PW, Bates ER, Green LA, Hand M, Hochman JS, Krumholz HM, Kushner FG, Lamas GA, Mullany CJ, Ornato JP, Pearle DL, Sloan MA, Smith SC Jr (2004) ACC/AHA guidelines for the management of patients with ST-elevation myocardial infarction: a report of the American College of Cardiology/ American Heart Association Task Force on Practice Guidelines. Writing Committee to revise the 1999 guidelines for the management of patients with acute myocardial infarction. *Journal of the American College of Cardiology* **44**(3): 671–719.

Bertrand ME, Simoons ML, Fox KAA, Wallentin LC, Hamm CW, McFadden E, De Feyter PJ, Specchia G, Ruzyllo W (2002) Management of acute coronary syndromes without persisting ST-segment elevation: the Task Force report on the Management of Acute Coronary Syndromes of the European Society of Cardiology. *European Heart Journal* **23**(23): 1809–1840.

Birhanyilmez M, Guray U, Guray T, Altay H, Demirkan B, Caldir V, Cay S, Refiker ME, Sasmaz H, Korkmaz SY (2005) Metabolic syndrome is associated with extension of coronary artery disease in patients with non ST segment elevation acute coronary syndromes. *Coronary Artery Disease* **16**(5): 287–292.

Boersma E, Maas ACP, Deckers JW, Simoons ML (1996) Early thrombolytic treatment in acute myocardial infarction: reappraisal of the golden hour. *Lancet* **348**(9030): 771–775.

Braunwald E, Antman EM, Beasley JW, Califf RM, Cheitlin MD, Hochman JS, Jones RH, Kereiakes D, Kupersmith J, Levin TN, Pepine CJ, Schaeffer JW, Smith EE III, Steward DE, Theroux P (2002) ACC/AHA 2002 Guideline update for the management of patients with unstable angina and non-ST-segment elevation myocardial infarction: a report of the American College of Cardiology/American Heart Association Task Force on Practice Guidelines (Committee on the Management of Patients with Unstable Angina). http://www.acc.org/clinical/guidelines/unstable/unstable.pdf (accessed 12th May 2006).

Brieger D, Eagle KA, Goodman SG, Steg PG, Budaj A, White K, Montalescot G, GRACE Investigators (2004) Acute coronary syndromes without chest pain, an under-diagnosed and undertreated high risk group: insights from the Global Registry of Acute Coronary Events. *Chest* **126**(2): 461–469.

British Heart Foundation (2005) Coronary heart disease statistics. http://www.heartstats.org (accessed 9th March 2006).

Burke AP, Tracy RP, Kolodgie F, Malcom GT, Zieske A, Kutys R, Pestaner J, Smialek J, Virmani R (2002) Elevated C-reactive protein values and atherosclerosis in sudden coronary death: association with different pathologies. *Circulation* **105**(17): 2019–2023.

Canto JG, Shlipak MG, Rogers WJ, Malmgren JA, Frederick PD, Lambrew CT, Ornatao JP, Barron HV, Kiefe CI (2000) Prevalence, clinical characteristics, and mortality among patients with myocardial infarction presenting without chest pain. *Journal of the American Medical Association* **283**(24): 3223–3229.

Chandra NC, Ziegelstein RC, Rogers WJ, Tiefenbrunn AJ, Gore JM, French WJ, William J, Rubison M, for the National Registry of Myocardial Infarction–I (1998) Observations of the treatment of women in the United States with myocardial infarction. *Archives of Internal Medicine* **158**: 981–988.

Channer K, Morris F (2003) Myocardial ischaemia. In Morris F, Edhouse J, Brady WJ, Camm J (Eds) *ABC of Clinical Electrocardiography*, pp. 37–41. London, BMJ Publishing Group.

Chew DP, White HD (2004) Pathophysiology, classification, and clinical features. In Bhatt DL, Flather DM (Eds) *Handbook of Acute Coronary Syndromes*, pp. 1–23. London, Remedica Publishing.

Dauerman HL, Lessard D, Yarzebski J, Furman MI, Gore JM, Goldberg RJ (2000) Ten-year trends in the incidence, treatment, and outcome of Q wave myocardial infarction. *American Journal of Cardiology* **86**(7): 730–735.

De Luca G, Suryapranata H, Ottervanger JP, Antman EM (2004) Time delay to treatment and mortality in primary angioplasty for acute myocardial infarction: every minute of delay counts. *Circulation* **109**(10): 1223–1225.

Department of Health (2000) *National Service Framework for Coronary Heart Disease – Modern Standards and Service Models*. Stationery Office, London.

Edwards N, Varma M, Pitcher D (2005) Changing names, changing times, changing treatments: an overview of acute coronary syndromes. *British Journal of Resuscitation*. **4**(1): 6–10.

Erhardt L, Herlitz J, Bossart L, Halinen M, Keltai M, Koster R, Marcassa C, Quinn T, van Weert H (2002) Task Force Report on the management of chest pain. *European Heart Journal* **23**(15): 1153–1176.

Fiegl EO, Schaper W (2002) Physiology of coronary circulation, Section 2. In Crawford MH, DiMarco JP (Eds) *Cardiology* pp. 1.1–1.8. London, Mosby.

Fox CS, Evans JC, Larson MG, Kannel WB, Levy D (2004) Temporal trends in coronary heart disease mortality and sudden cardiac death from 1950 to 1999: the Framingham Heart Study. *Circulation* **110**(5): 522–527.

Fox KA (2004) Management of acute coronary syndromes: an update. *Heart* **90**(6): 698–706.

Ghuran A, Uren N, Nolan J (2003) *Emergency Cardiology: An Evidence-based Guide to Acute Cardiac Problems.* London, Arnold.

Goff DC Jr, Howard G, Wang CH, Folson AR, Rosamond WD, Cooper LS, Chambless LE (2000) Trends in severity of hospitalized myocardial infarction: The Atherosclerosis Risk in Communities (ARIC) study 1987–1994. *American Heart Journal* **139**(5): 874–880.

Goodacre S, Nicholl J, Dixon S, Cross E, Angelini K, et al. (2004) Randomised controlled trial and economic evaluation of a chest pain observation unit compared to routine care. *British Medical Journal* **328**: 254–260.

Grundy SM, Brewer HB Jr, Cleeman JI, Smith SC Jr, Lenfant C (2004) Definition of metabolic syndrome: Report of the National Heart, Lung, and Blood Institute. *Circulation* **109**(3): 433–438.

Hansson GK, Nilsson J (2002) Pathogenesis of atherosclerosis, Section 1. In Crawford MH, DiMarco JP (Eds) *Cardiology*, pp. 1.1–1.12. London, Mosby.

Hellermann JP, Reeder GS, Jacobsen SJ, Weston SA, Killian JM, Roger VL (2002) Longitudinal trends in the severity of acute myocardial infarction: a population study in Olmsted county, Minnesota. *American Journal of Epidemiology* **156**(3): 246–253.

Hill J, Timmis A (2003) Exercise tolerance testing. In Morris F, Edhouse J, Brady WJ, Camm J (Eds) *ABC of Clinical Electrocardiography*, pp. 41–45. London, BMJ Publishing Group.

Himbert D, Klutman M, Steg G, White K, Gulba DC – the GRACE Investigators (2005) Cigarette smoking and acute coronary syndromes: a multinational observational study. *International Journal of Cardiology* **100**(1): 109–117.

Hochman JS, Sleeper LA, Webb JG, Sanborn TA, White HD, Talley JD, Buller CE, Jacobs AK, Slater JN, Col J, McKinlay SM, LeJemtel TH (1999) Early revascularization in acute myocardial infarction complicated by cardiogenic shock. SHOCK Investigators. Should we emergently revascularize occluded coronaries for cardiogenic shock. *New England Journal of Medicine* **341**(9): 625–634.

Horne R, James D, Petrie K, Weinman J, Vincent R (2000) Patients' interpretation of symptoms as a cause of delay in reaching hospital during acute myocardial infarction. *Heart* **83**(4): 388–393.

International Diabetes Federation (2005) www.idf.org/home/index (accessed 15th May 2006).

Jaffe AS, Davidenko J (2002) Diagnosis of acute myocardial ischaemia and infarction, Section 2. In Crawford MH, DiMarco JP (Eds) *Cardiology*, pp. 12.1–12.19. London, Mosby.

James SK, Lindahl B, Wallentin LC (2005) Biomarkers for risk stratification in non-ST segment elevation acute coronary syndromes: what is their relation to classical clinical characteristics? In Ferrari R, Hearse DJ (Eds) *Dialogues in Cardiovascular Medicine – Acute Coronary Syndromes* **10**(3): 153–162.

Jamrozik K (2002) Epidemiology of atherosclerotic disease, Section 1. In Crawford MH, DiMarco JP (Eds) *Cardiology*, pp. 2.1–2.14. London, Mosby.

Keeley EC, Boura JA, Grines CL (2003) Primary angioplasty versus intravenous thrombolytic therapy for acute myocardial infarction: a quantitative review of 23 randomised trials. *Lancet* **361**(9351): 13–20.

Khot UN, Khot MB, Bajzer CT, Sapp SK, Ohman EM, Brener SJ, Ellis SG, Lincoff AM, Topol EJ (2003) Prevalence of conventional risk factors in patients with coronary heart disease. *Journal of the American Medical Association* **290**(7): 898–904.

Lindahl B, Toss H, Siegbahn A, Venge P, Wallentin L (2000) Markers of myocardial damage and inflammation in relation to long-term mortality in unstable coronary artery disease. FRISC Study Group. Fragmin during instability in coronary artery disease. *New England Journal of Medicine* **343**(16): 1139–1147.

Macleod J, Munro J, Edwards CRW (Eds) (1995) *Clinical Examination*, 10th edition. London, Churchill Livingstone.

Malmberg K, Ryden L, Wedel H, Birkeland K, Bootsma A, Dickstein K, Efendic S, Fisher M, Hamsten A, Herlitz J, Hildebrandt P, MacLeod K, Laakso M, Torp-Pedersen C, Waldenstrom A, DIGAMI 2 Investigators (2005) Intense metabolic control by means of insulin in patients with diabetes mellitus and acute myocardial infarction (DIGAMI 2): effects on mortality and morbidity. *European Heart Journal* **26**(7): 650–661.

Menozzi A, Vignali L, Solinas E, Ardissino D (2005) Should all patients presenting with ST-segment elevation myocardial infarction undergo primary percutaneous coronary intervention? In Ferrari R and Hearse DJ (Eds) *Dialogues in Cardiovascular Medicine – Acute Coronary Syndromes* **10**(3): 168–173.

Morris F, Edhouse J, Brady WJ, Camm J (Eds) (2003) *ABC of Clinical Electrocardiography*. London, BMJ Publishing Group.

National Institute for Clinical Excellence (2001) Prophylaxis for patients who have experienced a myocardial infarction: drug treatment, cardiac rehabilitation and dietary manipulation. Inherited Clinical Guideline A. Issued April 2001. www.nice.org.uk/page.aspx?0=16479 (accessed 12th May 2006).

National Institute for Clinical Excellence (2004) Clopidogrel in the treatment of non-ST-segment-elevation acute coronary syndrome. Technology Appraisal number 80. Issued July 2004. www.nice.org.uk/TAO80guidance (accessed 12th May 2006).

Neunteufl T, Heher S, Kostner K, Mitulovic G, Lehr S, Khoschsorur G, Schmid RW, Maurer G, Stefenelli T (2002) Contribution of nicotine to acute endothelial dysfunction in long term smokers. *Journal of American Cardiology* **39**(2): 251–256.

Newby D, Cockcroft J, Wilkinson I (2005) *Coronary Heart Disease: Your Questions Answered.* London, Churchill Livingstone.

Rogers WJ, Canto JG, Lambrew CT, Tiefenbrunn AJ, Kinkaid B, Shoultz DA, Frederick PD, Every N (2000) Temporal trends in the treatment of over 1.5 million patients with myocardial infarction in the US from 1990 through 1999: the National Registry of Myocardial Infarction 1, 2 and 3. *Journal of the American College of Cardiology* **36**(7): 2056–2063.

Rosengren A, Wallentin L, Simoons M, Gitt A, Behar S, Battler A, Hasdai D (2005) Cardiovascular risk factors and clinical presentation in acute coronary syndromes. *Heart* **9**(9): 1141–1147.

Ryan CJ, DeVon HA, Zerwic JJ (2005) Typical and atypical symptoms: diagnosing acute coronary syndromes accurately. *American Journal of Nursing* **105**(2): 34–36.

Sano T, Tanaka A, Namba M, Nishibori Y, Nishida Y, Kawarabayashi T, Fukuda D, Shimada K, Yoshikawa J (2003) C-reactive protein and lesion morphology in patients with acute myocardial infarction. *Circulation* **108**(3): 282–285.

Scottish Intercollegiate Guideline Network (SIGN) (2002) *Cardiac Rehabilitation. A Quick Reference Guide.* Supported and endorsed by the British Association of Cardiac Rehabilitation. SIGN Executive, Royal College of Physicians, 9 Queen Street, Edinburgh, Scotland, UK. www.sign.ac.uk (accessed 12th May 2006).

Silber S, Albertsson P, Aviles FF, Camici PG, Colombo A, Hamm C, Jorgensen E, Marco J, Nordrehaug J-E, Ruzyllo W, Urban P, Stone GW, Wijns W (2005) Guidelines for Percutaneous Coronary Interventions. The Task Force for Percutaneous Coronary Interventions of the European Society of Cardiology. *European Heart Journal* **26**: 804–847.

Van de Werf F, Ardissino D, Betriu A, Cokkinos DV, Falk E, Fox KAA, Julian D, Lengyel M, Neumann F-J, Ruzyllo W, Thygesen C, Underwood R, Vahanian A, Verheugt FWA, Wijns W (2003) Management of acute myocardial infarction in patients presenting with ST-segment elevation: Task Force Report on the Management of Acute Myocardial Infarction of the European Society of Cardiology. *European Heart Journal* **24**(1): 28–66.

Wallentin L, Bertil L, Siegbahn A (2002) Unstable coronary artery disease Section 2. In Crawford MH, DiMarco JP (Eds) *Cardiology*, pp. 13.1–13.19. London, Mosby.

Wood D, Wray R, Poulter N, Williams B, Kirby M, Patel V, Durrington P, Reckless J, Davis M, Sivers F, Potter J (2005) JBS2: Joint British Societies Guidelines on prevention of cardiovascular disease in clinical practice. *Heart* **91**(Suppl. V): v1–52.

Websites

www.acc.org/clinical/guidelines
www.escardio.org/knowledge/guidelines
http://www.heartstats.org
www.dh.gov.uk
www.nice.org.uk/page.aspx?0=cardiovascular&View=All&template=diseasetax.aspx
www.sign.ac.uk

Chapter 7

Analysing the presentation of women with chest pain and other symptoms associated with coronary heart disease and myocardial infarction

John W. Albarran

Aims

The aim of this chapter is to review the complexities of symptoms described by women that may not include chest pain but are associated with an acute manifestation of coronary heart disease. The challenges of establishing a differential diagnosis in women with chest pain, the need for acute and long-term strategies promoting early symptom recognition by staff and patients, and the importance of improving the lifestyle and overall management of such women is also addressed. The chapter concludes that difficulties in assessing women with a traditional description of chest pain as a primary symptom are less problematic; the real challenge lies in diagnosing those who present without chest pain or have atypical symptoms. The development of gender-sensitive approaches to risk assessment and clinical investigation of women should lead to improved survival and recovery outcomes.

Learning outcomes

Following the completion of this chapter, the reader will have:

- A detailed understanding of mortality and morbidity patterns among women with coronary heart disease.
- An appreciation of the specific risk factors for coronary heart disease and how these apply to women deemed vulnerable.
- An increased awareness of the abnormal/atypical presentations of women who are subsequently diagnosed with either myocardial ischaemia or infarction.
- A developed insight into the role of clinical presentation, history taking, clinical examination and investigations as applied to women with a suspected myocardial infarction.

- An appreciation of the importance of a gender-sensitive approach to the assessment and management of women with undifferentiated chest symptoms suggestive of coronary heart disease.

Background

In the past two decades, a substantive body of evidence has been amassed suggesting that, compared with men, women experience higher death rates due to cardiovascular disease, particularly beyond the age of 65 years. Specifically, gender-based differences associated with coronary heart disease exist in respect of clinical presentation, diagnostic measures, response to interventions and adverse outcomes.

For most of the last century, coronary heart disease (CHD) has been viewed as only affecting Caucasian middle-class high-achieving men (Lockyer and Bury 2002; Wenger 2004). International evidence, however, suggests that death rates among women with CHD are increasing and in some instances are higher than in men, particularly after the age of 75 years (European Heart Network 2005; Petersen et al. 2005). Recent United Kingdom data for 2004 reveal that 47,287 women died from CHD (BHF 2004). Similarly, in the United States, CHD is also the principal cause of death among women, with over half a million being affected annually (American Heart Association (AHA) 2002). This represents 41.3% of all deaths, more than from all cancer types, and equates to one woman dying from CHD each minute (AHA 2002). Additionally, of sudden deaths associated with CHD, nearly two-thirds of women will experience no symptoms (Wenger 2004). It is not only elderly women who are affected. In the US, over 9000 American women below 45 years of age sustain a myocardial infarction annually. One study also concluded that women under 50 years of age who have sustained an MI are twice as likely to die when compared with men with MI of equal age (Vaccarino et al. 1999). Recent evidence also suggests that the high incidence of stable angina is comparable between the genders. However, the presence of stable angina in women is associated with increased coronary mortality compared with women in the general population (Hemingway et al. 2006).

Contributory factors for trends in mortality and morbidity of CHD

There are specific reasons accounting for the high prevalence of CHD among women. Primarily, the onset of coronary heart disease in women lags between 10 and 20 years behind that of men (Chandra et al. 1998). The clinical manifestations may occur at a time when women have other comorbidities, including symptoms of the menopause, heart failure, diabetes and hypertension. This places them at an increased risk for acute MI or sudden death. More women than men delay seeking help following the onset of acute cardiac symptoms (see Table 7.1). This means that women may not benefit from early coronary artery reperfusion with thrombolytic therapy (Boersma et al. 1996). Additionally, women will experience a greater number of recurrent infarctions and higher

Table 7.1 Reasons why women with coronary heart disease delay seeking urgent healthcare.

- Symptom character: the initial presentation of CHD symptoms for many women can be intermittent, vague and indeterminate. Consequently these undifferentiated symptoms may be ignored or dismissed as not serious
- Symptom attribution: women, particularly those with a chronic condition, may attribute CHD symptoms to a chronic illness (arthritis) or factors such as ageing, being overweight, cigarette smoking and physical exertion
- Symptom expectations: women expect the symptoms of MI to be dramatic, and to involve loss of consciousness and sudden death. Where the symptoms are at odds with their experiences, they are unlikely to seek medical help
- Perceptions around candidacy: women generally believe that it is men who are most at risk of MI and CHD
- Understanding and knowledge of CHD: awareness of the risk factors for heart disease is poor but lower in women younger than 45 years of age
- Perceptions of hospital staff: women might be embarrassed about reporting unspecific symptoms which may not be taken seriously and fear that they may be chastised for previous or current negative lifestyle behaviours
- Consultation process: following the onset of symptoms, women, more than men, tend to delay seeking health advice because they consult family members and friends before making their decision. Women from ethnic minority groups have longer delays in seeking help
- Lack of health advice: health messages have not been well communicated to women and hence they have a low awareness of CHD
- Access to public transport and financial factors are known to influence decisions to seek healthcare advice (Dempsey et al. 1995; Dracup and Moser 1997; Ruston et al. 1998; Meischke et al. 1999; Finnegan et al. 2000; Horne et al. 2000; Miller 2000; Perry et al. 2001; Rosenfeld 2001; Brink et al. 2002; Richards et al. 2002; Mosca et al. 2004a; Hart 2005; Lockyer 2005; Albarran et al. in press)

rates of mortality after their MI (AHA 2002). Although there has been a reduction in mortality from CHD in men worldwide, this decline has not been reproduced in women. This is because CHD in women has been largely underrecognised, underdiagnosed and undertreated (Grady et al. 2003; Miller 2003; Naidoo and Fox 2006). To address these disparities and trends in morbidity and mortality, the BHF (2003) and the European Society of Cardiology (ESC, *Women at heart initiative*, 2005) have launched a series of gender-specific initiatives that aim to raise public awareness and improve the provision of cardiac services for women.

Causes

Although the potential for developing atherogenic risk factors is similar between the sexes, it is the relative weighting and the effects of each that are different. Specifically, women differ from men in relation to the use of contraceptives, hormonal differences, cholesterol metabolism, hypertension and rates of diabetes (Wenger 1997; Edmunds and Lip 2000; Stangl et al. 2002; Collins 2006). In the areas of smoking and exercise levels, new differences are emerging.

Menopause

Post-menopausal women have a heightened risk of death due to MI. A deficiency of female reproductive hormones is believed to precipitate atherogenic risk factors but can be reduced in some women by taking hormone therapy (Halm and Penque 1999). The speculated benefits of oestrogen on lipid profiles, in reducing platelet aggregation and in promoting coronary vasodilatation have led to the use of hormone replacement therapy in eligible women. However, the use of hormone therapy remains controversial and should be used with other lipid-lowering drugs.

Cholesterol

The relationship between raised cholesterol concentrations and the risk of coronary heart disease is well established. In pre-menopausal women total cholesterol (TC) and low-density-lipoprotein cholesterol (LDL-C) levels are decreased, accounting for the lower risks of CHD when compared with men (Stangl et al. 2002; Collins 2006). Following the menopause this advantage is lost, resulting in elevation of TC and LDL-C levels; as women tend to have a higher percentage of body fat, their vulnerability for developing CHD is amplified.

Hypertension

Hypertension is another serious atherogenic risk factor. Hypertensive women are 3.5 times more likely to experience CHD and have more adverse cardiovascular events than normotensive females (Stangl et al. 2002). When combined with other known CHD risks, the incidence of death rises.

Diabetes and glucose intolerance

These two conditions are leading cardiovascular risk factors in both women and men and their prevalence is increasing in younger people. The presence of diabetes affects acute and long-term outcomes following an MI, and in addition the detrimental effects of the disease are more pronounced in women than in men of the same age. Moreover, the number of women having coronary artery bypass grafts or revascularisation procedures is highest among those with diabetes.

Smoking

Smoking is a well recognised risk factor for atherogenesis and other circulatory disorders. Women smokers using oral contraceptives, who are older than 40 years of age, have increased risks of thromboembolic events than non-smokers. Additionally women smokers are, on average, 19 years younger at the time of their first MI, when compared with non-smoking females (Hardesty and Trupp 2005). There is also growing concern that, compared with boys, the prevalence of smoking in younger women is increasing, thereby reducing the age at which CHD develops (Petersen et al. 2005).

Physical inactivity

Lack of regular exercise is an independent risk factor for CHD in women. A recent survey suggests that only one in four women in the UK engages in frequent physical activities and 25% never exercise (Clark 2003). Many women either lack the motivation or perceive that they do not have the time because of work, family and domestic pressures (Hart 2005). Others are reluctant to attend gym or rehabilitation classes owing to feelings of embarrassment, economic factors and the limitations placed by advanced age and chronic illnesses. With a third of the population being currently diagnosed as overweight and one in four classified as obese, promoting physical activity has become a national priority (Collins 2006).

Pathophysiology

The presence of the known risk factors for CHD (see Chapter 6) can accelerate or modify complex and chronic inflammatory processes, which ultimately manifest as fibrous atherosclerotic plaques within the intimal layer of a coronary artery. It is also speculated that circulating inflammatory processes such as C-reactive protein play a major role in predisposing individuals towards developing ACS (Libby and Theroux 2005).

Anatomical nuances between men and women also appear to account for gender differences in relation to cardiovascular disease. For example, women have smaller hearts, coronary arteries and cardiac muscle fibres (Naidoo and Fox 2006). Because of the reduced size of coronary arteries, cardiac invasive procedures are more precarious and less successful. Differences in cardiac remodelling processes may also be attributed to the size of vessels, which may cause a decrease in left ventricular performance (Miller 2002). Women also have higher resting heart rates, stroke volumes and ejection fractions, but lower end-diastolic pressures and volumes. Lower blood volume and oxygen saturation are also not uncommon, but are factors that may explain the false-negative results that occur in women during exercise tests (Jensen and King 1997).

Clinical presentation

The diagnosis of cardiac ischaemia is difficult in some women because many of their symptoms (refer to Table 7.2) differ from the 'classic' normative presentation. Some women may have unspecific chest pain, while in others the discomfort can be located outside the chest region, whereas the elderly and those with diabetes may not experience chest pain at all (Then et al. 2001).

Within the area of cardiac symptoms, recognition of a gendered construction of CHD is being accepted. Historically, women have been excluded from many clinical (and pharmaceutical) trials for safety reasons related to female

Table 7.2 Comparison of frequently reported acute symptoms by women with coronary artery disease.

Symptom	Penque et al. 1998 (n = 51)	Ashton 1999 (n = 57)	Milner et al. 1999 (n = 90)	McSweeney et al. 2001 (n = 76)	McSweeney et al. 2003 (n = 515)	DeVon and Zerwic 2003 (n = 50)
Central chest pain	94%	79%	70%	54%	57%	100%
Shortness of breath	66%	55%	50%	59%	57.9%	74%
Weakness				47%	54.8%	74%
Unusual fatigue	71%			59%	42.9%	64%
Nausea	48%	31%	30%	44%	35.5%	42%
Dizziness	56%	31%	21%	42%	39%	

reproduction. Many of the diagnostic processes and treatment interventions currently offered to women have been derived from the extrapolation of research findings conducted on Caucasian men with CHD (Lockyer and Bury 2002; Grady et al. 2003; O'Donnell et al. 2004). This under-representation in research has been detrimental to women (Wenger 2006). For example, when women's symptoms do not match the accepted normative criteria (derived from these male populations), these are likely to be defined as abnormal and 'atypical'. This means that women may be less likely to receive thrombolytic therapy or to undergo investigations or interventions.

Gender-specific cardiac symptoms

Prodromal symptoms

As many as 95% of women with CHD experience prodromal symptoms in the weeks or months prior to MI, but their role as early warning signs is unclear (Miller 2000; McSweeney et al. 2003). Women can experience a range of prodromal symptoms prior to their MI and those with the greatest number are likely to experience more acute symptoms. The most commonly cited prodromal symptoms are listed in Table 7.3. Because of the unspecific and erratic manifestation of their cardiac symptoms, women may have particular difficulties interpreting their significance. It is hypothesised that physiological differences, comorbidities and the late onset of CHD result in a so-called 'atypical' symptom profile in women (Hochman et al. 1999; Rosenfeld 2001; Then et al. 2001).

Acute symptoms

Generally, over 50% of women report the more conventional symptoms of CHD; however, in those with less typical primary symptoms, the potential for misdiagnosis is high (Canto et al. 2000; Pope et al. 2000; Miller 2003). Misdiagnosis is increased in younger women presenting with breathlessness as their primary symptom with a normal or non-diagnostic electrocardiogram (ECG) and also in

Table 7.3 Commonly cited prodromal symptoms experienced by women more than a month prior to their MI.

Shortness of breath	Exhaustion
Unusual fatigue	Central chest pain
Sleep disturbances	Indigestion
Ankle oedema	Anxiety
Dizziness	

those with underlying chronic conditions. Because ascertaining the diagnosis of CHD in women is challenging, the threshold of suspicion should be raised, particularly in the presence of risk factors.

Presence/absence of chest pain

Whether crushing sub-sternal chest pain is the most frequently reported symptom by men and women alike, as part of their cardiac event, is a topic of controversy. The debate, in part, has been fuelled by concerns about how symptoms are recorded and classified. For example, one of the difficulties in assessing women with a suspected MI is that many use terms other than 'chest pain' to communicate discomfort across the chest, including cramps, heaviness and tightness, stabbing and burning sensations. These terms are often associated with specific non-cardiac diagnoses and therefore differential diagnosis in women poses particular problems. Studies comparing men's and women's symptoms for MI identify the onset of chest pain as the most common reason for seeking urgent treatment (for example Penque et al. 1998; Milner et al. 1999). However, researchers tend to classify all accounts of discomfort within the thoracic area as episodes of 'chest pain'. This inevitably leads to over-reporting of chest pain as a primary symptom of CHD and reinforces gender neutrality of the disease. On this basis, the presence of chest pain as a reliable indicator of MI is becoming questionable (McSweeney et al. 2005).

Patterns of pain radiation among men and women with CHD differ. In women with MI, feelings of discomfort can extend or be confined to the upper limbs, neck, jaw and stomach. In particular, distribution to the dorsal region has been found to be significantly higher in a third of women with MI, when compared with men with the same diagnosis (Everts et al. 1996; Penque et al. 1998; Milner et al. 1999; Albarran et al. 2002). Reported sensations can include chest spasm, cramp, or pins and needles in the shoulder and upper limbs, further confounding differential diagnosis.

Between 30 and 50% of women who are subsequently diagnosed with MI present without chest pain. Typically those who present with silent ischaemia are:

- Women over 70 years of age
- Long-term diabetics
- Women with heart failure (Hochman et al. 1999; Canto et al. 2000; Dorsh et al. 2001)

A label of silent ischaemia can be unhelpful and disadvantage women. Generally, patients presenting without discomfort in the chest area may be diagnosed through subsequent ECG analysis as having had a silent ischaemic attack (Halm and Penque 1999). Since women experience varying patterns of pain radiation that are not confined to the thoracic region, there is a strong possibility that, in the absence of crushing central chest pain, their other symptoms will be misinterpreted.

Breathlessness

A presentation of breathlessness and/or shortness of breath (SOB) can be an initial symptom of many women with underlying CHD. This explains why women under 55 years of age with acute SOB as a primary event may be mismanaged (Pope et al. 2000). Since women present with a variety of symptoms that fall outside the normative model of CHD, the process of history taking and clinical examination must be comprehensive to discriminate between those with ischaemic events and those with non-cardiac causes. These stages should also be underpinned by a gender-sensitive model of healthcare.

History taking

In addition to the factors discussed in Chapters 3 and 6, history taking in relation to women presenting with symptoms suggestive of cardiac ischaemia should specifically attend to:

- Age of patient
- Family history
- Evidence of hypertension
- Menopausal status
- Levels of physical exercise, frequency and duration
- History of other comorbidities (such as gastric problems, diabetes mellitus, and heart failure)

History taking should go beyond focusing solely on the presence or absence of traditional chest pain symptoms; instead women should be invited to describe their symptom history. Indeed chest pain may not be the most worrisome symptom from a woman's perspective (Miller 2002) and clinicians should elicit the chief complaint as perceived by the patient. Open-ended questions generate more background information, and the application of terms used by patients to describe their feelings of discomfort helps to strengthen relationships. An initial complaint of breathlessness associated with or without exertion may be of relevance in patients suspected of having an MI or unstable angina, whereas reports of pain in the shoulders, upper limbs, neck, jaw and back need further investigation. Use of a framework such as the PQRST mnemonic can systematically guide the collection of data (Albarran 2002) by focusing on:

P – Precipitating factors
Q – Quality
R – Region and radiation
S – Associated symptoms
T – Time that the symptoms lasted, and treatments used to relieve symptoms

Formal discussion of symptoms with patients is crucial, otherwise women may misinterpret the actions of hospital personnel as suggesting there is nothing seriously wrong or that their symptoms are doubted. The way in which health professionals respond to reported symptoms can influence the future actions and behaviours of women.

Clinical examination

A detailed guide is given in Chapter 4, but preparation should include maintaining privacy during the examination and being sensitive to cultural issues. A structured approach to the examination will help in consolidating an understanding of the nature of symptoms triggering help-seeking behaviours. Together with history-taking data, the role of the clinical examination should support distinguishing between those with cardiac ischaemia and those with other differential diagnoses.

In respect of palpation of the chest to feel the PMI (see Chapter 4) or apex beat in a woman, this must involve placing the palm of the right hand directly beneath the patient's left breast such that the edge of the index finger rests against the inferior surface of the breast. The rationale for the procedure should be explained to the patient prior to palpating the chest. With advancing age, tissue litheness diminishes causing the breasts to hang below the level of the heart.

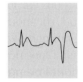

Initial investigations

Most of the immediate investigations in those with an acute episode of chest pain and suspicions of ACS have been discussed in Chapter 6. However, specific tests are particularly important in aiding diagnosis in women.

Electrocardiogram

Because of the limiting value of symptom reports and the fact that many women have a non-diagnostic 12-lead ECG, the role of laboratory and other non-invasive techniques is vital. Not all patients who develop myocardial ischaemia or necrosis exhibit ECG changes, but this does not rule out a diagnosis of MI. Generally there are fewer ST elevations but higher rates of ST depression and T-wave inversions in the ECG of women, making cardiac diagnoses more unreliable (Elsaesser and Hamm 2004).

Laboratory tests

Cardiac troponin assays are currently the enzyme markers of choice in evaluating evidence of irreversible myocardial cell death in the blood. Use of cardiac troponin measures has revolutionised the classification of acute coronary syndromes and has helped to identify those who would benefit most from early aggressive management. Other laboratory tests should include fasting lipid levels, fasting blood sugars, serum biochemistry, C-reactive protein and full blood count as these will help to establish a differential diagnosis.

Differential diagnosis

Because of the terminology used by patients with sudden onset of chest pain or other symptoms, the potential for misdiagnosis is high. Indeed many descriptions of symptoms associated with CHD might be attributed to pulmonary disease or to aortic or musculoskeletal injury. One important role of the preliminary physical survey is to eliminate life-threatening causes such as MI, ruptured oesophagus, aortic dissection, pneumothorax, and pulmonary embolism (Kanojia and Salih 2000). Possible causes of discomfort across the chest can also be associated with eating, movement or coughing, or be triggered by an empty stomach. In addition, pain might be referred, caused by exertion, and episodic in nature. Skill in establishing a differential diagnosis requires competence in history taking, clinical examination, appropriate weighting of existing risk factors and listening to the cues that patients present.

Immediate management and interventions

The immediate management of a patient with symptoms and ECG criteria indicative of MI should be along the guidelines described in Chapter 6. In women with abnormal or atypical symptoms the emphasis must be on rapid diagnosis, early risk stratification and management of acute symptoms such as relief of pain, breathlessness and anxiety. Risk should be estimated and relevant therapies implemented. In the acute phase, patients classified as intermediate or at high risk (see Table 7.4) are vulnerable and therefore need to be managed aggressively (Mosca et al. 2004b). Wenger (2004) suggests that specific challenges for clinical staff should focus on providing rapid and appropriate access to care, to diagnosis and to evidence based therapies. In order to reverse the current trend of delayed referrals to both investigations and treatment for women with atypical symptoms, clinicians need to maintain a high degree of suspicion for possible underlying cardiac causes based on a risk assessment.

Further investigations

The number of non-invasive investigations has grown over the years, but because most were designed and developed from data extrapolated from studies of Caucasian males with heart disease, low levels of disease detection and accuracy have resulted when used in women.

Table 7.4 Guidelines for the prevention of coronary heart disease according to a woman's risk group. Adapted from Mosca et al. (2004b).

High-risk women (>20% CHD risk) (Established CHD and CVD, diabetes mellitus, aortic aneurysm, peripheral vascular disease)	Intermediate-risk women (10–20% risk) (Multiple risk factors, FH with early onset of CHD)	Low-risk women (<10% CHD risk) (May include women with multiple risk factors, metabolic syndrome, or one or no risk factors)
Class I recommendations • Smoking cessation • Physical activity • Diet therapy • Weight maintenance/reduction • Blood pressure control • Lipid control/statin therapy • Glycaemic control in diabetics • Aspirin therapy • Beta-blocker therapy • ACE inhibitor therapy *Class IIa recommendation* • Assess/treat depression *Class IIb recommendations* • Omega 3 fatty acid supplement • Folic acid supplements	*Class I recommendations* • Smoking cessation • Physical activity • Dietary modification • Weight management/reduction • Blood pressure control • Lipid control *Class IIa recommendation* • Aspirin therapy	*Class I recommendations* • Smoking cessation • Physical activity • Dietary modification • Weight management/reduction • Treat individual risk factors according to guidelines

CHD, coronary heart disease; CVD cardiovascular disease; FH, family history.

Exercise stress testing

This inexpensive technique is routinely used for evaluating patients who present with chest pain, those who have chest pain on exertion and those with known ischaemic heart disease and at risk of cardiac events. However, being of advanced age can limit the capacity of women to sustain prolonged periods exercising on the treadmill/stationary bicycle. Additionally, compared with 10% of men who have false-positive test results, these occur in 25% of women. Exercise stress testing therefore has limited detection rates for CHD in women (Scordo 2005).

A negative exercise stress test in women has high predictive value for the absence of CHD and should be sufficient to guide further management. Deaton et al. (2001) agree that in women with normal resting ECG and with an adequate exercise capacity, an exercise test can be performed provided that gender-specific criteria are developed as part of the evaluation. For women with an abnormal resting ECG, an echocardiogram and nuclear imaging investigations are more appropriate. Guidance issued by the National Institute for Clinical Excellence (NICE 2003) recommends that myocardial perfusion scintigraphy should be part of the diagnostic strategy for investigating women suspected of CHD or future cardiac events due to the unreliable results associated with exercise testing.

Echocardiography (physical/pharmacological)

Echocardiography has gained popularity in recent years as it is more specific and reliable than standard ECG exercise testing. It can be used in women with an intermediate risk of CHD, who are symptomatic and have an abnormal resting ECG. In particular, stress echocardiography has been found to be more predictive than exercise ECG for women with typical or atypical angina and other at-risk groups (Deaton et al. 2001; Scordo 2005). Pharmacological stress echocardiography with drugs such as dobutamine can be used to produce ischaemic changes in women who are functionally impaired and unable to exercise for a number of reasons, including a recent MI, severe hypertension or rhythm disorders. Furthermore, compared with a stress ECG, a positive pharmacological stress test in women is more accurate in detecting evidence of CHD and in predicting potential cardiac complications, whereas a negative finding in those with chest pain carries a good prognosis. When the results are inconclusive or where there is a positive stress test, women should be referred for coronary angiography.

Medium- to long-term management plan

A central aspect of management involves categorising women as low, intermediate or high risk for adverse events based on risk assessment (ESC 2003; Mosca et al. 2004b; Wenger 2004). The degree of invasive interventions will be guided by the extent to which the patient has been defined as being at risk (see Table 7.4). Elderly women are more likely to be classified at high risk and will be candidates for coronary angiography. The assessment of patients should determine the level of viable myocardial tissue and their risk of lethal dysrhythmias. Those at the low end of the spectrum will be managed according to their symptomatic status.

Generally, the medium- and long-term management of women revolves around pharmacological therapies (anti-thrombotic agents, beta-blockers, calcium antagonists, nitrates, angiotensin converting enzymes, and lipid-lowering agents) and targeting modifiable risk factors in order to reduce the incidence and progression of CHD. Apart from assessing women's conceptions of health risks, the application of evidence based guidelines like those developed by the AHA can effectively reduce the threat of cardiovascular disease and secondary complications (Mosca et al. 2004b; Hardesty and Trupp 2005).

Lifestyle interventions

Tobacco smoking

Decreasing cigarette consumption is a global priority (Mosca et al. 2004a), and various studies have confirmed that smoking cessation can significantly attenuate the incidence of and risks for CHD (Hardesty and Trupp 2005). The availability of support from smoking-cessation clinics, the use of group and self-help techniques as well as hypnotherapy, acupuncture and nicotine patches can be effective in aiding women to stop smoking. NICE (2006a) has recently recommended the increased involvement of health staff in delivering brief opportunistic advice which is sensitive and individualised to help people stop smoking, and if appropriate in referring them to specialist support services.

Dietary

Dietary advice should be directed at increasing the consumption of vegetables, fruit, oily fish and fibre, and reducing the intake of saturated and total fat. Foods low in saturated fat and high in polyunsaturated fats are recommended for lowering cholesterol levels. A reduction of dietary salt intake to less than 0.6 g/day is beneficial in preventing cardiovascular complications. Moderate alcohol consumption is associated with a small reduction in coronary events, but a high intake and binge drinking can result in weight gain and cardiovascular complications. Women should adhere to the recommended intake of 14 units per week and have alcohol-free days.

Increased physical activity and weight management

A moderate amount of regular physical activity can help individuals maintain or reduce weight. Brisk walking for 25–30 minutes three to five times a week has a beneficial impact on health. Supervised gym classes can also increase physical activity levels as they provide women with support and opportunities to socialise, which in turn can assist some in maintaining regular exercise. NICE (2006b) has recently proposed that healthcare professionals should target inactive people and provide specific advice to encourage them to exercise more regularly based on their preferences and abilities. Additionally, national introduction of low-cost strategies including exercise referral schemes, the use of pedometers and community-based exercise programmes to increase physical activities such as walking and cycling is recommended (NICE 2006b). The emphasis should be placed on sustained performance and increasing functional capacity over time. A well balanced diet low in cholesterol in combination with a reduction of alcohol consumption will enhance weight loss and improve patients' quality of life and self-esteem. Those who are deemed overweight should aim for a waist of 35 inches (89 cm) or less, with a recommended ideal body mass index of between 20 and 25 kg/m^2 (Williams et al. 2004). Underlying causes of obesity need to be investigated and dieting should be guided by health professionals.

Major health interventions

Blood pressure control/maintenance

Routine checking of women who may develop hypertension due to lifestyle factors or because of a strong family history is essential. According to guidance from NICE (2004), patients with systolic blood pressure in the range 140–159 mmHg or with a diastolic blood pressure of 90–99 mmHg, with or without cardiovascular disease, with possible target organ damage and with an estimated risk of developing cardiovascular disease of more than 20%, should commence treatment. In those with diabetes, which typically includes elderly women, treatment should be instigated if they have a sustained systolic of greater than 140 mmHg and/or a sustained diastolic greater than 90 mmHg (Wegner 2006). In those with borderline hypertension, a combination of low calorie diet, reduced alcohol intake and regular exercise can decrease the need for drug therapy and/or enhance the benefit of antihypertensive therapy (NICE 2004; Williams et al. 2004).

Lipid analysis control/maintenance

Generally, women greater than 55 years of age tend to have higher total cholesterol than men. Since post-menopausal women lose the LDL-C lowering benefits associated with oestrogen, regular checks should be pursued in women identified at risk for CHD. For women with modest risk of CHD, dietary and alcohol advice together with physical activity and weight loss or maintenance should be encouraged, in the first instance, as a means of reducing serum cholesterol. Those at high risk for CHD or with elevated LDL cholesterol and triglycerides may need to be managed with lipid-lowering therapy, ideally with a statin as well as by adopting lifestyle interventions (Hardesty and Trupp 2005).

Diabetic control/maintenance

Since diabetes is more common in women, regular health checks are essential, particularly as silent MI is more common in these individuals. In those with diabetes, control of blood sugars through advice on adherence of dietary factors and prescribed medication is vital in optimising well-being. Weight reduction is also important, and obese patients should be closely monitored and supported in increasing their levels of exercise activity, reducing their intake of saturated fats and taking responsibility for lifestyle options.

Aggressive educational strategies

The findings of BHF (2003), Mosca et al. (2004a) and Hart (2005) suggest that women, particularly those below 45 years and from ethnic groups, are less aware of the risks of CHD and have a misplaced perception that they are at greater risk of death from cancer. Educational strategies therefore should be targeted at young women in schools, in higher education and in the workplace, focusing on primary prevention. The media industry also needs to work closely with health professionals to ensure that messages about how to prevent CHD reach women. According to the BHF (2003) survey, only a small minority of women were familiar with the effects of heart disease as a result of reading about it. Women's magazines and newspapers need to be dedicated to changing women's misconceptions, raising awareness about the major risks associated with CHD, and encouraging recognition of and response to symptoms. Television dramas need to include women experiencing symptoms of CHD to raise awareness about varied symptom presentation and challenge existing perceptions about those most at risk. The use of the World Wide Web is also another medium that could be used to convey health messages particularly aimed at younger women. Wenger (2004) believes that increasing the public's awareness is one of the major challenges facing health professionals in the fight against gender-based disparities in the cardiovascular care and outcomes of women.

Key learning points

- Women, particularly above 65 years of age, have higher rates of mortality and morbidity due to coronary heart disease when compared with men.
- Women with CHD can present with classical and atypical symptoms, but a small minority will experience silent ischaemia.
- The initial symptom in at least half of the women presenting with a myocardial infarction can be shortness of breath; consequently they may be overlooked and mismanaged.
- In women presenting with discomfort across the chest, a high index of suspicion for CHD should be considered until proven otherwise; such individuals should be offered immediate and appropriate access to care, diagnostic interventions and gender-specific evidence based therapies.
- Mixed methods should be used to convey key messages to women about how to decrease the risks and prevent CHD, as well as cardiac symptom recognition and the need for an urgent response.

References

Albarran JW (2002) The language of chest pain. *Nursing Times* **98**(4): 38–40.

Albarran JW, Durham B, Gowers J, Dwight J, Chappel G (2002) Is the radiation of chest pain a useful indicator of myocardial infarction? A prospective study of 541 patients. *Accident and Emergency Nursing* **10**(1): 2–9.

Albarran JW, Clarke B, Crawford J (In press) 'It was not really chest pain, I can't explain it!' – an exploratory study on the nature of symptoms experienced by women during their myocardial infarction. *Journal of Clinical Nursing*.

American Heart Association (2002) *Heart Disease and Stroke Statistics – 2003 Update*. Dallas, American Heart Association.

Ashton K (1999) How men and women with heart disease seek care: the delay experience. *Progress in Cardiovascular Nursing* **14**: 53–60, 74.

Boersma E, Maas ACP, Deckers JW et al. (1996) Early thrombolytic treatment in acute myocardial infarction: reappraisal of the golden hour. *Lancet* **348**: 771–775.

Brink E, Karlson B, Hallberg L (2002) To be stricken with acute myocardial infarction: a grounded study of symptom perception and care-giving behaviour. *Journal of Health Psychology* **7**(5): 533–543.

British Heart Foundation (2003) *Take Note of Your Heart: a Review of Women and Heart Disease in the UK*. London, British Heart Foundation.

British Heart Foundation Heart Statistics (2004) *Numbers Dying from CVD and CHD*. http://www.heartstates.org/temp/Tabsp1.2spweb06.xls (accessed 13th June 2006).

Canto J, Shlipak M, Rogers W, Malmgrem J, Frederick P, Lambrew C, Ornato J, Barron H, Kiefe K (2000) Prevalence, clinical characteristics, and mortality among patients with myocardial infarction presenting without chest pain. *Journal of the American Medical Association* **283**(4): 3223–3229.

Chandra NC, Ziegelstein RC, Rogers WJ, Tiefenbrunn AJ, Gore JM, French WJ, William J, Rubison M, for the National Registry of Myocardial Infarction – I (1998) Observations of the treatment of women in the United States with myocardial infarction. *Archives of Internal Medicine* **158**: 981–988.

Clark J (2003) Women too busy to exercise. *British Medical Journal* **326**: 467.

Collins P (2006) Risk factors for cardiovascular disease and hormone therapy in women. *Heart* **92**(Suppl. III): iii24–iii28.

Deaton C, Kunik C, Hachamovitch R, Redberg R, Shaw L (2001) Diagnostic strategies for women with suspected coronary artery disease. *Journal of Cardiovascular Nursing* **15**(3): 39–53.

Dempsey J, Dracup K, Moser D (1995) Women's decision to seek care for symptoms of acute myocardial infarction. *Heart and Lung* **24**: 444–456.

DeVon HA, Zerwic JJ (2003) The symptoms of unstable angina: do women and men differ? *Nursing Research* **52**(2): 108–118.

Dorsh M, Lawrance R, Sapsford R, Durham N, Oldham J, Greenwood D, Jackson B, Morrell C, Robinson M, Hall A, for the EMMACE study group (2001) Poor prognosis of patients presenting with symptomatic myocardial infarction without chest pain. *Heart* **86**(5): 494–498.

Dracup K, Moser D (1997) Beyond sociodemographics: factors influencing the decision to seek treatment for symptoms of acute myocardial infarction. *Heart and Lung* **26**(4): 253–262.

Edmunds E, Lip G (2000) Cardiovascular risk in women: The cardiologist's perspective. *Quarterly Journal of Medicine* **93**(3): 135–145.

Elsaesser A, Hamm C (2004) Acute coronary syndrome: the risk of being female. *Circulation* **109**: 565–567.

European Heart Network (2005) *European Cardiovascular Disease Statistics* 2005. http://www.ehnheart.org/files/EurCVDstat2000-112408A.pdf.

European Society for Cardiology (2003) Task Force for the management of acute myocardial infarction of the European Society of Cardiology. *European Heart Journal* **24**: 28–66.

European Society for Cardiology (2005) *Women at Heart Initiative.* www.escardio.org/initiatives/WomenHeart/WaH_Initiative/ (accessed 9th March 2006).

Everts B, Karlson B, Warborg P, Hedner T, Herlitz J (1996) Localisation of pain in suspected myocardial infarction in relation to final diagnosis, age, sex and type of infarction. *Heart and Lung* **35**: 430–437.

Finnegan J, Meischke H, Zapka J, Leviton L, Meschack A, Benjamin-Garner R, Estabrook L, Hall N, Schaeffer S, Smith C, Weitzman E, Raczynski J, Stone E (2000) Patient delay in seeking care for heart attack symptoms: findings from focus groups conducted in five US regions. *Preventative Medicine* **31**: 205–213.

Grady D, Chaput L, Kristof M (2003) Results of systematic review of research on diagnosis and treatment of coronary heart disease in women. *Evidence Report/Technology Assessment Number 80 Agency for Healthcare Research and Quality (AHRQ) Publication number 03-E034*, Rockville, Washington, United States Department of Health and Human Services, Public Health Services.

Halm M, Penque S (1999) Heart disease in women. *American Journal of Nursing* **99**(4): 26–31.

Hardesty P, Trupp R (2005) Prevention: the key to reducing cardiovascular disease in women. *Journal of Cardiovascular Nursing* **20**(6): 433–441.

Hart PL (2005) Women's perceptions of coronary heart disease: an integrative review. *Journal of Cardiovascular Nursing* **20**(3): 170–176.

Hemingway H, McCallum A, Shipley M, Manderbacka K, Martikainen P, Keskimaki I (2006) Incidence and prognostic implications of stable angina pectoris among women and men. *Journal of the American Medical Association* **295**: 1404–1411.

Hochman JS, Tamis JE, Thompson TD, Weaver D, White H, Van Der Werf FR, Aylward P, Topol E, Califf RM for the Global Use of Strategies to Open Occluded Coronary Arteries in Acute Coronary Syndromes IIb Investigators (1999) Sex, clinical presentation, and outcome in patients with acute coronary syndromes. *New England Journal of Medicine* **341**: 226–232.

Horne R, James D, Petrie K, Weinman J, Vincent R (2000) Patient interpretation of symptoms as a cause of delay in reaching hospital during acute myocardial infarction. *Heart* **83**: 388–393.

Jensen L, King K (1997) Women and heart disease: the issues. *Critical Care Nurse* **17**(2): 45–53.

Kanojia A, Salih AA (2000) Recent advances in evaluation of chest pain. *British Journal of Cardiology* **7**: 123–130.

Libby P, Theroux P (2005) Pathophysiology of coronary artery disease. *Circulation* **111**: 3481–3488.

Lockyer L (2005) Women's interpretation of their coronary heart symptoms. *European Journal of Cardiovascular Nursing* **4**: 29–35.

Lockyer L, Bury M (2002) The construction of a modern epidemic: the implications of gendering coronary heart disease. *Journal of Advanced Nursing* **39**(5): 432–440.

McSweeney JC, Cody M, Vrane PB (2001) Do you know them when you see them? Women's prodromal and acute symptoms of myocardial infarction. *Progress in Cardiovascular Nursing* **15**(3): 26–38.

McSweeney JC, Cody M, O'Sullivan P, Elberson K, Moser D, Garvin B (2003) Women's early warning symptoms of acute myocardial infarction. *Circulation* **108**: 2619–2623.

McSweeney JC, Lefler LL, Crowder BF (2005) What's wrong with me? Women's coronary heart disease diagnostic experiences. *Progress in Cardiovascular Nursing* **20**(2): 48–57.

Meischke H, Yutaka Y, Kuniyuki A, Bowen D, Andersen R, Urban N (1999) How women label and respond to symptoms of myocardial infarction: responses to hypothetical symptom scenarios. *Heart and Lung* **28**(4): 261–269.

Miller C (2000) Cue sensitivity in women with cardiac disease. *Progress in Cardiovascular Nursing* **15**: 82–89.

Miller C (2002) A review of symptoms of coronary artery disease in women. *Journal of Advanced Nursing* **39**(1): 17–23.

Miller C (2003) Symptom reflections of women with cardiac disease and advanced practice nurses: a descriptive study. *Progress in Cardiovascular Nursing* **18**(2): 69–76.

Milner A, Funk M, Richards S, Wilms RM, Vaccarino V, Krumholz HM (1999) Gender differences in symptom presentation associated with coronary heart disease. *American Journal of Cardiology* **84**(4): 396–399.

Mosca L, Ferris A, Fabunmi R, Robertson RM (2004a) Tracking women's awareness of heart disease: an American Heart Association National Study. *Circulation* **109**: 573–579.

Mosca L, Appel L, Benjamin EJ, Berra K, et al. (2004b) Evidence based guidelines for cardiovascular disease prevention in women. *Journal of the American College of Cardiology* **43**(5): 900–921.

Naidoo VV, Fox KM (2006) Fashioning a new approach to coronary care in women. *Heart* **92**(Suppl. III): iii1.

National Institute for Clinical Effectiveness (2003) *Myocardial Perfusion Scintigraphy for the Diagnosis and Management of Patients with Angina and Myocardial Infarction*. London, NICE.

National Institute for Clinical Effectiveness (2004) *Management of Hypertension in adults in Primary Care*. http://www.nice.org.uk/pdf/CG018NICEguideline.pdf.

National Institute for Health and Clinical Effectiveness (2006a) *Brief Interventions and Referral for Smoking Cessation in Primary and Other Settings*. London, NICE.

National Institute for Health and Clinical Effectiveness (2006b) *Four Commonly Used Methods to Increase Physical Activity: Brief Interventions in Primary Care, Exercise Referral Schemes, Pedometers and Community-based Exercise Programmes for Walking and Cycling*. London, NICE.

O' Donnell S, Condell S, Begley CM (2004) 'Add women & stir' – the biomedical approach to cardiac research. *European Journal of Cardiovascular Nursing* **3**: 119–127.

Penque S, Halm M, Smith M, Deutsch J, Van Roekel M, McGlaughlin L, Dzubay S, Doll N, Beahrs M (1998) Women and coronary disease: relationship between descriptors of signs and symptoms and diagnostic treatment and course. *American Journal of Critical Care* **7**: 175–182.

Perry K, Petrie K, Ellis C, Horne R, Moss-Morris M (2001) Symptom expectations and delay in acute myocardial infarction patients. *Heart* **86**(1): 91–92.

Petersen P, Peto V, Scarborough P, Rayner M (2005) *Coronary Heart Disease Statistics 2005* (13th edition). London, British Heart Foundation. www.heartstats.org (accessed 9th March 2006).

Pope J, Aufderheide T, Ruthazer R, Woolard R, Feldman J, Beshanski J, Griffith J, Selker H (2000) Missed diagnoses of acute cardiac ischaemia in the emergency department. *New England Journal of Medicine* **342**: 1163–1170.

Richards HM, Reid ME, Wyatt GC (2002) Socioeconomic variations in responses to chest pain: qualitative study. *British Medical Journal* **324**: 1308–1312.

Rosenfeld R (2001) Women's risk decisions delay in acute myocardial infarction: implications for research and practice. *AACN Clinical Issues* **12**(1): 29–39.

Ruston A, Clayton J, Calnan M (1998) Patients' action during their cardiac event: qualitative study exploring differences and modifiable factors. *British Medical Journal* **316**: 1060–1063.

Scordo KA (2005) Noninvasive diagnosis of coronary artery disease in women. *Journal of Cardiovascular Nursing* **20**(6): 420–426.

Stangl V, Baumann G, Stangl K (2002) Coronary atherogenic risk factors in women. *European Heart Journal* **23**: 1738–1752.

Then KL, Rankin JA, Fofonoff DA (2001) Atypical presentation of acute myocardial infarction in three age groups. *Heart and Lung* **30**(4): 285–293.

Vaccarino V, Parsons L, Every NR, Barron HV, Krumholz HM and participants in the National Registry of Myocardial Infarction 2 (1999) Sex based differences in early mortality after myocardial infarction. *New England Journal of Medicine* **341**: 217–225.

Wenger N (1997) Coronary heart disease: an older woman's major health risk. *British Medical Journal* **315**: 1085–1090.

Wenger N (2004) You've come a long way, baby: cardiovascular health and disease in women – problems and prospects. *Circulation* **109**: 558–560.

Wenger N (2006) Coronary heart disease in women: highlights of the past two years – stepping stones, milestones and obstructing boulders. *Nature Clinical Practice Cardiovascular Medicine* **3**(4): 194–202.

Williams B, Poulter NR, Brown MJ, Davis M, McInnes GT, Potter JF, Sever PS and McG Thom S (2004) Guidelines for the management of hypertension: report of the fourth working party of the British Hypertension Society, 2004 – BHS IV. *Journal of Human Hypertension* **18**: 139–185.

Useful websites

www.escardio.org/initiatives/WomenHeart/WaH_Initiative/
http://www.bhf.org.uk/news/uploaded/bhf_take_note_of_your_heart.pdf
http://www.goredforwomen.org/
http://circ.ahajournals.org/cgi/reprint/106/25/3143.pdf (lipids)
http://www.escardio.org/knowledge/guidelines/Guidelines_list.htm?hit=quick
http://www.ash.org.uk/html/factsheets/html/fact06.html

Assessing and managing the patient with chest pain due to either acute pericarditis or myocarditis

John W. Albarran

Aim

A number of patients seek urgent health advice when experiencing an acute episode of chest pain although in many instances this may not always be associated with a life-threatening condition. Chest pain produced either by pericarditis or myocarditis presents an unusual challenge for busy clinicians. The aim of this chapter is to examine the specific characteristics, diagnostic and management strategies of patients presenting with chest pain due to either pericarditis or myocarditis. The chapter will consider the aetiology and pathophysiology of each condition as well as evaluating the acute and long-term management of these patients.

Learning outcomes

Following the completion of this chapter, the reader will have:

- An understanding of mortality and morbidity patterns in patients with acute pericarditis and myocarditis.
- An appreciation of the causes resulting in acute pericarditis or myocarditis.
- An increased awareness of the distinguishing features of acute pericarditis and myocarditis with particular reference to chest pain and electrocardiographic changes.
- A developed understanding of specific clinical investigations related to these conditions.
- An appreciation of the main forms of acute and long-term treatment for individuals diagnosed with acute pericarditis or myocarditis.

ACUTE PERICARDITIS

Background

According to recent statistics covering the period 2004–2005, a total of 1654 episodes of acute pericarditis were reported and treated in NHS hospitals across England. Of those most affected, 76% were men, 70% were between the ages of

15 and 59 years and the mean age of hospitalised patients with acute pericarditis was 47 years. The average length of stay was 4.5 days (Department of Health, DH, 2005). Carter and Brooks (2005) acknowledge that pericarditis is a complication of myocardial infarction (MI), but this only affects 15% of these patients. Mortality is rare in acute and idiopathic pericarditis but can reach 100% in untreated purulent forms (Gentlesk and McCabe 2005).

Causes

The pericardium is a thin, fibrous membrane that surrounds the heart and consists of an inner (visceral) layer and an outer (parietal) layer. In health, there are 15–20 ml of fluid separating these two layers which serve to decrease friction and lubricate cardiac motion (Carter and Brooks 2005).

Inflammation in any of these layers may result in pericarditis as either a primary condition or a secondary condition due to a systemic disease. In response to inflammation, excess fluid can accumulate between the layers and produce a pericardial effusion (Holcomb 2004). The causes of pericarditis are diverse (see Table 8.1) but in many cases it is a complication of a viral infection.

Table 8.1   Causes of pericarditis.

Cardiac complications
- Post-myocardial infarction: occurs over 2–4 days after MI
- Post-cardiac surgery, develops within days or months
- Dressler's syndrome, occurs 2–10 weeks after a myocardial infarction

Infection
- Viral infections: a recent viral infection often precedes pericarditis in young people; viruses include influenza, hepatitis B, Coxsackie A or B, and Epstein–Barr virus (most common cause)
- Bacterial infections, such as gram-positive and gram-negative organisms
- Fungal infections, occur mainly in immunocompromised patients (such as *Candida* and *Aspergillus*)

Auto-immune
- Rheumatoid arthritis and lupus
- Rheumatic fever
- Systemic lupus erythematosus

Drugs
- Anticonvulsive agents (phenytoin)
- Antihypertensives (hydrallazine)
- Penicillin
- Isoniazid

Other causes
- Radiation to the lungs or breast stimulates inflammatory responses
- Chest trauma associated with injury to the chest from a steering wheel
- Malignant disease: secondary breast and lung malignancies can cause inflammation and irritation of pericardial layers
- Uraemic pericarditis (Goyle and Walling 2002; Swanton 2003; Carter and Brooks 2005)

Table 8.2 Classification of pericarditis. Adapted from Goyle and Walling (2002).

- Acute pericarditis (<6 weeks): effusive or fibrous
- Subacute pericarditis (6 weeks to 6 months)
- Chronic pericarditis (>6 months): effusive, adhesive, effusive–adhesive and constrictive

Pathophysiology

Acute pericarditis

In acute pericarditis, the response to acute inflammation results in the production of serous fluid, pus or a dense fibrinous mesh (Goyle and Walling 2002). Viral pericarditis is the most common infectious disease of the pericardium (caused by adenovirus, enterovirus, cytomegalovirus and influenza virus). There is a gradual accumulation of serous fluid, which often resolves without intervention. The body is able to adjust to the change and so the patient may experience mild symptoms or be asymptomatic. However, with a sudden build-up of pericardial fluid between the pericardial layers, there is a rise of intrapericardial pressure compromising cardiac output. In this situation, cardiovascular collapse will ensue secondary to cardiac tamponade which should be treated as a medical emergency (Carter and Brooks 2005).

Chronic constrictive pericarditis

In some instances, pericarditis may progress to a chronic state. Here excess fluid within the pericardial layers, caused by repetitive episodes of inflammation, turns into a thickened coating (which may calcify), resulting in the obstruction of flow of blood within the coronary vessels and restricting wall motion. Moreover, the pericardial sac can adhere to muscle fibres, thereby constricting and squeezing the heart, a process that is associated with 'chronic constrictive pericarditis' (Goyle and Walling 2002). Eventually, it impairs filling of the ventricles and ventricular functioning. Acute pericarditis is currently classified according to the underlying pathophysiologic processes (see Table 8.2).

Clinical presentation

The primary feature of pericarditis is the unexpected onset of chest pain, which is also the reason why patients seek help. The pain may be substernal and radiate to the left shoulder, neck and back, but rarely to the left arm. However, radiation to the left trapezius muscle is usual and highly indicative of pericarditis. The pain can be persistent and described as sharp, stabbing and with a piercing quality. Because of these features, chest pain reports can be confused for ischaemic pain or myocardial infarction (MI), particularly if there are electrocardiographic (ECG) changes involving ST segment elevation. However, unlike other forms of chest pain, it is unrelieved by nitrates and the pericarditic pain is made worse:

- During deep inspiration and when coughing
- While lying flat or on the left side
- When changing body position

Generally patients prefer to lie still or to sit/lean forward to ease their discomfort. Since the pericardium is attached to the great vessels, sternum and diaphragm, deep inspiration causes the diaphragm to move downwards and pull on the pericardium which precipitates a sharp stabbing sensation (Carter and Brooks 2005). Patients may also present with dyspnoea, which may be attributed to a reluctance to take deep breaths. Other symptoms may include non-specific fever, dry cough, tachypnoea and sweating.

In those with chronic pericarditis, the typical signs of pericardial friction rub, pericardial effusion and ECG features may be less noticeable when compared with their initial event. Pericardial pain may remain the only symptom noted, but this will decrease in severity over time (Soler-Soler et al. 2004).

History taking

The aim of history taking should be to identify the underlying cause of the patient's symptoms. Areas of inquiry should focus on a description of sensations in the chest, onset, intensity and duration of other symptoms, as well as factors which alleviate or precipitate chest pain and respiratory rate. Questions around recent medical illnesses, episodes of trauma to the chest, and whether patients are currently receiving hospital treatments are especially important and should help inform differential diagnoses. For example, around 5% develop acute pericarditis between 2 and 10 weeks after their MI, also known as Dressler's syndrome (Gentlesk and McCabe 2005). However, the incidence of this syndrome has fallen with the introduction of thrombolytic therapy and other medications (Karim and Jerôme 2004).

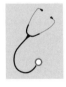

Clinical examination

The process of clinical examination needs to proceed along the systematic guidelines outlined in Chapter 4. On examination, the patient may be young and appear distressed and anxious. The individual may be feverish, tachycardic and taking shallow breaths which will not be associated with exertion. Depending on the cause of pericarditis, some patients may exhibit the presence of a rash which may be itchy; this finding may suggest an underlying cause. The exact localisation of sharp sensations to the left and back trapezius muscle by the patient is suggestive of pericarditis (Carter and Brooks 2005).

One of the most important physical findings in acute pericarditis is a pericardial friction rub, but this will only be present in half of cases. The rub is caused by the movement of the inflamed pericardial layers against each other. Using the diaphragm of the stethoscope, a pericardial friction rub is best heard at the left lower sternal border or between the 4th and 5th intercostal spaces. In the patient with pericarditis, a high pitched scratching and grating sound may be heard. The rubs that are heard are triphasic and comprise (1) an atrial systolic rub that precedes S1, (2) a ventricular systolic rub between S1 and S2 and coincident with the peak carotid pulse, and (3) an early diastolic rub after S2 (Gentlesk and McCabe 2005). Because pericardial friction rubs are intermittent and soft/faint, it may be difficult to hear them at the first attempt. It may also be mistaken for a systolic murmur. During chest auscultation, the most effective way to hear the rub is to have the patient sitting up, leaning forward and holding their breath. A pericardial rub can be heard immediately after exhalation, regardless of whether an effusion is present (Spondick 2003). It is important to be mindful that a pericardial friction rub is not exclusive to primary acute pericarditis, as it may also be evident with large transmural myocardial infarctions (Wang et al. 2003).

In constrictive pericarditis, the heart sounds are different from acute pericarditis and usually include a high-pitched sound heard in the 4th and 5th intercostal spaces with the patient learning forward (Carter and Brooks 2005). Note, however, that a slow progressive accumulation of pericardial fluid may produce dullness to percussion in the scapular region due to the left lung being compressed.

Since cardiac tamponade and constrictive pericarditis are serious adverse events, an important sign to look for is a raised jugular venous pressure (JVP, see Chapter 4). In the presence of tamponade, the resultant haemodynamic changes are transmitted across the pericardial and cardiac walls, eventually causing a rise in right atrial pressure and within the superior vena cava (Goyle and Walling 2002). Jugular vein distension is best seen during inspiration, with the patient positioned in bed at a 45° angle. The outcome of the haemodynamic changes can also produce a fall in systolic blood pressure of 10 mmHg or more during inspiration leading to signs of *pulsus paradoxus*. A systolic fall in blood pressure during each inspiration, pulsus paradoxus is a trademark of cardiac tamponade, (but not of constrictive pericarditis) and is detected in around 70–80% of cases and in about a third of those with pericarditis. If unrecognised, the outcome for the patient is fatal. Patients with suspected cardiac tamponade will exhibit distended neck veins, the presence of profound hypotension, muffled heart sounds, tachycardia, pulsus paradoxus and tachypnoea (Maisch and Ristic 2003).

Initial investigations

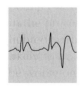

Diagnostic procedures will depend on the individuals' aetiology but typically these include four main components: ECG characteristics, echocardiography, chest x-ray, and laboratory investigations (Maisch and Ristic 2003).

Table 8.3 Key electrocardiographic features of pericarditis (Maisch and Ristic 2003; Carter and Brooks 2005).

Stages	Duration	ECG changes
Stage I	Up to 2 weeks	Concave ST segment elevation in all leads except AVR
		PR segment deviates opposite to P wave polarity
		There is no ST depression (or reciprocal changes)
Early stage II	Several weeks	All ST segments return to baseline; PR segment is deviated
Late stage II		T waves progressively flatten and invert
Stage III	Several weeks	Generalised T wave inversion across most or all leads
Stage IV	Up to 3 months	ECG trace returns to pre-pericarditis level

Electrocardiogram

In 90% of patients with pericarditis and without an effusion, a diffuse 'saddle-shaped' ST segment elevation will appear across all leads except AVR (Holcomb 2004). Because of this, the 12-lead ECG trace may be incorrectly interpreted as an acute MI. Unlike an MI, where the ST segment elevation is convex, in acute pericarditis the ST segment has an upward concave shape but this rarely exceeds 5 mm. In addition, there are no reciprocal changes or T wave inversion and the PR segment is depressed due to abnormal atrial depolarisation (Goyle and Walling 2002; Wang et al. 2003; see Figure 8.1).

The ECG changes of acute pericarditis, like those of an acute MI, are also time dependent (see Table 8.3). Normally, the pattern of diffuse ST elevation typical of pericarditis may have a 2- to 3-day onset and remain present for up to 2 weeks before the segment returns to the baseline (see Table 8.3). After this period, the T waves become inverted but these will gradually resolve (Maisch and Ristic 2003; Spondick 2003; Carter and Brooks 2005). It is worth noting that, with acute pericarditis, both the sub-epicardial layers of the ventricular and atrial walls are affected by inflammatory changes and these account for the pattern of ST segment elevation and depression of the PR segment. Atrial dysrhythmias, in particular atrial fibrillation, are typical of patients with acute pericarditis (Goyle and Walling 2002).

Patients with acute pericarditis, in the absence of heart disease, will never present with Q wave abnormalities, dysrhythmias or conduction disorders. These changes are more characteristic of myocardial ischaemia (Spondick 2003). It is important to be aware that reliance on the software of ECG machines is hazardous since they are programmed to diagnose infarction, therefore caution is required in evaluating the 12-lead trace (Spondick 2003). Likewise, good practice demands that the ECG must be interpreted in the context of the clinical symptoms and findings. In patients with cardiac tamponade, *electrical alternans* may also be present. This is characterised by beat-to-beat variability in the size of QRS complexes due to excessive cardiac movement (Carter and Brooks 2005; Gentlesk and McCabe 2005).

Radiography

The chest x-ray plays a minimal role in evaluating patients with suspected acute pericarditis. However, a volume of 250 ml within the pericardial sac may stand

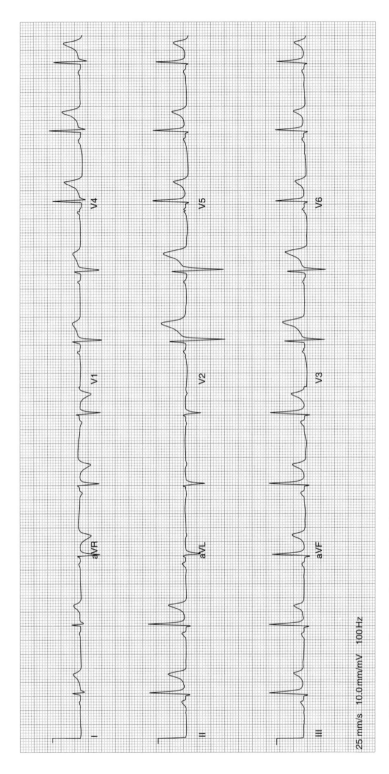

Figure 8.1 Electrocardiogram of acute pericarditis.

out as an enlarged cardiac silhouette or 'water-bottle' shape (Maisch and Ristic 2003) but with smaller effusions a normal sized heart will be present. Pleural effusions may manifest with conditions that trigger the onset of pericarditis such as cancer, infections and trauma to the chest. In constrictive pericarditis, calcification may be observed around the heart.

Echocardiography

An echocardiogram with Doppler studies is of help for patients suspected of acute pericarditis in confirming the presence and size of a pericardial effusion, as well as to differentiate this from ascites, pleural fluid and atelectasis. Echocardiograms also enable assessment of the potential haemodynamic changes and regional wall abnormalities caused by cardiac tamponade and constrictive pericarditis. It is also possible to detect the presence of fibrin, clot, tumour, calcium and air (Maisch and Ristick 2003). Trans-oesophageal echocardiography is also valuable in gauging the size of the effusion and the extent to which left ventricular function is limited.

Laboratory investigations

The tests below may help identify the suspected source of pericarditis and to exclude other possible causes:

- Cardiac enzymes, e.g. troponin
- Serum chemistry
- Liver function tests
- Full blood count
- Viral titres
- Serum reactive protein
- Blood cultures
- Blood clotting
- Immune complex titres
- Erythrocyte sedimentation rate

Where appropriate, throat swabs, sputum and faecal samples may be necessary as will studies into fungal infections (Swanton 2003). The choice of tests will be determined by the clinical history and primary symptoms. Sensitivity and confidentiality is a priority when screening patients for human immunodeficiency virus or hepatitis B as a cause for their pericarditis.

Differential diagnosis

These can be divided into cardiac and non-cardiac, as illustrated below. Commonly, acute pericarditis is confused with MI and therefore skill in ECG interpretation, analysis of symptoms and results from cardiac enzymes can assist in the preliminary differential diagnosis.

Cardiac
Myocardial infarction
Myocardial ischaemia
Aortic dissection
Coronary artery vasospasm

Non-cardiac
Oesophageal rupture and spasm
Oesophagitis
Gastric ulceration

Immediate management and interventions

If a patient's haemodynamic status is stable, admission to hospital or a critical care setting will not be necessary. Depending on the underlying condition, treatment will be tailored to the specific aetiology. For example, for infective pericarditis, antibiotics will be based on the micro-organisms from samples obtained. Bed rest and analgesia form the mainstay of clinical interventions and this can often be managed at home. To relieve the pain and inflammation accompanying pericarditis the following may be prescribed:

- A 2-week course of non-steroidal anti-inflammatory drugs (NSAIDs) such as indomethacin (Indocin) is the standard treatment.
- Ibuprofen 6–8 hourly may a preferable alternative due to minimal side effects.
- Soluble aspirin is a useful adjunct/alternative for relieving symptoms of pain and fever (Goyle and Walling 2002; Maisch and Ristric 2003; Swanton 2003).

According to Maisch and Ristic (2003) pericarditis may resolve within a 2-week period, but recurs in 50% of occasions. Acute hospital management may be necessary in the patient who is tachycardic and hypotensive and has distended neck veins and muffled heart sounds. In addition to cardiac monitoring, oxygen therapy and pain control, emergency aspiration of pericardial effusion (pericardiocentesis) in a controlled environment is normally undertaken to alleviate the symptoms of cardiac tamponade. But fluid aspiration may also be performed for diagnostic purposes. Patients with chronic pericarditis and large pericardial effusions may be asymptomatic, although they too can suddenly develop cardiac tamponade.

Medium- to long-term management plan

Patients failing to respond to NSAIDs may require a short course of oral steroids, commencing with prednisolone 45–60 mg daily decreasing over 2 weeks. In patients unable to tolerate or reacting to NSAIDs and steroids, colchicine is an effective substitute that is well tolerated (Goyle and Walling 2002; Holcomb 2005). Colchicine may also be used to minimise recurrent episodes of pericarditis and for avoiding long-term steroid use.

Where pericardial effusion recurs despite pericardiocentesis, a pericardial window may be surgically performed, most commonly in patients with uraemic, malignant or bacterial pericardial effusions (Goyle and Walling 2002). In patients with chronic constrictive pericarditis, a pericardiectomy may be undertaken.

Patients with sudden chest pain caused by acute pericarditis might be anxious that they may be at risk from coronary heart disease. Holcomb (2004) advises that these patients need to be reassured that their chest pain is not indicative of coronary heart disease and informed that the symptoms of pericarditis may take weeks to resolve. It is also important, if appropriate, to avoid vigorous activities until symptoms disappear. Understanding the role of medications and managing symptom recurrence is part of equipping the patient to manage their care.

MYOCARDITIS

Background

The incidence of acute myocarditis is much lower than that of pericarditis, with only 157 hospital episodes reported for the period 2004–2005. Typically 71% of those affected are men, and 73% are aged 15–59 years, with a mean age of 36 years (DH 2005). The average length of stay is 6.4 days. Myocarditis is difficult to recognise because many patients are asymptomatic, and in some instances diagnosis after sudden death is only confirmed during autopsy examination (Howes and Booker 2005). Some studies report an annual mortality of 20% for the first year, rising to 56% at four years (Kearney et al. 2001). Egred and Davis (2005) also add that myocarditis has been identified in 20–30% of patients who died from cocaine abuse, confirmed in the biopsy findings of chronic users (see Chapter 15).

Causes

The causes responsible for myocarditis are many (see Table 8.4) and in some cases unknown. However, enteroviral infections, such as Coxsackie B virus, are commonly to blame.

Pathophysiology

Acute myocarditis is a rare disorder involving inflammation of the myocardium, triggered by infectious, autoimmune or toxic aetiologies and carrying a poor prognosis if untreated. It affects adults and children, although the focus here is on the former. Classically, the majority of cases develop following pulmonary or gastrointestinal infections, but the rarity of this disease makes it difficult to assess, diagnose and treat (Kühl 2002; Howes and Brooker 2005). Usually a third of patients will recover, a similar number will have some residual scarring and a further third will go on to develop dilated cardiomyopathy (DCM). In this latter group, myocarditis may be responsible for coronary artery thrombosis, coronary ischaemia, cardiac arrhythmias, DCM and sudden death (Holcomb 2005).

Myocarditis can develop during or just after experiencing a viral throat, chest or gastric infection or can be in response to having influenza. It is hypothesised that the development of myocarditis is mediated by a person's immune response to infection and viral cytotoxic mechanisms which induce myocardial cell destruction (Kearney et al. 2001). In myocarditis, leucocytes, lymphocytes and macrophages infiltrate the myocardium causing inflammation and interstitial fibrosis in this muscle (Holcomb 2005). Consequently, blood flow around the

Table 8.4 Causes responsible for triggering acute myocarditis.

Viral infections
- Coxsackie type A and B
- Adenoviruses
- Influenza
- Hepatitis
- Human immunodeficiency virus (1 in 10 HIV patients develop myocarditis)
- Rubella
- Cytomegalovirus

Bacterial infections
- Salmonella typhi
- Streptococci
- Meningococci
- Staphylococci
- Diphtheria

Fungal infections

Chemicals, toxins and drugs
- Chemotherapy, carbon monoxide, arsenic, excess alcohol
- Radiation
- Wasp and spider stings
- Antibiotics, lithium
- Cocaine misuse

Tropical diseases
- Chagas disease
- Parasites

Auto-immune diseases
- Lupus
- Rheumatoid arthritis
- Scleroderma (Holcomb 2005; Howes and Brooker 2005)

heart is reduced, with areas of local or global myocardial necrosis developing and causing a decrease in myocardial contractility and a fall in cardiac output. If the latter is sustained, left ventricular functioning deteriorates and the patient may die. In less extreme situations the patient remains at risk for complications or death as a result of dilated cardiomyopathy (Holcomb 2005).

Clinical presentation

Patients with myocarditis are likely to be young men (aged 45 years or less) who present with tight chest pain, tachycardia, palpitations, shortness of breath/dyspnoea and early signs of heart failure (Kearney et al. 2001). These authors suggest that only 35% of patients experience chest pain, which is normally described as squeezing, sharp, or stabbing. The chest discomfort is localised to either the precordial area or the substernal region. This combination of characteristics makes the overall presentation suspicious of cardiac ischaemia. Non-specific signs and symptoms including fever, generalised fatigue and myalgia should alert the practitioner to consider other causes. A minority of patients may exhibit symptoms of congestive heart failure; however, a larger majority may be asymptomatic due to cardiac changes being self-limiting.

History taking

A detailed history may reveal that in the days or weeks preceding the onset of chest pain the patient had flu-like symptoms. This finding is typical of 60% of patients with myocarditis (Kearney et al. 2001). Episodes of fever, abdominal pain, dizzy spells, palpitations and myalgia may also be described.

Clinical examination

Clinical examination may identify the presence of a fever, respiratory chest infection, tachycardia and tachypnoea, although in some instances there will be no abnormal findings. However, the patient may be cold, cyanosed and hypotensive if they are in the advanced stages of left ventricular failure (Howes and Booker 2005). Altered or diminished heart sounds and pulmonary congestion may reflect a failing heart, and the presence of DCM will be evidenced by aortic and/or tricuspid murmurs on cardiac auscultation. Jugular vein distension, peripheral oedema and shortness of breath at rest will also be indicative of heart failure. Should the inflammation spread to other layers of the heart, this may stimulate the development of a pericardial effusion as well as a pericardial and pleural friction rub.

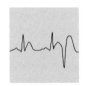

Initial investigations

Unlike acute pericarditis, evaluation for the presence of suspected myocarditis involves ECG analysis, chest x-ray review, echocardiography, and laboratory tests.

Electrocardiogram

The characteristics of the ECG in myocarditis are distinctive from acute pericarditis specifically in that the patient may have sinus tachycardia and the changes shown in Table 8.5. Complete heart block can occur but this usually resolves without a need for a permanent pacemaker. Resolution of ECG changes to normal may take 8 weeks (Kearney et al. 2001; Howes and Booker 2005).

Radiography

The chest x-ray may reveal a normal cardiac silhouette or an enlarged heart with either alveolar oedema or distended blood vessels (Holcomb 2005). Pleural and pericardial effusions are also not uncommon in this group of patients.

Table 8.5 ECG characteristics of patients with acute myocarditis.

- Diffuse ST segment elevation without reciprocal T wave depression and may be confused with MI
- Decreased QRS amplitude
- Transitory Q wave evolvement
- Complete atrioventricular block (in 20% of patients with myocarditis)
- Atrial and ventricular dysrhythmias
- Left or right bundle branch block is typical (in 20% of myocarditis patients)
- Supraventricular tachyarrhythmias
- Ventricular tachyarrhythmias

Echocardiography

This may reveal impairment of left ventricular systolic and diastolic functioning, abnormal wall movements, and reduced ejection fraction. A pericardial effusion and cardiac chamber and valvular disorders can also be observed in some patients. Tissue biopsy through cardiac catherisation has been a traditional diagnostic technique. However, due to the patchy distribution of myocarditis, accuracy in obtaining a sample is problematic. Varghese et al. (2004) have recently suggested that magnetic resonance imaging is a safer method of detecting myocarditis and differentiating it from myocardial ischaemia.

Laboratory investigations

A broad range of investigations, including throat and nose swabs, are required to identify the cause of myocarditis, viral titres being particularly important. The three main changes found with myocarditis include raised cardiac enzymes. In particular, troponin concentration may be elevated due to myocite damage that accompanies myocarditis. It is therefore vital to rule out cardiac ischaemia and to consider other laboratory data, ECG and clinical examination findings (Wong and White 2002). A raised erythrocyte sedimentation rate is common in around 60% and an elevated white cell count (leukocytes) is noted in one out of every four patients with myocarditis.

Differential diagnosis

Because many patients presenting with symptoms of acute myocarditis are men between the ages of 30 and 40 years, it will be vital to exclude cardiac ischaemia, myocarditis and the use of recreational drugs such as cocaine (see Chapter 15) as possible causes of chest pain. Other conditions to consider include:

- Acute coronary syndrome
- Aortic dissection

- Myocardial infarction
- Congestive cardiac failure
- Pulmonary embolism
- Oesophageal rupture/spasm
- Pneumonia

Immediate management and interventions

Identifying the underlying cause of myocarditis and initiating early treatment is important, although in a great number of instances myocarditis is mild and does not require treatment. Currently, there is no evidence for the use of immunosuppressant agents in this group of patients, but immune globulin may offer some benefits (Kearney et al. 2001). For those who need hospitalisation owing to a compromised haemodynamic status, the goals of management (see Table 8.6) are directed at recognising and treating dysrhythmias, optimising myocardial performance and avoiding the development of heart failure and/or DCM (Holcomb 2005). Medical therapy for those with heart failure secondary to myocarditis should include loop diuretics, angiotensin converting enzymes, β-adrenoceptor blockers and spironolactone (Kearney et al. 2001). In the case of tachyarrhythmias these should be aggressively treated by agents without negative inotropic effects.

Minor residual wall changes may be present in some patients. In others their condition may be severe and they will need referring to specialist centres for cardiac transplantation (Holcomb 2005).

Table 8.6   Acute management of the patient with myocarditis.

Monitoring measures	Interventions
Assess for pain and score intensity on a regular basis	Administer analgesia to relieve chest and other muscular pains. Record pain scores regularly
Maintain baseline observations of pulse, blood pressure, respiratory rate, oxygen saturation and temperature	Oxygen therapy to alleviate respiratory distress and enhance oxygenation. Keep on bed rest to reduce myocardial oxygen consumption
Dysrhythmias are common in early stages, therefore cardiac monitoring is essential	In patients with Mobitz II heart block or complete heart block, pacemaker placement is essential
Careful management of fluid status, restrict sodium intake and if possible record daily weight	In patients with signs of heart failure, angiotensin converting enzymes and intravenous administration of diuretics are commonplace. Anticoagulants may be used to minimise the development of thrombosis or emboli

Key learning points

Acute pericarditis

- Pericarditis is mainly induced by viral infections and affects men between the ages of 15 and 59 years.
- Cardiac tamponade and constrictive pericarditis are both serious conditions which can depress myocardial functioning.
- Patients with acute pericarditis present with substernal sharp and stabbing chest pain that radiates to left shoulder, neck and jaw; additionally deep breathing and upper body movement can aggravate discomfort.
- Diffuse concave ST elevation across the 12-lead ECG, the presence of pericardial friction rub and a pericardial effusion are key findings of acute pericarditis.
- A 2-week course of non-steroidal anti-inflammatory drugs such as indomethacin is recommended in the first instance.

Acute myocarditis

- Myocarditis is a rare condition, mainly induced by viral infections and affecting patients between the ages of 30 and 40 years.
- In most instances myocarditis is self-terminating, although a small number of patients may go on to develop dilated cardiomyopathy.
- Myocarditis patients may present with substernal chest pain and diffuse ST elevation that may suggest cardiac ischaemia.
- Early recognition and treatment are vital in influencing long-term outcomes.
- The objectives of treatment involve monitoring cardiovascular function and preventing adverse events.

References

Carter T, Brooks CA (2005) Pericarditis: inflammation or infarction. *Journal of Cardiovascular Nursing* **20**(2): 239–244.

Department of Health (2005) *Hospital Episodes Statistics Data 2004–05*, http://www.dh.gov.uk/PublicationsAndStatistics/Statistics/HospitalEpisodeStatistics/fs/en (accessed 31 March 2005).

Egred M, Davis G (2005) Cocaine and the heart. *Postgraduate Medical Journal* **81**: 568–571.

Gentlesk P, McCabe J (2005) Acute pericarditis. *Emedicine* http://www.emedicine.com/med/topic1781.htm (accessed 14th April 2006).

Goyle K, Walling A (2002) Diagnosing pericarditis. *American Family Physician* **66**(6): 1695–1702.

Holcomb SS (2004) Recognizing and managing pericarditis. *Nursing* **34**: 32cc1–35cc1.

Holcomb SS (2005) Recognizing and managing different types of carditis. *Nursing* **35**: 6–11.

Howes D, Brooker E (2005) Pericarditis. *Emedicine*. http://www.emedicine.com/emerg/topic326.htm (accessed 16th April 2006).

Karim B, Jerôme P (2004) Is Dressler's syndrome dead? *Chest* **126**(5): 1680–1682.

Kearney MT, Cotton J, Richardson P, Shah AM (2001) Viral myocarditis and dilated cardiomyopathy: mechanisms, manifestations, and management. *Postgraduate Medical Journal* **77**(903): 4–10.

Kühl U (2002) Virus induced myocarditis and inflammatory cardiomyopathy. *E-Journal of Cardiology Practice* **1**(11): 1. http://www.escardio.org/knowledge/cardiology_practice/ejournal_vol1/Vol1_no11.htm (accessed 16th April 2005).

Maisch B, Ristic A (2003) Practical aspects of the management of pericardial disease. *Heart* **89**: 1096–1103.

Soler-Soler J, Sagrista-Sauleda J, Permanyer-Miralda G (2004) Relapsing pericarditis. *Heart* **90**: 1364–1368.

Spondick DH (2003) Acute pericarditis: current concepts and practice. *Journal of the American Medical Association* **289**(9): 1150–1153.

Swanton RH (2003) *Cardiology*. Oxford, Blackwell Publishing.

Varghese A, Davis S, Pennell DJ (2004) Diagnosis of myocarditis by cardiovascular magnetic resonance. *Heart* **91**: 567.

Wang K, Asinger RW, Marriott HJ (2003) ST-segment elevation in conditions other than acute myocardial infarction. *New England Journal of Medicine* **349**: 2128–2135.

Wong CK, White HD (2002) Recognising 'painless' heart attacks. *Heart* **87**: 3–5.

Useful websites

http://www.emedicine.com/emerg/topic326.htm
http://www.emedicine.com/med/topic1781.htm
http://www.merck.com/mmhe/sec03/ch030/ch030b.html
http://www.utmem.edu/cardiology/articles/Acute%20Pericarditis.ppt#5

Chapter 9

Assessing and managing the patient with chest pain due to an aortic dissection

Helen Cox

Aims

This chapter aims to explore the diagnosis and management of patients presenting with chest pain who are subsequently diagnosed as having an acute aortic dissection. Specifically the incidence, causes, clinical presentation, management and treatment of patients presenting with a suspected aortic dissection will be considered. The profile of those who are at risk of developing an aortic dissection and the unique characteristics of presentation will be emphasised. A significant guide for the management and treatment of aortic dissection is available from the European Society of Cardiology (ESC 2001).

Learning outcomes

On completion of this chapter, the reader should be able to:

- Understand the incidence and causative factors associated with the development of aortic dissections.
- Have increased awareness of the pathophysiology of aortic dissections.
- Recognise the specific clinical features associated with an aortic dissection and include these in differentiating between patients presenting with chest pain.
- Appreciate the role of clinical presentation, history taking, clinical examination and clinical investigations in patients suspected of having an aortic dissection.
- Discuss the management and treatment options for these patients.

Background

Cardiovascular disease is the leading cause of death in western society, with aortic diseases contributing to the overall high mortality rates (Tsai et al. 2005) However, in recent years there has been growing awareness that patients presenting with clinical presentation suggestive of aortic dissection need prompt assessment, diagnosis and management (Tsai et al. 2005).

Acute aortic dissection is a clinical emergency, which carries a high incidence of mortality. Each year there are approximately 3000 people diagnosed with aortic dissection across Europe and 2000 in the United States with the incidence of aortic dissection being approximately 2.6 to 3.5 cases per 100,000 person years (Tsai et al. 2005). Gender appears to be a significant factor. In a review of 1078 patients from the International Register of Acute Aortic Dissection (IRAD) (Hagan et al. 2000), two-thirds of the sample comprised men with a mean age of 63 years. Among women, the incidence of aortic dissection is much lower; however, they tend to be slightly older (mean age 67 years). Women also tend to be managed medically and are less likely to be given immediate treatment due to difficulties in diagnosis. In-hospital complications are greater for women with aortic dissection, resulting in increased in-hospital mortality compared with men with the same condition (Neinaber et al. 2004).

Causes

Mechanisms which lead to the degeneration and weakening of the medial layers of the aorta can cause higher wall stress and predispose individuals to aneurysm formation and aortic dissection. Results from the IRAD suggest that evidence of atherosclerosis may also be present in approximately one-third of all patients and highlight the commonest predisposing factor to be hypertension (72%), which may result in ruptured aneurysms in 85% of cases (Hagan et al. 2000; ESC 2001).

In health, the diameter of the aorta of an adult is 3 cm at its source, decreasing to 2.5 cm in the descending thoracic aorta and 1.8–2 cm in the abdominal aorta (Beese-Bjurstrom 2004). However, the width of the aorta in adulthood is dependent on factors such as age, gender and workload. The normal aorta wall thickness is 4 mm but under certain circumstances it can reach an upper limit of 7 mm. When the aortic diameter enlargement exceeds 50% of the normal range, this represents ectasia and is a precursor to aneurysm formation.

There are different four different forms of aortic aneurysm (Erbel and Eggebrecht 2006):

- True aneurysm: this involves enlargement of the inner lumen
- False aneurysm or pseudoform aneurysm is associated with perforation of the vessel wall forming an outer sac
- Circumscript aneurysm: here only segments of the aorta are involved
- Diffuse aneurysm entails enlargement of parts of the whole aorta

Patients who have identified chronic aortic aneurysms tend to become symptomatic with the possibility of rupture within 5 years of diagnosis (ESC 2001). Other causes for aortic dissection are rarer and can be divided into three groups: traumatic, inflammatory diseases and hereditary disorders.

Traumatic and iatrogenic

Aortic aneurysm formation and rupture may result from surgical and invasive cardiac procedures including insertion of an intra-aortic balloon pump and cross-clamping of the aorta during cardiac surgery. Blunt chest trauma (as discussed in Chapter 11), and deceleration trauma following a car accident and falling from a great height can cause aortic dissections (Yee 2004; Tsai et al. 2005; Erbel and Eggebrecht 2006). Toxic substances such as cocaine and amphetamines can weaken the wall of the aorta leading to aneurysm formation and possible dissection (Erbel and Eggebrecht 2006). Aortic dissection can also occur in the third trimester stage of pregnancy due to an increased production of hormones, which work on smooth and connective tissue necessary for uterine growth, and an increase of 50% in circulating blood volume. Both cause undue stress on vessel walls (Yee 2004).

Inflammatory diseases

The structure of the aorta can change due to inflammatory processes that destroy the medial layers of the aortic wall (ESC 2001). Aortitis is a common cardiovascular manifestation of syphilis, leading to aortic wall thickening and aneurysm formation in the ascending aorta (Bossert et al. 2004). Similarly, auto-immune diseases such as Tayayasu arteritis and Ormond's disease can cause inflammatory lesions. These diseases cause aortic wall changes due to inflammatory infiltrate of smooth muscle and fibrosis of the vessel wall (Tavora et al. 2005). Rheumatoid arthritis can also lead to aortitis, although dissections in rheumatoid arthritis are unusual.

Inherited diseases

Whilst aortic aneurysm and dissection are more prevalent in people over 60 years of age, young persons (less than 40 years of age) may also be affected due to its associations with Marfan's syndrome, Ehler-Danlos syndrome or other congenital cardiac abnormalities, including coarctation of the aorta (Tsai et al. 2005).

There is an estimated incidence of Marfan's syndrome being present in 1/5000 of the population. This syndrome involves not only the aorta but also the skeletal, ocular, pulmonary and vascular systems. Current evidence indicates that mutations of the fibrillin 1 gene account for approximately 6–9% of all known dissections due to this condition (Erbel and Eggebrecht 2006). In this syndrome, the aneurysm formation is commonly within the ascending aorta and it is suggested that Marfan patients who have a bicuspid aortic valve have a nine-fold higher risk of dissection than those with a tricuspid aortic valve (Burks et al. 1998; Yee 2004; Erbel and Eggebrecht 2006).

Ehler–Danlos is a heterogeneous group of inheritable connective tissue disorders with an estimated incidence of 1/5000 births. Tissue fragility, skin hyperextensibility and articular hypermobility are key findings. The disease is caused by structural defects in the pro a-I (III) chain of collagen type III. There are eleven categories of this syndrome but aortic involvement is primarily seen in Ehler-Danlos type IV (ESC 2001).

Annulo-aortic ectasia and familial aortic dissections account for 5–10% of patients undergoing aortic valve replacement for aortic regurgitation. Familial gender-linked aggregation with a possible existence of genetic heterogeneity is thought to be responsible (Erbel and Eggebrecht 2006). Histological examination reveals loss of elastic fibres and medial degeneration similar to that seen in Marfan's syndrome (Neinaber and Eagle 2003).

Pathophysiology

Atherosclerosis is the main cause of aortic aneurysm formation leading to aortic dissection. The identifiable risk factors for atherosclerosis include cigarette smoking, dyslipidemia, diabetes mellitus and drug abuse, predominately cocaine. All of these influence the development of atherosclerotic plaques and loss of arterial elasticity. Atherosclerosis leads to thickening of the intima, which increases the distance between the endothelial layer and the media; this may compromise nutritional and oxygen supplies, which results in medial thickening and then necrosis (see Chapter 6). Changes in the elasticity of the medial wall may also lead to vessel stiffness. With the inability to maintain elastic potency, the linings are predisposed to the formation of aneurysms and dissections due to shear wall stress (Neinaber and Eagle 2003). The rapid development of an intimal flap can result in a true and false lumen. The dissection can spread antegradely or retrogradely and, depending on the position of the lesion, patients may present with a variety of clinical manifestations including chest pain due to coronary insufficiency, aortic regurgitation, syncope, and cardiac tamponade (ESC 2001).

Historically, aortic dissections have been classified in many ways, but generally on the basis of their location (see Figure 9.1):

- DeBakey I, II and III
- Stanford type A and B
(European Society of Cardiology (2001))

A Stanford type A dissection indicates that it is located within the ascending and possibly the descending aorta. A Stanford type B dissection suggests that it is confined to the descending segments of the aorta. This is unlike DeBakey I, which in-dicates the whole aorta is dissected, whereas DeBakey II and III suggest that the dissection may have involved the ascending and descending segments respectively.

Dissection involving the ascending aorta has a significant mortality risk of between 1 and 2% of presenting patients per hour after symptom onset. Medically managed dissections of the ascending aorta carry a mortality rate of 24% within the first 24 hours, 29% by 48 hours and 49% by 14 days. Although slightly lower figures are seen with surgical repair, the mortality rate continues to reach 20% at 14 days post-operatively. However, survival outcomes are dependent on other factors, for example the age of the patient, renal failure and further complications such as cardiac tamponade (Tsai et al. 2005).

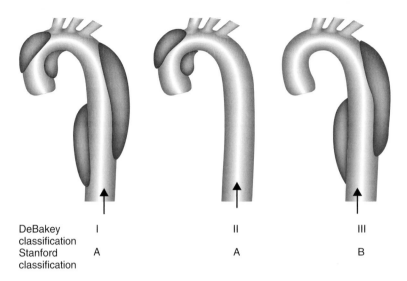

| DeBakey classification | I | II | III |
| Stanford classification | A | A | B |

Figure 9.1 Stanford and DeBakey classification of aortic dissection.

Dissection of the descending aorta is less lethal, having 10% mortality at 30 days. The mortality rate is dependent on specific variables, for example ischaemic complications, renal failure or subsequent aortic rupture, which often may require surgical intervention (Tsai et al. 2005).

More recently, the ESC (2001) has proposed a new classification of aortic dissections on the basis of evidence from new studies demonstrating that intramural haemorrhage, haematoma and ulceration are signs of evolving dissections. Accordingly, aortic intramural haematoma is seen as a precursor to aortic dissection and follows the classic signs of an aortic dissection. There are two types of intramural haematoma and haemorrhage. Type I is classified as a smooth inner aortic lumen with a diameter usually less than 3.5 cm with a haematoma formation. Typically, type II occurs with aortic atherosclerosis. Consequently the aorta dilates to a width greater than 3.5 cm, with the longitudinal extent of the haematoma similar to that of type I, which is approximately 11 cm. Acute intramural haematoma progressing to aortic dissection occurs in approximately 28–47% of presentations and to aortic rupture in 21–47% of cases. Regression of the haematoma is seen in only approximately 10% of cases (Neinaber et al. 1995; Shimizu et al. 2000; Neinaber and Eagle 2003).

A diagnosis of aortic dissection cannot be made purely on clinical examination. Advanced imaging techniques are necessary to confirm the diagnosis. Intramural haemorrhage of the ascending aorta carries a prognosis similar to Stanford type A dissection, and conversely intramural haemorrhage of the descending aorta carries a similar prognosis to Stanford type B (Tsai et al. 2005); consequently the new classification reflects this new evidence (Table 9.1).

Table 9.1 Classification of aortic dissections based on the European Society of Cardiology (2001) proposals.

Class 1:	Classical aortic dissection with an intimal flap between true and false lumen
Class 2:	Medial disruption with formation of intramural haematoma/haemorrhage
Class 3:	Discrete/subtle dissection without haematoma, eccentric bulge at tear site
Class 4:	Plaque rupture leading to aortic ulceration, penetrating aortic atherosclerotic ulcer with surrounding haematoma, usually subadventitial
Class 5:	Iatrogenic and traumatic dissection

Clinical presentation

The clinical presentation of a patient with aortic dissection will include shock, anxiety and a feeling of 'impending doom'. The patient may complain of dyspnoea and may be cyanosed. According to Yee (2004), in the early stages patients may present with an elevated blood pressure. A normal or reduced systolic blood pressure on admission may signal volume depletion, which may be caused by blood sequestration in the false lumen, or the pericardial or pleural space, warranting further investigation (ESC 2001). Syncope is also a common manifestation, often indicating the development of serious complications (for example, obstruction to cerebral vessels, cardiac tamponade and neurological impairment). Results from the IRAD highlighted that syncope was present in up to 20% of patients with aortic dissection and that such individuals were at greater risk of in-hospital mortality (Hagan et al. 2000).

Traditionally, notions of ripping/tearing sensations and retrosternal chest or back pain of sudden onset have been associated with aortic dissections. However, such sensations are apparently quite rare, as typically patients describe their pain as sharp and severe. Additionally, 4.5% of patients denied having any chest pain, which in itself may be indicative of chronic aortic dissection (Hagan et al. 2000; ESC 2001). Some patients may also initially report abdominal pain (Hagan et al. 2000). Gender-related differences in presentation for acute aortic dissections are not uncommon. A study by Neinaber et al. (2004) demonstrated that women diagnosed with aortic dissections were significantly older and tended to present later than men. Coma and altered mental status were typical of women's presentation, whereas pulse deficit was less common. The diagnosis of aortic dissection in women was often delayed due to differing clinical presentations (see Chapter 7).

Reports of chest pain are generally more common in patients when the dissection involves the ascending segment of the aorta, whereas back pain and abdominal pain are typical in those with descending aorta involvement (Hagan et al. 2000). It is further suggested that patients presenting with predominant abdominal pain have a higher mortality, which may be associated with a delay in diagnosis (Hagan et al. 2000; Tsai et al. 2005). Dependent on the level of the dissection and any other arteries involved, an array of other clinical symptoms may also be present. For example, some patients may be admitted with paraplegia due to the involvement of the intercostal arteries, and with oliguria associated with the renal arteries being compromised (Beese-Bjurstrom 2004).

History taking

Since rates of mortality are highest during the first hour of symptom onset, prompt assessment is vital. Collection of patient data should consist of the history of events, presenting symptoms and physical examination, which should include inspection, palpation, auscultation and percussion (Hudak et al. 1997; Bates 2003). Determining the origin of chest pain and whether it is life-threatening depends on obtaining appropriate patient data to eliminate other differential diagnoses. A systematic review of chest pain characteristics utilising the aid of a mnemonic tool may aid in confirming the pain's origin (Newberry et al. 2005). Risk factors for coronary artery disease should be identified, and specifically a history of hypertension.

Clinical examination

A comprehensive clinical physical examination is imperative in determining the presence and origin of the aortic dissection. Auscultation of the chest, for example, may reveal the presence of a diastolic murmur, which is indicative of aortic regurgitation. This finding occurs in approximately 50% of patients with proximal aortic dissection (ECS 2001). In aortic regurgitation the aortic valve fails to close completely during diastole, and blood regurgitates back into the left ventricle. The murmur can be heard loudest between the 2nd and 4th left intercostal spaces. This is best heard when the patient is sitting and leaning forwards. S3 plus S4 sounds suggest severe regurgitation. Two other murmurs may also be present: a midsystolic murmur from increased flow across the aortic valve and a mitral diastolic murmur (Austin Flint murmur) (Bates 2003). Alternatively, if there is involvement of the pericardium, a pericardial rub may be heard as a high pitched scratchy sound located in the 3rd left intercostal space (Bates 2003).

The presence of a pleural effusion, caused by rupture of the aorta into the pleural space, may be identified during auscultation of the lungs. Percussion sounds will be dull to flat over the effusion and there may be decreased or absent breath sounds over the affected area (Bates 2003). A raised jugular venous pressure and/or a paradoxical pulse (refer to Chapter 8) may also be evident which may be a sign of pericardial involvement (ECS 2001; Bates 2003).

Patients with a suspected dissection of the descending aorta must be examined for signs of abdominal rigidity, tenderness and evidence of a palpable mass. The aorta may be palpated by pressing firmly on the upper abdomen slightly to the left of the midline. The width of the aorta may be assessed by pressing deeply with one hand on each side of the aorta. A periumbilical or upper abdominal mass with increased pulsations is suggestive of an aortic aneurysm and warrants further investigation (Bates 2003).

Other potential findings include a difference in pulse and blood pressures in upper or lower extremities caused by the obstruction of the peripheral vessels at the level of the dissection. Therefore both radial, femoral and poplitial pulses, in addition to recording the blood pressure from the right and left arms, need to be monitored regularly. This finding is common in around 30% of patients with a Stanford type A aortic dissection, as compared with 21% of individuals with Stanford type B aortic dissection (Hagan et al. 2000). As discussed previously, depending on the level of the lesion, oliguria and paraplegia may also be present.

Initial investigations

Electrocardiogram

An electrocardiogram (ECG) should be acquired in all patients although the interpretation needs to be considered with caution. Depending on the location and severity of the aortic dissection, signs of myocardial ischaemia or infarction may be evident on the 12-lead ECG trace. Approximately 20% of patients with Stanford type A dissections have evidence of acute myocardial infarction, although most patients will have non-specific ST and T wave changes (Kamp et al. 1994; Tsai et al. 2005). If dissection of the aortic root occurs, this may affect coronary artery blood flow and the patient may exhibit signs of a myocardial infarction. However, this is secondary to the aortic dissection (Yee 2004).

Radiography

A routine chest X-ray may show widening of the upper mediastinum, a sign that is suggestive of aortic dissection and is present in approximately 60–80% of patients (ESC 2001). More advanced imaging techniques may be more reliable in producing diagnostic images and can be performed more rapidly. These include echocardiography, computerised tomography (CT) and cardiac magnetic resonance imaging (MRI) to confirm diagnosis and guide treatment options by localising tears and the extent of the dissection (Tsai et al. 2005).

TTE, TOE, CT and MRI

Transthoracic echocardiography (TTE) and transoesophageal echocardiography (TOE) can be used in the emergency or operating department settings. In particular, TTE has a sensitivity and specificity of approximately 80% and 96% respectively for identifying the involvement of the ascending aorta, although its visualisation of the descending aorta is limited. The most widely used diagnostic tool, however, is the computerised tomography scan (CT scan), which has a sensitivity of greater than 90% and a specificity of 85%. In contrast, magnetic resonance imaging (MRI) is quick and safe, albeit its value is limited in the emergency setting but it has an accuracy level of approximately 100% for visualising the aorta (ESC 2001; Tsai 2005).

Biochemical markers

The use of conventional biochemical markers has limited applicability in the diagnosis of aortic dissection, although assay of circulating myosin that is released from aortic medial muscle and rises in the first 3 hours following aortic dissection appears promising (Suzuki et al. 1996). Studies into the value of D-dimers have also been the subject of continuing research, and a negative result makes the presence of aortic dissection unlikely (Weber et al. 2003). The roles of C-reactive protein, fibrinogen and serum elastin continue to be explored. Beyond the acute situation, further laboratory tests would need to consider genetic family studies and mutation identification. Blood samples should be taken for urea and electrolytes, full blood count, group and cross-match, and blood gas analysis to plan future management (Yee 2004).

Differential diagnosis

Due to the variety of presentations of an acute aortic dissection, other differential diagnoses need to be ruled out. A common manifestation of patients presenting with aortic dissection is back and chest pain. ECG changes and clinical presentation may initially guide the clinician to a variety of differential diagnoses including pulmonary embolism and myocardial infarction, whose management and treatment with thrombolysis may have dire consequences (Beese-Bjurstrom 2004). Indeed the clinical picture may be confused with patients presenting with chest pain and ECG changes indicative of acute coronary syndromes, pulmonary embolism, perforated duodenal ulcer and aortic stenosis. As discussed in the previous chapters, each differential diagnosis of chest pain will have its own unique presentation. However, the differential diagnosis of acute aortic dissection should always be considered in patients presenting with unexplained syncope, acute left ventricular failure, cerebral vascular accident or ischaemia of the extremities, even when chest pain is not the major symptom.

Immediate management and interventions

The immediate management of a patient presenting with suspected acute aortic dissection, regardless of type of dissection, is medical stabilisation and reduction of arterial blood pressure. This reduces the force of the left ventricular ejection pressure, which affects the degree of dissection extension and consequent rupture (Tsai et al. 2005). The lowest tolerable blood pressure should be achieved whilst maintaining other vital organ perfusion (Beese-Bjurstrom 2004), the ideal target range being a systolic of between 100 and 120 mmHg (Yee 2004; Tsai et al. 2005).

- The first-line pharmacological therapy of choice with the ability to reduce both the force of left ventricular ejection and blood pressure is beta-blockers (for example, metoprolol and labetolol). Consideration must also be given to the half-life of any medication.

- In patients unable to tolerate beta-blockers, such as asthmatics, a test of esmolol may be given due to its short half-life (ESC 2001; Tsai et al. 2005).
- In the event of intolerance or other contraindications, calcium channel blockers may be an alternative option, although there is a lack of clinical data supporting their use in this way (ESC 2001).
- Vasodilators as a monotherapy are contraindicated as they increase the force of left ventricular ejection; however, in patients in whom hypertension cannot be controlled, vasodilators with beta-blockers as a combination therapy can be used (ESC 2001). In severe cases other blood-pressure-lowering drugs may be used, for example sodium nitroprusside.

In patients who present with an initial low or near normal blood pressure, volume depletion may be due to haemorrhage into the false lumen. These patients will require urgent fluid resuscitation and diagnostic imaging prior to surgical intervention (Tsai et al. 2005).

Whilst lowering the blood pressure may result in some relief of pain as a result of the reduction of the pressure of the walls of the aorta, the patient may need pain relief and reassurance. Morphine sulphate may be used and should be administered in conjunction with an anti-emetic to prevent further aortic trauma due to vomiting (Beese-Bjurstrom 2004). Once the patient's blood pressure has been reduced, diagnostic imaging techniques can then be undertaken to confirm the presence and location of the aortic dissection.

Patients with a Stanford type A (ascending) or DeBakey I and II dissection are deemed surgical emergencies, and treatment will help prevent aortic rupture and the development of pericardial effusion which may lead to cardiac tamponade. Medical management alone is associated with increased mortality (ESC 2001).

The most appropriate surgical technique to be used is dependent on the size of the aortic root and the condition of the aortic valves. If the ascending aorta and aortic dimensions are normal with no detachment of aortic valve leaflets, a tubular graft may be anastomosed to the sinotubular ridge (ESC 2001). However, when the aortic valve needs attention, the valve may need to be replaced or repaired prior to insertion of a graft. The standard approach is via a median sternotomy. The creation of a leak-proof and firm graft is achieved by the use of Teflon felt, tissue adhesive usually in the form of gelatine resorcinol formaldehyde glue (GRF-glue), or both. The glue anastomoses the dissected layers forming a leather-like texture and obliterates dead spaces between the graft and the aorta. Treatment continues to cause debate where the aortic arch has been affected in Stanford type A and DeBakey I and II dissection. Aortic arch tears occur in 30% of patients with aortic dissections. Depending on the level of the dissection, sub-total or total arch placement may be necessary. Choice of treatment from the great variety of surgical procedures that exist is dependent on patient presentation, on cardiac and genetic abnormalities, and on the experience and accessibility of the surgical centre (ESC 2001). Should the dissection involve the coronary arteries, a coronary artery bypass graft may also be considered (Yee 2004).

In Stanford type B (descending) and DeBakey III dissections the indications for surgery continue to be an area of debate. Uncomplicated dissections historically have been treated conservatively with pain relief, beta-blockers and other antihypertensive agents. There appears to be no conclusive evidence to support the superiority of surgical intervention by stent grafting or medical therapy. However, time is of the essence and surgical intervention carries an in-hospital mortality as high as 89% when associated with peripheral vascular ischaemic complications such as renal and mesenteric ischaemia. The indications for surgery are dependent on persistent chest pain, aortic expansion, haematoma formation and ischaemic branch vessel involvement. However, mortality rates for elective surgery are approximately 27% and exceed 50% in the emergency setting (Eggebrecht et al. 2005).

Endovascular repair offers a less invasive treatment and at times replaces the need for open surgical procedures. Two methods can be used depending on whether there is static or dynamic obstruction of the aortic branch arteries: percutaneous stenting is the preferred method for static obstruction whereas percutaneous balloon fenestration with or without stenting is used for obstruction to the aortic branch arteries. The goal of percutaneous balloon fenestration is to create a tear in the dissection flap that separates the true from the false lumen, and a stent may be needed to ensure the lumen remains patent. However, stent graft placement only seals the bleeding from the luminal side and so fatal rebleeding may occur (ESC 2001). Endovascular repair of type B aortic dissections provides a short-term response to a life-threatening condition. Further medical and surgical intervention will be necessary in the long term (Eggebrecht et al. 2005).

Further investigations

Identification of patients at risk of dissection has proven to be difficult. Whilst it is acknowledged that familial thoracic aneurysms and dissections (TAAD) occur as a complication of known syndromes (e.g. Marfan's syndrome), 20% of patients presenting with thoracic aneurysms and dissections who do not have Marfan's syndrome have a first-degree relative with the disease, this being inherited in an autosomal dominant manner. Researchers are attempting to determine the genetic components that predispose to aortic dissections, and future research will endeavour to identify those at risk (Hasham et al. 2003; Wung and Aouizerat 2004).

Medium- to long-term management plan

All patients should receive lifelong blood pressure management treatment to minimise aortic wall stress, with a recommended goal of <120/80 mmHg. Pharmacological agents include beta-blockers, calcium channel blockers and other antihypertensive agents such as angiotensin-converting enzyme inhibitors (Yee 2004). Regular assessment of the aorta should be performed, looking for signs of aneurysm formation, aortic expansion and leaks from any anastomosis or stent sites. These should be performed at 1, 3, 6 and 12 months following the acute event, then yearly thereafter. MRI appears to be the diagnostic technique of choice as this permits a large field of visualisation at neighbouring anatomical structures; however, CT imaging is the method most frequently observed (ESC 2001). Re-operation may be necessary for approximately 10% of survivors at 5 years and 40% at 10 years, with a higher incidence in patients with Marfan's syndrome (ESC 2001; Tsai et al. 2005).

Preventative measures include the identification and modification of risk factors for coronary heart disease to prevent the development of atherosclerotic plaques, which would predispose to aneurysm formation and dissection. For example, the management of hypertension is vital to prevent added aortic wall stress (ESC 2001). In Marfan patients, prophylactic replacement of the aortic root should be considered when an aortic diameter of 5.5 cm has been reached, although a smaller threshold may apply for younger patients (ESC 2001).

Key learning points

- Factors that affect the elasticity of the vessel wall and predispose to plaque formation should be monitored and treated appropriately, e.g. hypertension and diabetes.
- Trauma, iatrogenic factors, and inflammatory and inherited diseases can contribute to aortic dissection.
- Patients with ascending aortic dissections may present with chest pain, which may be described as severe; others may complain of abdominal discomfort.
- Aortic dissection can be life threatening: a number of victims may present in a collapsed state.
- Depending on the location of the dissection, the patient may present with other symptoms which include paraplegia or back pain.
- Initial treatment is immediate blood pressure control with beta-blockers
- Surgical treatment is the recommended strategy for Stanford type A and DeBakey I and II dissections

References

Bates B (2003) *Guide to Physical Examination*. Philadelphia, Lippincott Williams and Wilkins.

Beese-Bjurstrom B (2004) Aortic aneurysms and dissections. *Nursing* **34**(2): 36–41.

Bossert T, Battellini R, Kotowicz V, Falk V, Gummert JF, Mohr FW (2004) Ruptured giant syphilitic aneurysm of the descending aorta in an octogenarian. *Journal of Cardiac Surgery* **19**(4): 356–357.

Burks J, Iles R, Keating E (1998) Ascending aortic aneurysms in young adults with bicuspid aortic valve; implications for echocardiographic surveillance. *Clinical Cardiology* **21**: 439–443.

Eggebrecht H, Lonn L, Herold U, Breuckmann F, Leyh R, Jakob H, Erbel R (2005) Endovascular stent graft placement for complications of acute type B aortic dissection. *Current Opinions in Cardiology* **20**: 477–483.

Erbel R, Eggebrecht H (2006) Aortic dimensions and the risk of dissection. *Heart* **92**: 137–142.

European Society of Cardiology Task Force Report (2001) Diagnosis and management of aortic dissection. *European Heart Journal* **22**: 1642–1681.

Hagan PG, Neinaber CA, Isselbacher EM, Bruckman D, Karavite DJ, Russman PL, Evangelista A, Fattoria R, Suzuki T, Oh JK, Moore AG, Malouf JF, Pape LA, Gaca C, Sechtem U, Lenferink S, Deutsch HJ, Diedrichs H, Marcs Y, Robles J, Llovet A, Gilon D, Das SK, Armstrong WF, Deeb GM, Eagle K (2000) The International Register of Acute Aortic Dissection (IRAD). New insights into an old disease. *Journal of the American Medical Association* **283**: 897–903.

Hasham SN, Willing MC, Guo D, Muilenburg A, Rumin He MD, Tran V, Scherer SE, Shete SS, Milewicz DM (2003) Mapping a locus for familial thoracic aortic aneurysms and dissections (TAAD2) to 3p 24–25. *Circulation* **107**(25): 3184–3190.

Hudak C, Gallo B, Morton D (1997) *Critical Care Nursing: A Holistic Approach*, 7th edition. Philadelphia, Lippincott Williams & Wilkins.

Kamp T, Goldschmidt-Clermont P, Brinker J, Resar J (1994) Myocardial infarction, aortic dissection and thrombolytic therapy. *American Heart Journal* **128**: 1234–1237.

Neinaber C, Eagle K (2003) Aortic dissection: new frontiers in diagnosis and management. Part 1 From etiology to diagnostic strategies. *Circulation* **108**: 628–635.

Neinaber C, Von Kodolitsch Y, Peterson B (1995) Intramural haemorrhage of the thoracic aorta: diagnostic and therapeutic implications. *Circulation* **92**: 1465–1472.

Neinaber C, Fattori R, Mehta R, Richartz B, Evangelista A, Petzch M, Cooper J, Januzzi J, Ince H, Scechtem U, Bossone E, Fang J, Smith D, Isselbacher E, Pape L, Eagle K (2004) On behalf of the International Register of Acute Aortic Dissection. Gender–related differences in acute aortic dissection. *Circulation* **109**: 3014–3021.

Newberry L, Barnett GK, Ballard N (2005) Clinical notebook. A new mnemonic for chest pain assessment. *Journal of Emergency Nursing* **31**(1): 84–85.

Shimizu H, Yohino H, Udagawa H (2000) Prognosis of intramural haemorrhage compared with classic aortic dissection. *American Journal of Cardiology* **85**: 792–795.

Suzuki T, Katoh H, Watanabe M, Kurabayashi M, Hiramori K, Hori S, Nobuyoshi M, Tanaka H, Kodoma K, Sato S, Tsuchio Y, Yazaki Y, Nagai R (1996) Novel biochemical diagnostic method for aortic dissection: results of a prospective study using an immunoassay of smooth muscle myosin heavy chain. *Circulation* **93**: 1244–1249.

Tavora F, Jeudy J, Gocke C, Burke A (2005) Takayasu aortitis with acute dissection and haemopericardium. *Cardiovascular Pathology* **14**(6): 320–323.

Tsai T, Neinaber C, Kin K (2005) Acute aortic syndromes. *Circulation* **112**: 3802–3813.

Weber T, Hogler S, Auer J, Berent R, Lassnig E, Kvas E, Eber B (2003) D-dimer in acute aortic dissection. *Chest* **123**(50): 1375–1378.

Wung S, Aouizerat B (2004) Newly mapped gene for thoracic aneurysm and dissection. *Journal of Cardiovascular Nursing* **19**(6): 409–416.

Yee C (2004) Aortic dissection: the tear that kills. *Nursing Management* **35**(2): 25–33.

Useful websites

http://www.escardio.org

http://www.surgical-tutor.org.uk/default-home.htm?system/vascular/dissection. htm~right

http://www.nice.org.uk/page.aspx?o=297798

Chapter 10
Assessing and managing the patient with chest pain due to pulmonary embolism

Jan Keenan

Aims

This chapter guides the reader through the rather muddy water of the diagnosis of pulmonary embolism (PE). This is a relatively unique condition with a high incidence and significant mortality, but one which is both under- and overdiagnosed in clinical practice. The chapter therefore seeks to raise awareness of risk factors for the development of venous thromboembolism (VTE), and explores ways in which the condition might be diagnosed and treated quickly. There are two significant guidelines relating to the management of PE, one from the British Thoracic Society (BTS 2003) and one from the European Society of Cardiology (ESC 2000); both are relevant. The reader's attention is drawn to these existing guidelines regarding the assessment, diagnosis and management of the patient presenting with suspected pulmonary embolism.

Learning outcomes

Having read the chapter and undertaken further reading where applicable in relation to the practice background, as well as having sought an appropriate level of supervised practice, the reader should be able to:

- Consider the presentation of pulmonary embolus and include it as a consideration for differential diagnosis in the patient with chest pain.
- Understand the risk factors for the development of venous thromboembolism.
- Discuss the pathophysiology of pulmonary embolism.
- Undertake the assessment of the patient and clearly identify those features of the history which suggest or refute a potential diagnosis of pulmonary embolism.
- Order and interpret, where appropriate, the results of diagnostic tests which may rule in, or out, the possibility of pulmonary embolism.
- Discuss the management of the patient presenting with minor, or massive, pulmonary embolism and the mainstays of treatment for the presentation.
- Discuss the need for further investigation, referral, or intervention.

- Describe the longer term management of the condition in relation to its potential recurrence.

Background

PE is a major international health problem with an annual estimated incidence of 65,000 cases among hospitalised patients in England and Wales alone. In written evidence to a House of Commons Select Committee on Health, Cohen (2004) estimated the cost of the total burden of VTE on health services in the UK to be up to £640 million. However, the diagnosis of PE is often difficult to obtain and frequently missed (ESC 2000). The annual incidence of deep vein thrombosis (DVT) and PE in the general population of the western world may be estimated at 1.0 and 0.5 per 1000 respectively. The BTS (2003) points out that large community studies show the overall incidence of PE to be 60–70 cases per 100,000, with half of these cases developing VTE while in hospital or in long-term care and the remainder of cases equally divided between idiopathic causes and those with recognised risk factors. However, the ESC Task Force on Pulmonary Embolism (2000) points out the difficulties in estimating the true incidence of the problem, given differences in diagnostic coding and criteria as well as discrepancies between clinical diagnosis and autopsy findings. They point out in addition that the incidence of unsuspected PE in patients at post mortem has not diminished, and that the number of clinically silent non-fatal cases cannot be determined.

PE develops when a blood-borne substance lodges in a branch of the pulmonary artery and obstructs blood flow. The embolism may consist of a thrombus, air that has been accidentally injected during an infusion, fat mobilised from bone marrow following a fracture, or amniotic fluid entering the maternal circulation at the time of delivery (Porth 2004). By far the majority of pulmonary emboli arise from the deep veins of the legs or pelvis, where thrombus is likened by Bourke (2003) to a beast that 'typically lurks . . . like a treacherous assassin lying in wait to claim the life of the victim by suddenly shooting off a major embolus to the lungs'. Goldhaber (1998a) considers that DVT and PE should be considered part of the same pathological process. A study by Moser et al. (1994) revealed that almost 40% of patients with DVT had evidence of PE on lung scanning. Because of the close association between DVT and PE, this chapter is concerned with both, referred to collectively in more recent literature as venous thromboembolism (VTE).

Causes

Among the factors that contribute to thrombus formation and propagation are venous stasis, venous endothelial injury and hypercoagulability states, known collectively as Virchow's triad (Turpie et al. 2003; see Table 10.1). Venous stasis tends to occur if a patient is immobilised, for example following surgery, or if a limb is immobilised in a plaster cast, where there is prolonged local pressure, or where there is venous obstruction. Stasis is common in congestive heart failure,

Table 10.1 Risk factors for venous thromboembolism (European Cardiac Society 2000; Bourke 2003; Porth 2004).

Venous stasis and venous endothelial injury	Immobility Prolonged bed rest Local pressure Venous obstruction Heart failure Myocardial infarction Spinal cord injury Dehydration Long distance travel Trauma, particularly hip or femur fracture Orthopaedic surgery Surgery for gynaecological cancer Previous thrombosis Inflammation Advanced age Chronic venous insufficiency Central venous catheters Obesity (BMI > 30)
Hypercoagulability states	Surgery Trauma/fractures Childbirth, pregnancy/puerperium Malignancy +/− chemotherapy Oral oestrogen contraceptives Smoking Nephrotic syndrome Sickle cell disease Polycythaemia vera
Specific abnormalities of the clotting system	Factor V Leiden deficiency (most commonly associated with VTE) Anti-thrombin III deficiency Protein S or C deficiency Anti-cardiolipin antibody disease Hyperviscosity Congenital dysfibrinogenaemia

shock, hypovolaemia, dehydration and varicose veins. Air travel has been implicated as a risk factor for VTE, with 100 cases of PE reportedly occurring after air travel in the past three decades (Lapostolle et al. 2001). These authors systematically reviewed all cases of PE requiring medical care on arrival at a single European airport over 7 years, noting that, of 135.29 million passengers during the study period, 56 had confirmed pulmonary embolism. The incidence was higher in passengers travelling more than 5000 km (1.5 cases per million) and higher still (4.8 cases per million) in those travelling further than 10,000 km, indicating that distance travelled is a significant contributing risk factor. Immobility is assumed to be responsible for the increase in risk. However, it has to be acknowledged that the researchers were unable to identify any cases which may have presented later, which may have considerably altered their calculation of risk.

Vascular endothelial injury can occur as a result of inflammation or by local trauma such as that associated with indwelling venous catheters, surgery, fractures or infection. Patients following gynaecological or orthopaedic surgery for fractures to the hip or femur are particularly vulnerable to DVT because of the risk of trauma to the femoral and iliac veins.

Intravascular coagulability of blood increases in several conditions, such as sickle cell disease and polycythaemia vera; in these conditions the viscosity of blood increases, favouring sluggish flow next to vessel walls (West 2001). Of various identified thrombophilias, the factor V Leiden mutation is most associated with VTE, with other disorders less commonly associated. A combination of disorders, however, further elevates the risk of VTE (Goldhaber 1998a). Cancers, particularly adenocarcinomas and metastatic cancers, can produce thrombin and synthesise procoagulation factors, increasing the risk of coagulation (Turpie et al. 2003). Use of oral contraceptives, pregnancy and hormone replacement therapy are thought to increase resistance to endogenous anticoagulants (Porth 2004), with the risk of PE among users of oral contraceptives approximately three times the risk of non-users, increasing significantly in women who smoke.

Pathophysiology

The pulmonary circulation moves blood through the lungs, creating a link with the gas exchange function of the respiratory system and the systemic circulation, which moves blood through the body (Porth 2004). It consists of the right heart, the pulmonary arteries, pulmonary capillaries, and pulmonary veins (see Figure 10.1).

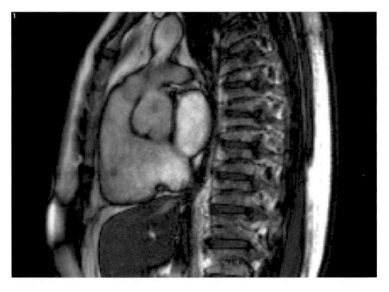

Figure 10.1 MRI of pulmonary artery tree.

Although the pulmonary and systemic circulations function similarly, they have important differences. The pulmonary circulation is a low pressure circuit with a mean arterial pressure of approximately 12 mmHg. Because of the low pressure, blood moves comparatively slowly through the lungs, which is important for gas exchange; blood flow at rest is around 6 litres per minute. Consistent with the low pressure in the circuit, the pulmonary vascular resistance is low (West 2001).

In the acute phase of DVT, once a thrombus is formed in veins it can resolve, extend proximally or embolise. Pulmonary embolism occurring following DVT is particularly common when thrombosis occurs in the proximal femoral or iliac veins, with a risk as high as 50% suggested by Ghuran et al. (2003), but is less likely when thrombosis is confined to the calf veins. Whilst most arise from deep veins in the legs, PE may occasionally arise from thrombus in the inferior vena cava, the right side of the heart or from indwelling catheters in the subclavian or jugular veins (Bourke 2003). PE may occur as a single event or in the form of successive episodes (ESC 2000), and in the acute phase a first attack may cause death, or produce mild or severe clinical consequences or no symptoms at all. However, anatomically large emboli generally pose a greater threat than small ones.

If an embolus blocks the flow of blood to one or more lobes of the lung, pulmonary vascular resistance rises. However, as West (2001) describes, the increase is less than might be expected because, as pulmonary arterial pressure rises, the pulmonary vascular pressure of non-embolised lung falls. This is because an increase in either pulmonary arterial pressure or venous pressure will result in an increase in capillary pressure, which triggers two mechanisms. First, under normal conditions some of the pulmonary vascular capillaries are closed; as the pressure rises within the capillary bed, these capillaries open, begin to conduct blood and thus lower overall resistance. This is termed *recruitment* (West 2001). Secondly, at higher capillary pressures *distension*, or increase in calibre of the capillaries, occurs, further reducing vascular resistance at relatively high vascular pressures. Whilst this development of what is effectively a collateral circulation serves to protect the pulmonary circulation, it has limited value in the presence of massive PE. Further distension of capillaries can lead to the development of pulmonary arteriovenous shunts and bronchopulmonary arterial anastomoses. Precapillary hypertension reduces the vascular bed and causes bronchoconstriction and arteriolar vasoconstriction (ESC 2000).

As a result of obstruction, there is local aggregation of platelets and release of vasoactive substances including thromboxane A_2 released by activated platelets, which induce vasoconstriction (Ghuran et al. 2003). Histamine, serotonin and prostaglandins are also released causing bronchoconstriction (Lea and Zierler 2000). The persistent obstruction and associated vasoconstriction and bronchoconstriction create a mismatch between ventilation (V) and perfusion (Q). Sustained VQ mismatch results in arterial hypoxia. In an attempt to compensate, respiratory rate increases and the partial pressure of arterial carbon dioxide ($PaCO_2$) falls. Rather than correcting the VQ mismatch, however, reduction in $PaCO_2$ induces further bronchoconstriction and vasoconstriction, thereby increasing the severity of the problem.

Haemodynamically, the consequences of PE may be profound. Decrease in arterial flow to the lungs increases both pulmonary artery and right heart pressures. Cardiac output eventually decreases as a consequence of right ventricular dilatation and overload, and lowered left ventricular preload results in systemic arterial hypotension. In acute PE, right ventricular dilatation may be constrained by the pericardium and there is a shift to the left of the interventricular septum, which also contributes to a reduction in cardiac output (ESC 2000). This sequence of events is more likely in acute PE because the right ventricle is not hypertrophied and therefore less able to overcome the increase in afterload. Embolism without pulmonary infarction is the general rule, and true pulmonary infarction is a relatively rare complication most likely to occur in patients with pre-existing left ventricular failure or pulmonary disease.

Clinical presentation

Both the magnitude of embolisation and the absence or presence of pre-existing cardiopulmonary disease are responsible for the haemodynamic consequences of PE (ESC 2000), and therefore the clinical presentation will be dependent on the size of the embolism as well as on the general condition of the patient prior to the event. The majority of texts classify PE in terms of clinical presentation, as either 'massive' or 'non-massive', although there is overlap between the different presentations. Massive PE is further subdivided in some texts into acute and subacute (see, for example, Bourke 2003). Moser et al. (1994) revealed that around 40% of patients with DVT who have no pulmonary symptoms have abnormal lung scintigrams indicating embolism; it is therefore possible that many minor PEs may remain asymptomatic or are clinically undetectable. Acute minor PEs present with dyspnoea, typically accompanied by pleuritic chest pain, and haemoptysis (Bourke 2003); the onset of massive PE may have been preceded in the last weeks by a number of smaller events and occurs as a result of acute occlusion of >50% of the pulmonary vascular bed (Ghuran et al. 2003). Most patients with PE, however, have mild signs and symptoms of cardiorespiratory distress but do not, at least initially, appear to have a life-threatening illness (Goldhaber 2003) and are often triaged into a medical assessment or clinical decision unit.

PE has a wide range of clinical presentations but should be considered in all patients presenting with sudden onset of shortness of breath where there is a clinical probability of PE based on risk factors (Bickley and Szilagyi 2003; see Table 10.1). Presenting symptoms include pleuritic chest pain (52–66% of patients), which is usually due to distal emboli causing pleural irritation, with dyspnoea (80%), tachypnoea (70%) and cough (20–37%). Substernal chest pain may occur in up to 12% of patients (ESC 2000).

Haemoptysis occurs in 11–13% of patients although this tends to be associated with pulmonary infarction (Bourke 2003). However, sudden onset dyspnoea may be the only presenting symptom, and is a confounding factor in patients with known pulmonary disease or heart failure, who may only notice an increase in shortness of breath. Isolated dyspnoea of rapid onset is usually due to a more central PE not affecting the pleura (ESC 2000), and may be associated with substernal, angina-like chest pain. Sweating, fear and apprehension are common (Swanton 2003) and there may be subtle changes in mental functioning or level of consciousness (Lea and Zierler 2000). There has been discussion regarding the extent to which fever may be caused by PE. Although it has been reported in several cases, the extent to which it is associated with PE rather than with associated disease was studied by Stein et al. (2000). They concluded that among patients with PE in whom recognised causes of fever were eliminated, 86% were afebrile, and pyrexia was no more frequent in patients with pulmonary haemorrhage or infarction. They concluded that, although most patients with PE are afebrile, a low-grade fever may occur, though a high fever which is not associated with any other coexisting disease is rare.

Massive PE presents clinically with shock or hypotension (systolic blood pressure <90 mmHg), or a sustained fall in blood pressure >40 mmHg for more than 15 minutes, where it is not known to be caused by arrhythmia, hypovolaemia or sepsis. In addition to the symptoms listed above, there may be such clinical signs as cyanosis (11%; ESC 2000), tachycardia (26%), a gallop rhythm, raised jugular venous pressure (JVP) or syncope (11%). Syncope and shock suggest a large central PE with severe haemodynamic effects, and may be accompanied by oliguria, acute right heart failure and shutdown of the peripheral circulation. PE can also present as cardiac arrest, with the most likely causes being non-ventricular fibrillation arrhythmias such as pulseless ventricular tachycardia or pulseless electrical activity.

History taking

PE is associated primarily with sudden onset of dyspnoea, and in 90% of cases suspicion of PE is raised by a history of dyspnoea, chest pain or syncope in combination or in isolation (ESC 2000).

The diagnosis of PE is made on the basis of clinical probability as well as associated clinical presentation and findings, and therefore a history should include or exclude likely risk factors. Turpie et al. (2003) base clinical probability on the suspicion of DVT or risk of its development in patients with related clinical features, recent surgery or prolonged immobility, active cancer or a history of prior VTE. DVT itself may not be clinically suspected, but its presence, along with thrombotic risk factors, will make the diagnosis more likely. The BTS (2003) highlights that the value of making an assessment of clinical probability is that it encourages good clinical assessment and allows better interpretation of the results of investigations. It advocates the use of a relatively simple model for assessing probability (see Figure 10.2; BTS guidance on assessment of probability).

None of the symptoms suggestive of PE are specific to the condition, and it is therefore important to establish very early the clinical probability of PE by identifying the incidence of risk factors (see Figure 10.2). With this in mind, onset of symptoms is sudden, with dyspnoea an early feature, though Swanton (2003)

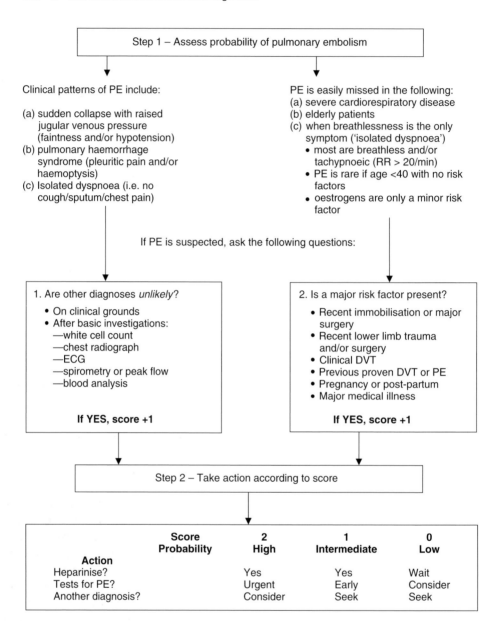

Figure 10.2 Initial assessment and actions in suspected PE (adapted from BTS 2003).

points out that, in retrospect, there may have been a history of mild dyspnoea in the preceding day or two. Location of chest pain is non-specific and, as highlighted earlier, in a few patients may be substernal (12%) although it is more likely to be pleuritic in nature. Pleuritic pain feels sharp and in particular will be worse on inspiration or be exacerbated by movement. In a few patients there may be radiation of the pain to the shoulder tip. Swanton (2003) explains this as association with involvement of the diaphragmatic pleura. A persistent dry cough is common.

Where there is a high suspicion of PE on the basis of clinical presentation and history, it is useful to consider early in the process of diagnosis whether a bleeding risk is present, as there are benefits from early anticoagulation which may help reduce mortality at an early stage.

Clinical examination

An initial survey suggests distress and anxiety, possibly shock, pain and breathlessness. The heart rate is likely to be elevated, and auscultation may reveal a gallop rhythm or murmur located in the pulmonary valve area, with an increase in intensity of the pulmonary component of the second heart sound. If there is right heart failure, the right heart may be palpable at the right sternal edge with a palpable heave and a 'rub' heard over the right ventricle, though cardiac anomalies may be difficult to identify in the presence of respiratory distress. An increase in jugular venous pressure, with bulging neck veins and a prominent 'v' wave, are also indicative of right heart failure (Goldhaber 1998b) and the patient may be cyanosed. The rhythm may be sinus tachycardia, sinus rhythm or atrial fibrillation.

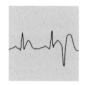

Initial investigations

Evaluating the likelihood of PE in an individual according to the clinical presentation is of the utmost importance in both the interpretation of diagnostic tests and the selection of an appropriate diagnostic strategy (ESC 2000). The progress of investigations will inevitably depend on the stability of the patient as well as the assessment of clinical probability of PE. Because of the difficulty in establishing a diagnosis of PE on clinical grounds alone, it is necessary to employ a combination of simple (ECG, X-ray, echocardiography, blood gases, D-dimer, troponin) and complex (V/Q scan, CT, MRI, angiography) investigations to confirm a clinical suspicion (Ghuran et al. 2003). Interest is growing in refining the number of diagnostic tests necessary to conclude the diagnosis, with a particular focus on a simple, fast strategy starting with a normal perfusion scan or a combination of normal D-dimer levels and low clinical probability, followed by the use of a reliable diagnostic method (Kruip et al. 2003).

Electrocardiogram

The value of the ECG in diagnosis of PE has been the subject of much discussion, although the patient will have a normal ECG in up to 27% of cases (Van Meigham et al. 2004). Submassive PE manifests a wide spectrum of non-specific changes on the surface ECG, ranging from no abnormality to multiple disturbances of rate, rhythm and conduction (Daniel et al. 2001). Typically, the ECG changes, if any, are those of a sinus tachycardia or atrial fibrillation with right heart strain (see Figure 10.3) although many ECG abnormalities have been reported (Conroy et al. 2004).

Van Meigham et al. (2004) quantify the abnormalities found in several studies, identifying rhythm disturbances, P wave abnormalities, QRS complex changes

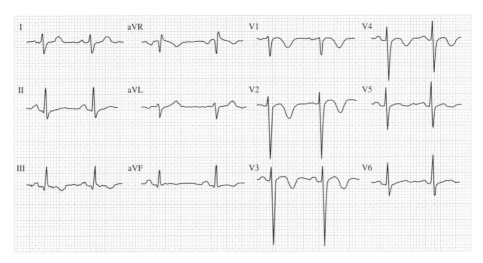

Figure 10.3 Electrocardiogram of changes seen in acute pulmonary embolism. Reproduced with permission from Harrigan & Jones (2002).

and ST segment or T wave abnormalities all as potential findings, none of which is specific to PE. Pre-existing cardiopulmonary disease can mimic several of the abnormalities associated with PE and this is therefore likely to further decrease the specificity of the ECG. The most common ECG finding in acute PE is T wave inversion in the anterior chest leads, particularly V_1–V_4, and these are probably reciprocal changes reflecting infero-posterior ischaemia due to compression of the right coronary artery by the right ventricle as a result of pressure overload (Goldhaber 1998b). The 'classical' '$S_1Q_3T_3$' (McGinn-White) pattern was identified as early as 1935, yet this reportedly occurs in only 11–50% of patients (Van Meigham et al. 2004). Although it has been considered to be very strongly associated with PE, a study by Chan et al. (2001) revealed that this pattern was equally prevalent in patients with and without PE. The ECG in Figure 10.2 was recorded from a patient presenting with sudden onset of shortness of breath accompanied by pleuritic pain, and reveals some of the findings associated with possible PE, including a right bundle branch block, the McGinn-White pattern ($S_1Q_3T_3$) and anterior T wave inversion suggesting right heart strain.

Right ventricular strain manifested on the ECG in acute PE is the single finding which is felt to have a high clinical importance (Daniel et al. 2001), as this evidence might predict the presence of pulmonary hypertension, which corresponds to the presence of right ventricular dysfunction and may therefore be correlated with outcome.

Radiography

In PE, the chest x-ray is often abnormal, although the common findings may be atelectasis and pleural effusion or elevation of a hemi-diaphragm, which are not specific to PE (ESC 2000). Decreased vascularity is uncommon (Ghuran et al. 2003). The clinical value of the chest x-ray is that it allows exclusion of other potential causes of dyspnoea and chest pain such as pneumonia, rib fracture or pneumothorax.

Arterial blood gases

Oxygen saturation monitoring is very insensitive and unlikely to be revealing. Arterial blood gases show evidence of hyperventilation and impaired gas exchange, with a reduction in PaO_2 due to ventilation/perfusion (V/Q) mismatch, and typical values will be less than 80 mmHg (<10.6 kPa), although Ghuran et al. (2003) point out that one study identified a PaO_2 of >11 kPa in 29% of patients younger than 40 compared with only 3% in older patients. Large pulmonary emboli result in severe hypoxia, hypocapnia and metabolic acidosis (Swanton 2003), and an increased alveolar–arterial oxygen gradient calculated from gases cannot accurately discriminate between those suspected of PE and those in whom no further investigation is required (Goldhaber 1998a). Therefore, whilst a mixed picture is likely to be present, arterial blood gases are not sufficiently revealing as to enable accurate diagnosis although they are of clinical value in raising the suspicion of PE.

D-dimer

D-dimer is a specific breakdown product released into the systemic circulation by endogenous fibrinolysis of cross-linked fibrin clot. D-dimers can be measured by an enzyme-linked immunosorbent assay (ELISA). A low plasma D-dimer (usually 0.5 mg/L) from a validated assay excludes the presence of thrombus and therefore has a 95% negative predictive value for VTE. However, because of the low specificity of the test, D-dimer concentrations greater than 0.5 mg/L do not rule in the diagnosis of VTE and indeed the ESC (2000) recommends that it be reserved for use in the emergency context because, in the elderly or inpatients, it is likely to be normal in less than 10% of patients. Fibrin is produced in a wide range of inflammatory conditions and a raised D-dimer may reflect other conditions such as myocardial infarction, stroke, sepsis, malignancy, recent surgery or trauma and advancing age (BTS 2003). Therefore plasma D-dimer is best used to exclude PE in patients with low clinical suspicion where there is no other systemic illness (Goldhaber 1998a), and it is not recommended that D-dimer should be performed in those with a high clinical probability of PE (BTS 2003).

Venous ultrasound and contrast venography

Lower limb ultrasound has the advantage that it is widely available and relatively inexpensive; compression ultrasonography of the legs can confirm the presence of DVT. Pressure is applied with an ultrasound transducer to compress opposing venous walls, with the primary diagnostic criterion that veins containing thrombus will be non-compressible. The presence of intraluminal echogenic thrombus, absence of a colour Doppler flow signal and loss of phases flow are secondary diagnostic criteria (Ghuran et al. 2003). However, the diagnostic accuracy is limited in pelvic and calf DVT, as well as in severe obesity or oedema, and therefore a single normal leg ultrasound cannot completely rule out the presence of subclinical DVT.

Troponin

Whilst traditional cardiac enzymes are of little or no value, a good deal of interest has been shown recently in the role of cardiac troponin. A relatively recent observation is that acute right heart strain in major PE can be detected by the release of cardiac troponin due to right ventricular muscle damage, and a troponin release may therefore offer prognostic information (ESC 2000). Goldhaber (2003) has suggested that cardiac troponin release in the context of acute PE is a promising tool for risk stratification. According to recent data from La Vecchia et al. (2004), an increased cardiac troponin 1 on admission predicts in-hospital mortality in acute pulmonary embolism. The troponin release is quantitatively small and far less than observed in ST-elevation myocardial infarction. However, given that troponin is released in acute coronary syndromes, myocarditis, myocardial trauma, ischaemic heart failure, ischaemic arrhythmia and PE (Conroy et al. 2004), it is of little independent diagnostic value.

Imaging: the V/Q scan

A V/Q scan is a non-invasive scan which has until relatively recently played a pivotal role in the diagnosis of PE (Giordiano and Angiolillo 2001). In PE, a defect can be identified in the perfusion portion of the scan in conjunction with a normal ventilation scan. However, the PIOPED investigators (1990), in a large multi-centre study, validated the ventilation/perfusion scan against pulmonary angiography or post mortem in acute pulmonary embolism, and found that PE could only be diagnosed or excluded reliably in a minority of patients by isotope lung scanning. PE was identified in the presence of non-diagnostic scans in 40% of cases. However, Goldhaber (1998b) argues that normal results are almost never associated with recurrent pulmonary embolism. With increasing background cardiorespiratory disease, the scan is less helpful, particularly with the presence of chronic obstructive pulmonary disease. However, in stable patients, the BTS (2003) recommends that a V/Q scan may be considered as the initial imaging investigation, providing facilities are available, chest radiograph is normal, there is no significant symptomatic concurrent cardiorespiratory disease, and standardised reporting criteria are used, with the proviso that the scan is interpreted in the context of clinical probability. The BTS (2003) also emphasises that further imaging is mandatory in all patients with an indeterminate scan or discordant clinical and scan probability.

Computerised tomographic pulmonary angiography

CT scanning allows rapid tomographic imaging during a single breath-hold and has the advantage of being rapid and generally widely available, particularly in the UK. The pulmonary vasculature can be visualised with a contrast dye injection (CT pulmonary angiography). This technique is increasingly being used as an adjunct to other imaging modalities and is clearly superior to ventilation perfusion isotope scanning (BTS 2003) although it remains limited by poorer visualisation of the peripheral areas of the upper and lower lobes (Ghuran et al. 2003). CTPA has the greatest sensitivity for emboli in the main, lobar or segmental pulmonary arteries but has a reduced sensitivity in the subsegmental arteries. However, thinner slice CT images may increase sensitivity. Figure 10.4 shows CTPA undertaken in a patient with an extensive clot in the pulmonary artery: the clot itself is surrounded by a 'halo' of bright contrast agent. Figure 10.5, from the same patient, shows a leak of contrast into the right ventricle, revealing right ventricular dilatation occurring as a result of the embolus.

Conventional pulmonary angiography has been considered to be the 'gold standard' in diagnosis against which other investigations have been evaluated. However, availability has been patchy at best, and the British Thoracic Society guideline asserts that conventional pulmonary angiography has largely been rendered obsolete by the advent of CTPA (BTS 2003), which is currently recommended as the initial lung imaging modality for non-massive PE.

Echocardiography

In suspected massive PE, transthoracic echocardiography is particularly useful. It is diagnostic in massive PE but allows firm diagnosis in a minority of others.

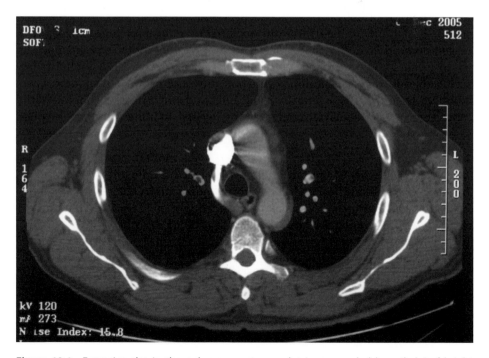

Figure 10.4 Extensive clot in the pulmonary artery – clot is surrounded by a 'halo' of bright contrast.

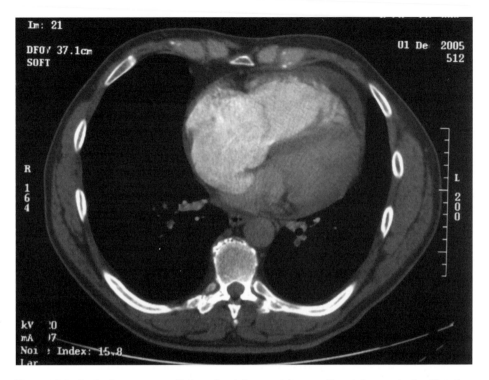

Figure 10.5 Leak of contrast media into the right ventricle, revealing right ventricular dilatation due to PE.

In addition, it can offer useful prognostic information, particularly the presence of right ventricular dysfunction. Detection of right ventricular hypertrophy suggests that the process is chronic (Goldhaber 1998a). It can often help identify conditions which may mimic PE such as myocardial infarction, aortic dissection or pericardial tamponade. Transoesophageal echocardiography offers the advantage of improving diagnostic accuracy by more reliably demonstrating the presence of thrombus, but other advantages over transthoracic echocardiography tend to be minimal (BTS 2003).

Differential diagnosis

The differential diagnoses for PE are extensive (see Table 10.2). However, a systematic approach to assessment and investigation assists both in ruling in the possibility of PE, and ruling out the possibility of conditions which may mimic PE. PE is both under- and overdiagnosed and it is likely that this is because it presents in a variety of ways and with such a broad spectrum of severity. The BTS (2003) has argued that careful assessment of clinical probability is the key to diagnosis, but although guidelines exist anecdotal evidence suggests that they are not generally followed well.

In the majority of patients the presentation is of sudden onset dyspnoea accompanied by pleuritic pain. Myocardial infarction is usually characterised

Table 10.2 Differential diagnosis for pulmonary embolism.

Cardiovascular	Non-cardiovascular
Myocardial infarction	Pneumonia, asthma
Exacerbation of heart failure	Exacerbation of COPD
New onset heart failure	Musculoskeletal pain
Acute pulmonary oedema	Pleurisy
Aortic dissection	Bronchogenic carcinoma

by a different pattern of onset and nature of symptoms, which will start suddenly but gradually increase in severity; in this context early investigation reveals more specific ECG changes suggestive of myocardial ischaemia or injury. Again the nature and pattern of pain are the features most likely to rule in, or out, aortic dissection as an alternative explanation. Pneumothorax or rib fracture will be visible on chest x-ray, which may also be useful in ruling out other causes of symptoms. The most difficult circumstances will be presented where there is significant coexisting cardiac or respiratory disease, particularly heart failure or chronic obstructive pulmonary disease where the patient presents with exacerbation of pre-existing shortness of breath. However, it is important to remember the assertion that sudden onset dyspnoea should always be regarded with suspicion and the diagnosis of PE ruled out if possible.

Patients with massive PE are a smaller proportion of those who present, but mortality is high and therefore early diagnosis is important. However, the clinical suspicion should be raised wherever there is a history of shortness of breath associated with syncope. In this respect the patient may be in a state of near collapse and the most important rule-outs are aortic aneurysm and myocardial infarction. Urgent availability of transthoracic echocardiography in the presence of cardiac signs, along with the ECG, should be sufficient to rule out the possibility of myocardial infarction or aortic aneurysm, and in this event the index of suspicion should be considerably raised and CTPA will confirm the diagnosis.

Immediate management and interventions

If left untreated, PE is associated with a high morbidity and mortality (Kruip et al. 2003) and it is advocated by both BTS and ESC guidelines that as soon as the clinical probability of PE has been established as intermediate or high, anticoagulation should be commenced (see Figure 10.2). The mainstay of treatment is reduction in both the development and propagation of venous thrombosis and the destruction of embolised clot. BTS guidance (2003) refers to the use of heparin as a first-line agent for anticoagulation in non-massive PE and mentions the role of low molecular weight heparin, though there is a sense that there is insufficient evidence to suggest that the onset of action of low molecular weight heparin is sufficiently rapid to begin the process of anticoagulation. There is now clearer evidence to suggest that fixed-dose low molecular weight heparin is as safe and as effective as dose-adjusted intravenous unfractionated heparin (Quinlan et al. 2004), although unfractionated heparin should still be considered in massive PE or when rapid reversal of effect may be needed.

In acute massive PE presenting with shock and/or severe hypoxia, or in PE with evidence of right ventricular dysfunction, the administration of thrombolysis with a bolus dose of 50 mg recombinant tissue plasminogen activator (r-TPA) is recommended. If clinical suspicion is high enough and cardiac arrest is imminent, BTS guidance supports the administration of thrombolysis on clinical grounds alone. However, thrombolysis in patients with sub-massive PE in the presence of right ventricular hypokinesia remains controversial (see Goldhaber 2005; Thabut and Logeart 2005). It is not indicated and therefore should not be used as first-line treatment in non-massive PE.

Oxygen supplementation will be necessary, and in the event of cardiorespiratory arrest associated with massive PE, supportive ventilation may be required. Haemodynamic support may also be initiated early in acute massive PE, with noradrenaline used in small doses to support the failing right heart only if the patient is in cardiogenic shock. Right heart filling pressure should be supplemented with carefully managed fluid replacement, although volume loading needs to be finely balanced against the potential for further dilatation and failure of the right ventricle.

In the absence of circulatory failure, a strategy of anticoagulation is required (Ghuran et al. 2003). Once VTE is confirmed, oral anticoagulation should be commenced with a target INR of 2.0–3.0, and only when this is achieved should the heparin be discontinued. BTS guidance suggests that the duration of anticoagulant treatment be determined by the underlying predisposition to VTE; in the case of temporary risk factors the duration of treatment should be 6 weeks; 3 months for first presentation of idiopathic VTE; and at least 6 months for any other identified potential source. In the presence of a persistent procoagulant stimulus such as malignant disease or where there is recurrent PE, treatment with warfarin should be prolonged further or should be lifelong (Ghuran et al. 2003).

Further investigations

Once treatment has been initiated it is appropriate to begin screening for any underlying pathological process such as carcinoma or metastatic disease, as well as for any previously unidentified coagulopathy. There is a considerable risk of recurrent PE, particularly during the first 4–6 weeks (ESC 2000).

Medium- to long-term management plan

Mortality in untreated PE is 25–30% but with adequate anticoagulant therapy the incidence of both fatal and non-fatal recurrent PE is reduced to less than 8% (ESC 2000). Mortality is influenced by cancer, advanced age, stroke and cardiopulmonary disease. Patients should be aware that having suffered VTE in the past increases the potential for VTE in the future.

Key learning points

- Pulmonary embolus is both under- and overdiagnosed, but the clinical suspicion should always be raised where there is sudden-onset dyspnoea.
- Classic symptoms of PE are pleuritic chest pain, dyspnoea and tachypnoea.
- The development of VTE is determined by Virchow's triad of local injury, hypercoagulability and stasis of venous blood flow.
- Clinical evidence of DVT is often not identified in patients presenting with PE.
- Systematic assessment of the patient according to a specified guideline such as BTS (2003) increases the probability of identifying PE.
- Many of the signs and symptoms suggestive of PE are non-specific.
- Assessment of clinical probability is the key to planning and interpretation of further investigations.
- Prognosis is improved by the early initiation of anticoagulation with low molecular weight heparin.
- Thrombolysis is only indicated in massive PE.

References

Bickley L, Szilagyi P (2003) *Bates' Guide to Physical Examination and History Taking*, 8th edition. Philadelphia, Lippincott Williams and Wilkins.

Bourke SJ (2003) *Lecture Notes on Respiratory Medicine*. Oxford, Blackwell Publishing.

British Thoracic Society (1997) Guideline for the diagnosis and management of pulmonary embolism. *Thorax* **52**(Suppl. 4): S2–S24.

British Thoracic Society (2003) British Thoracic Society guidelines for the management of suspected acute pulmonary embolism. *Thorax* **58**: 470–484.

Chan T, Vilke G, Pollack M et al. (2001) Electrocardiographic manifestations: pulmonary embolism. *Journal of Emergency Medicine* **21**: 263–270.

Cohen D (2004) Written evidence to the Select Committee on Health http://www.publications.parliament.uk/pa/cm200405/cmselect/cmhealth/99/99we07.htm

Conroy S, Kamal I, Cooper J (2004) Troponin testing: beware pulmonary embolus. *Emergency Medical Journal* **21**: 123–124.

Daniel K, Courtney M, Kline J (2001) Assessment of cardiac stress from massive pulmonary embolism with 12-lead ECG. *Chest* **120**: 474–481.

European Society of Cardiology (ESC) (2000) Task Force Report: Guidelines on diagnosis and management of acute pulmonary embolism. *European Heart Journal* **21**: 1301–1336.

Ghuran A, Uren N, Nolan J (2003) *Pulmonary embolism*. In *Emergency Cardiology: an Evidence Based Guide to Acute Cardiac Problems*, pp. 172–190. London, Arnold.

Giordiano A, Angiolillo D (2001) Current role of lung scintigraphy in pulmonary embolism. *Quarterly Journal of Nuclear Medicine* **45**: 294–301.

Goldhaber S (1998a) Clinical overview of venous thromboembolism. *Vascular Medicine* **3**: 35–40.

Goldhaber S (1998b) Pulmonary embolism. *New England Journal of Medicine* **339**(2): 93–105.

Goldhaber S (2003) Cardiac biomarkers in pulmonary embolism. *Chest* **123**(6): 1782–1784.

Goldhaber S (2005) Debate: Thrombolytic therapy for patients with pulmonary embolism who are haemodynamically stable but who have right ventricular dysfunction – pro. *Archives of Internal Medicine* **165**: 2197–2199.

Kruip M, Leclercq M, van der Heul C, Prins M, Buller H (2003) Diagnostic strategies for excluding pulmonary embolism in clinical outcome studies; a systematic review. *Annals of Internal Medicine* **138**: 941–951.

Lapostolle F, Surget V, Borron S, Desmaizieres M, Sordelet D, Lapandry C, Cupa M, Adnet F (2001) Severe pulmonary embolism associated with air travel. *New England Journal of Medicine* **345**(11): 779–783.

La Vecchia L, Ottani F, Favero L, Spadaro GL, Rubboli A, Boanno C, Mezzena G, Fontenelli A, Jaffe AS (2004) Increased cardiac troponin I on admission predicts in-hospital mortality in acute pulmonary embolism. *Heart* **90**: 633–637.

Lea H, Zierler BK (2000) *Hematopoiesis and coagulation.* In: Woods SL, Froelicher ES, Motzer S (Eds) *Cardiac Nursing*, 4th edition, pp. 109–131. Philadelphia, Lippincott Williams & Wilkins.

Moser KM, Fedullo P, Littlejohn J, Crawford R (1994) Frequent asymptomatic pulmonary embolism in patients with deep vein thrombosis. *Journal of the American Medical Association* **271**: 223–225.

PIOPED Investigators (1990) Value of the ventilation/perfusion scan in acute pulmonary embolism. *Journal of the American Medical Association* **263**(20): 2753–2759.

Porth CM (2004) *Essentials of Pathophysiology; Concepts of Altered Health States.* Philadelphia, Lippincott Williams and Wilkins.

Quinlan D, McQuillan A, Eikelboom J (2004) Low molecular weight heparin compared with intravenous unfractionated heparin for treatment of pulmonary embolism; a meta analysis of randomized controlled trials. *Annals of Internal Medicine* **140**: 175–183.

Stein P, Afzal A, Henry J, Villareal C (2000) Fever in acute pulmonary embolism. *Chest* **117**(1): 39–42.

Swanton R (2003) *Pocket Consultant: Cardiology*, 5th edition. Oxford, Blackwell.

Thabut G, Logeart D (2005) Debate: Thrombolysis for pulmonary embolism in patients with right ventricular dysfunction – con. *Archives of Internal Medicine* **165**: 2200–2203.

Turpie A, Chin B, Lip Y (2003) *Venous thromboembolism: pathophysiology, clinical features, and prevention.* In: Lip G, Blann A (Eds) *ABC of Antithrombotic Therapy.* London, BMJ Books.

Van Meigham C, Sabbe M, Knockaert D (2004) The clinical view of the ECG in non-cardiac conditions. *Chest* **125**: 1561–1576.

West JB (2001) *Pulmonary Physiology and Pathophysiology: An Integrated Case-Based Approach.* Philadelphia, Lippincott Williams and Wilkins.

Useful websites

http://www.patient.co.uk/showdoc/40001322
http://www.brit-thoracic.org.uk/
http://www.emedicine.com/med/topic1958.htm
http://www.merck.com/mmhe/sec04/ch046/ch046a.html

Chapter 11

Assessing and managing the patient with chest pain due to trauma

Simon Binks and Jonathan R. Benger

Introduction

Chest pain due to trauma can range from minor chest wall bruising to life-threatening vital organ disruption. Patients may present to first responders, primary care providers or emergency department staff. Sometimes the injury will be all too obvious, but at other times only careful history taking, clinical examination and specific investigations will clarify the diagnosis.

Aim

This chapter aims to discuss the diagnosis, investigation and management of a broad spectrum of chest injuries that cause chest pain.

Learning outcomes

After studying this chapter, the reader should be able to:

- Discuss the types and causes of chest injury.
- Demonstrate a structured approach in assessing the injured patient with chest pain.
- Recognise key signs and symptoms associated with chest injury.
- List the most appropriate initial investigations to be performed.
- Discuss the management options for patients with chest pain due to trauma.

Background

Trauma is a common and significant cause of mortality and morbidity throughout the world. Injury is the leading cause of death worldwide for people younger than 60 years of age (World Health Organization Department of Injuries and Violence Prevention 2000). After head injury, chest trauma is the most fatal type of injury (Demetriades et al. 2004), and in the UK the most common cause of chest trauma is road traffic collision (RTC). RTCs are the ninth leading cause of death worldwide, and the leading cause of death in 15–29 year olds in high income countries. Over one million people die on the world's roads every year, with 20–50 million injured at a global cost of $518 billion (World Report on Road Traffic Injury Prevention 2002). In an effort to reduce the burden of road deaths and injuries, the World Health Organization's road safety initiatives are central to its injury prevention programme.

The assessment of a patient with chest pain due to trauma is relevant not only to ambulance personnel and emergency department staff, but also to healthcare providers in primary care, who need to be able to distinguish a minor injury from a major one and to recognise the need for referral to an emergency department. These decisions will be based on the history and clinical findings.

This chapter will focus on selected conditions resulting from trauma where chest pain may occur as one of the key presenting features. The inclusion selection is by no means exhaustive but intended to guide the reader towards a likely diagnosis by a thorough assessment of symptoms and signs. A more specific review of initial investigations required for the selected conditions is presented in the later sections of the chapter.

Causes of chest trauma

Chest injuries may be classified as either blunt or penetrating. The mechanism of injury is important because each group of injuries has different pathophysiologies, and often different clinical courses (American College of Surgeons Committee on Trauma 2004).

Blunt injury

Most blunt injuries are managed non-operatively with interventions such as intubation and ventilation or chest drain insertion. Diagnosis of blunt injury may be more difficult and require additional investigations such as computerised tomography (CT) scanning. However, blunt trauma occurs as a consequence of road traffic collisions (involving drivers, passengers or pedestrians), falls, assault, sporting activities and industrial accidents.

Penetrating injuries

These are more likely to require operation, and complex investigations are required less often. Patients with penetrating trauma may deteriorate rapidly and recover much faster than patients with blunt injury. Most penetrating injuries are the result of assault with stabbing weapons or firearms.

Physiology

The age of the patient with a chest injury will influence the type and degree of injuries seen. Children and the elderly are more likely to be injured as pedestrians in a road traffic collision. A pedestrian child's size is such that the chest may be the point of impact with a car bumper, as opposed to the legs or pelvis in an adult. Children, particularly infants, may be subject to intentional chest injury.

The elastic or compliant nature of the paediatric thoracic skeleton means that rib fractures are rare, and significant internal injuries can occur in their absence, whereas the elderly frequently suffer sternal, costal cartilage or rib fractures. Indeed multiple rib fractures are common following even relatively minor trauma such as a fall from standing. This can cause significant pain with reduced lung ventilation and the risk of secondary complications such as atelectasis, pneumonia and respiratory failure (hypoxia) or ventilatory failure (hypercapnia). Additionally, elderly patients are more likely to have comorbidities, such as chronic obstructive pulmonary disease, which may complicate the clinical picture and add to the challenge of assessment.

Significant chest injury may initially be overlooked where other problems are obvious, such as drowning or burns. However, burns may coexist with blast injuries, and patients jumping from tall burning buildings may sustain chest injuries from the fall, whereas diving injuries may precede near-drowning.

Clinical presentation

Patients with significant chest injuries usually present immediately complaining of chest pain and associated shortness of breath. In blunt injuries the pain is commonly pleuritic due to chest wall injury and rib fracture, whilst patients with penetrating injuries will have pain at the site of the wound or wounds. Dyspnoea ranges from mild to severe, and may be associated with abnormal respiratory movements or increased work of breathing.

History taking

A history of major trauma, such as a road traffic collision or a fall from a height, should raise the suspicion of severe injury. If a patient presents some time after the initial injury, this may be reassuring, although a thorough assessment must be carried out regardless. Patients who are elderly or have underlying chest disease have less respiratory reserve and are therefore less able to cope with an injury that may be minor in a fit and healthy patient.

When assessing the trauma patient, precise and concise history taking is very important as intervention and further management may be time critical. Where major trauma is suspected it is sometimes necessary to examine and resuscitate the patient first, completing a 'primary survey' before a full history is taken. A useful aid to history taking often used by emergency practitioners is the 'AMPLE' mnemonic (ACSCT 2004):

A Allergies
M Medications
P   Past illnesses (particularly chest disease)/pregnancy

L   Last meal
E   Events/environment related to the injury

A history of events relating to the accident or assault is particularly important. Information from first-hand witnesses and attendees at the scene or pre-hospital personnel can aid in the prediction and assessment of injuries. Details of a road traffic collision such as the types of vehicle involved, use of seatbelt, deployment of airbag, deformation of the vehicle's exterior (side of impact, depth, etc.) and interior (steering wheel, dashboard) help to visualise the patient at the time of impact. Speed of impact, extrication time, ejection from the vehicle and other fatalities at the scene are predictive of the severity of injury and subsequent risk of death (ACSCT 2004).

Physical examination

Physical examination is the principal tool for diagnosis of acute chest injury. However, in a noisy emergency department, or in pre-hospital care, an adequate physical examination may be very difficult. Even under ideal conditions, signs of significant thoracic injury may be subtle or even absent. It is also important to understand that the effects of chest injury develop over time.

Significant chest injury is more likely, and referral should be considered, if there is abnormal breathing, abnormal circulation or significant tenderness on chest palpation. Signs of abnormal breathing include increased respiratory rate, reduced oxygen saturation, abnormal air entry, significant swelling/bruising or abnormal chest movement.

Advanced life support courses such as ATLS (Advanced Trauma Life Support for Doctors: ACSCT 2004) and APLS (Advanced Paediatric Life Support: Advanced Life Support Group 2005) advocate a systematic assessment of an injured patient that prioritises systems and injuries. This allows the identification and treatment of life-threatening injuries in the order that they endanger the patient.

ABCDE examination by 'looking, listening and feeling' can be applied to all aspects of the primary survey (see Table 11.1). Clinical examination of the chest is discussed in detail in Chapter 4. Life-threatening conditions are treated as they are identified, so that resuscitation is performed concurrently with assessment. Should the patient's condition change, the assessment is recommenced at the airway.

Injuries

Pneumothorax

Pneumothoraces occur when air enters the pleural space, causing the lung to collapse to a greater or lesser extent. They indicate injury to the pleura, and frequently the lung, and can follow blunt or penetrating trauma. A pneumothorax causes dyspnoea and pleuritic chest pain on the side of the injury, but the pain is rarely severe. If a patient with trauma to the chest presents with severe pain,

Table 11.1   Examination of chest injuries by ABCDE – look, listen and feel.

	Look for . . .	Listen for . . .	Feel for . . .
A	• Fogging of oxygen face mask • Foreign bodies/vomit in the mouth • Signs of airway obstruction (i.e. increased effort or see-saw/paradoxical breathing)	• Breath sounds at the mouth • Added noises (e.g. bubbling, stertor/snoring, stridor or wheeze)	• Breathing at the mouth • Subcutaneous emphysema
B	• Pallor or cyanosis • Chest wall asymmetry or paradoxical movement • Accessory muscle use • Bruising, seat belt marks, penetrating wounds	• Normal, equal breath sounds on both sides of the chest including the apices and axillae • Percuss both sides of the chest for dullness or increased resonance	• Tracheal deviation • Chest wall tenderness or crepitus, indicating rib fractures • Subcutaneous emphysema, indicating pneumothorax
C	• Pallor • Significant haemorrhage from any site • Check the capillary refill time centrally at the sternum	• Listen for normal heart sounds (a new murmur might indicate injury to the heart or aorta) • Check the blood pressure	• Radial pulse for rate and character – is it weak or thready? (In severe shock only the central pulses such as carotid or femorals may be palpable)
D	• Pupils for size, equality and reactivity • Abnormal limb posture (flexion or extension)	• Establish the patient's level of consciousness on the AVPU scale (**A**lert, responds to **V**oice, responds to **P**ain, **U**nresponsive)	
E	• Expose the patient fully to allow further assessment • Check the patient's temperature and blood sugar		

this is unlikely to be due to a simple pneumothorax, and other causes should be sought. In the past, chest drain insertion has been recommended for all traumatic pneumothoraces, but this practice is now being challenged. Small traumatic pneumothoraces, particularly those which are only detected on CT and not visible on standard chest x-ray, may be managed under close observation in a hospital setting. In such cases, air within the pleural space is ultimately absorbed into the circulation. Alternatively, aspiration of small pneumothoraces may be considered. Patients with a pneumothorax who require tracheal intubation and positive pressure ventilation are more likely to have a chest drain inserted because the risk of an enlarging, or tension, pneumothorax is increased. Two types of pneumothorax are life-threatening and require immediate treatment. These are described below.

Tension pneumothorax

A tension pneumothorax is the accumulation of air under pressure within the pleural space, usually due to a lung laceration, which allows air to escape into the pleural space but not to return. Positive pressure ventilation may exacerbate this 'one-way valve' effect leading to a more rapid onset. In the spontaneously breathing patient, tension may develop more insidiously (McRoberts et al. 2005).

Progressive build-up of pressure in the pleural space leads to circulatory collapse and cardiac arrest (typically pulseless electrical activity) if not treated promptly.

Causes

Tension pneumothorax may follow blunt or penetrating trauma. In blunt trauma it is usually associated with one or more rib fractures. In penetrating trauma the initial injury causes a pneumothorax, which then develops tension. A common misconception is that a penetrating injury cannot produce a tension pneumothorax because air under pressure will escape through the original wound. However, the tissues of the chest wall effectively seal most penetrating wounds soon after injury has occurred, allowing a subsequent tension pneumothorax to develop.

Clinical presentation

Patients are tachycardic and tachypnoeic, and may be hypoxic and hypotensive. These signs are common in patients with major trauma, and need to be differentiated from other possible causes. Unfortunately the 'classic' signs of a tension pneumothorax, though often quoted, are rarely clear and are difficult to elicit in practice (Leigh-Smith and Harris 2005). These are:

- Deviation of the trachea away from the side of the tension pneumothorax
- Hyper-resonant percussion on the affected side
- Reduced chest movement and air entry on the affected side

Absence of these signs does not exclude tension pneumothorax, and where suspicion is high, particularly in a patient who is rapidly deteriorating, immediate intervention is required.

Unexplained tachycardia, hypotension and a rise in airway pressure are strongly suggestive of a developing tension pneumothorax. Patients who require higher pressures for adequate ventilation, either due to pre-existing disease (such as asthma or chronic obstructive airways disease) or acute injury (pulmonary contusion), are at greater risk of developing pneumothoraces (Bersten 2003).

Immediate management

If suspected clinically in a compromised patient, a needle thoracocentesis should be immediately performed to decompress the tension pneumothorax. In the presence of shock, hypoxia, rapid deterioration and clear clinical signs, needle decompression is potentially life-saving (ACSCT 2004). This should be immediately followed by insertion of a definitive chest drain on the affected side (see Figure 11.1).

However, in the absence of haemodynamic compromise or desaturation, and in a relatively stable patient, it may be prudent to wait for the results of an immediate chest x-ray prior to intervening as needle decompression can be associated with complications, especially if the diagnosis is mistaken and a pneumothorax is not present. Lung laceration, pneumothorax, injury to the great vessels and laceration of an intercostal artery are serious complications that have all been described (Leigh-Smith and Harris 2005). Also, other conditions such as upper lobe collapse can cause hypoxia and tracheal deviation, mimicking a tension pneumothorax on the opposite side.

Needle thoracocentesis may be ineffective in relieving a tension pneumothorax, either because the thickness of the patient's chest wall prevents the needle from reaching the pleural space (Britten and Palmer 1996), or because the inserted

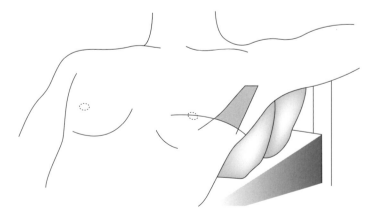

Figure 11.1 The safe triangle for chest tube insertion.

needle or cannula blocks or kinks before decompression can occur. Therefore the absence of a rush of air on needle insertion does not exclude the presence of tension pneumothorax, and if strong clinical suspicion persists a chest drain should immediately be inserted.

Open pneumothorax

An open pneumothorax occurs when air accumulates within the pleural space in the presence of a penetrating chest wound, such that the pneumothorax communicates with the exterior.

Causes

Following a penetrating chest injury, air may enter the chest cavity not through the trachea but through the hole in the chest wall during inspiration, when negative intrathoracic pressure is generated. If the size of the chest wall defect is greater than one-third of the diameter of the trachea, air preferentially enters through the hole. The consequences are loss of lung expansion, a progressive build-up of air within the pleural space and therefore inadequate ventilation.

Clinical presentation

The mechanism, timing and nature of injury give important clues regarding the potential extent of damage. In low velocity chest wounds, a penetrating object may remain embedded in the chest wall, which usually acts to seal the wound. Higher velocity wounds, such as those caused by explosions or some firearms, may leave foreign bodies within the chest as well as two or more open chest wounds and extensive internal injury.

An open chest wound that appears to be 'sucking air' and may be visibly bubbling is diagnostic. Depending on the size of the associated pneumothorax, the patient may be tachypnoeic and tachycardic and have increased work of breathing. There will be reduced expansion, accompanied by reduced breath sounds and an increased percussion note on the affected side. Occasionally, an open pneumothorax may tension if a flap of tissue acts as a valve that allows air into the chest cavity but not out (see previous section).

Immediate management

The immediate management of open pneumothorax is to place a three-sided dressing over the wound and insert a chest drain through a separate incision on the affected side. Consideration should be given to intubation when oxygenation or ventilation is inadequate: the accompanying change from spontaneous to assisted ventilation prevents open chest wounds from sucking in atmospheric air and improves the mechanics of ventilation. Foreign bodies should normally be left in place until formal exploration and removal can occur in an operating theatre.

A chest x-ray, or sometimes CT scanning, is used to determine the track, depth and anatomical location of foreign bodies within the chest prior to definitive surgery.

Flail chest

A flail chest occurs when a segment of the thoracic rib cage becomes separated and moves independently from the rest of the chest wall. This is usually defined as at least two fractures per rib in at least three ribs (Bjerke 2002). A flail segment does not expand with the rest of the chest wall and the underlying lung does not ventilate. Large flail segments may involve both sides of the chest and sternum. In these cases, disruption of normal pulmonary mechanics may be enough to require mechanical ventilation.

Causes

A flail chest is caused by blunt injury, and always associated with an underlying lung injury or pulmonary contusion. In most cases, it is the severity of the lung injury that determines the clinical course and requirement for intervention.

Clinical presentation

The history is usually of significant blunt trauma to the chest, such as a pedestrian or cyclist in collision with a car, or a fall from a considerable height. In the elderly patient a flail segment may occur following less severe trauma, such as a fall on to a kerb or the edge of a table. The patient will present with significant chest pain and dyspnoea. Large flail segments also cause hypoxia and hypercapnia. There is a high likelihood of other serious injuries.

Flail segments may have only subtle clinical signs and are easily missed unless the chest is carefully examined. Pain, increased on inspiration, and hypoventilation may initially splint a mobile segment so that the characteristic paradoxical movement is not visible (a flail segment usually moves inwards on inspiration and outwards on expiration). Palpation reveals the crepitus associated with broken ribs. Conscious patients will complain of severe pain. Respiratory compromise may develop with time as underlying lung contusion progresses.

Immediate management

The management of a flail segment is the same as that of any chest wall injury. The goal is to protect the underlying lung, and ensure adequate oxygenation, ventilation and pulmonary clearance (coughing) to prevent the complication of pneumonia. While a young fit patient will often recover easily from one or two rib fractures, the same injury in an elderly patient is regarded as major and may lead to pneumonia and respiratory failure if not appropriately managed.

Rib fractures associated with a flail segment may be missed on chest x-ray, but the associated contusion may be seen as patchy consolidation in one or both lungs.

Analgesia is the mainstay of therapy for flail segments and rib fractures. While strapping the chest to splint rib fractures may seem like a good idea, it impedes chest wall movement and prevents adequate inspiration and clearance of secretions, predisposing to pneumonia. Opioid analgesics are essential, but at high doses may produce respiratory depression – especially in the elderly. Advanced analgesic techniques such as patient controlled analgesia (PCA), epidural infusion or intercostal nerve blocks may be required (Dunitz 2002).

Intubation and mechanical ventilation are rarely indicated for chest wall injury alone. Where ventilation is necessary, it is usually for hypoxia due to underlying pulmonary contusions. Positive pressure ventilation may be required for severe chest wall instability, resulting in inadequate spontaneous ventilation. Intubation and ventilation may be required when anaesthesia is necessary to provide immediate and adequate analgesia and allow further assessment and management. Ventilation is usually necessary only until the resolution of the pulmonary contusion.

Pulmonary contusion

Blunt injury to the lung results in blood and interstitial fluid filling the alveoli, and preventing gas exchange in the affected area of lung. These changes can take hours or even days to develop, and may therefore be underestimated during an initial assessment. Pulmonary contusion is the commonest significant chest injury in children, because the elastic nature of the chest wall makes rib fractures relatively rare.

Causes

Pulmonary contusion follows blunt chest injury, for example an RTC where a driver's chest has struck the steering wheel, or a patient who has been kicked by a horse. Pulmonary contusion often underlies rib fractures or a flail segment.

Clinical presentation

Patients with pulmonary contusion present with increasing dyspnoea, hypoxia and hypercapnia. Pulmonary contusions are, in themselves, painless, but patients may complain of pain from overlying rib fractures, chest wall injury or involvement of the pleura. The presence of a pulmonary contusion indicates that a patient has sustained significant trauma, and other injuries should be actively sought. On examination, there will be reduced air entry in the affected area, and inspiratory crepitations may be heard. The overlying chest wall is likely to be tender, with evidence of injury and possible crepitus from rib fractures and/or surgical emphysema.

Immediate management

Treatment is supportive. Depending on the degree of contusion and previous lung disease, the patient may require anything from supplemental oxygen to intubation and ventilation. Complications of pulmonary contusion include adult respiratory distress syndrome (ARDS), respiratory failure, atelectasis and pneumonia (Cohn 1997).

Early chest x-ray following pulmonary contusion may be normal, with patchy opacification developing over hours to days. CT scanning allows more accurate assessment of the extent of pulmonary contusion (www.trauma.org).

Haemothorax

A haemothorax is a collection of blood in the pleural space, and may be caused by blunt or penetrating trauma. Massive haemothorax can lead to rapid exsanguination and is a life-threatening condition.

Causes

Most haemothoraces occur as a result of rib fractures, lung or minor venous injuries, and are self-limiting. Less commonly there is an arterial injury or major vessel disruption that is more likely to require definitive surgical repair.

Clinical presentation

With significant blood loss into the chest, the patient may have signs of hypovolaemic shock such as tachycardia, poor peripheral perfusion, decreased blood pressure, sweating or agitation. Blood in the pleural space can cause chest discomfort, but if pain is a dominant feature this is more likely to be due to associated injuries than the haemothorax itself.

Most small or moderate haemothoraces cannot be detected by clinical examination, and will be identified on chest x-ray. However, a 'massive' haemothorax, where at least 1500 ml or one-third of the patient's circulating volume accumulates rapidly in the chest, can be clinically recognised, allowing prompt treatment before an x-ray is taken.

Physical examination of the chest may demonstrate the presence of external bruising, lacerations or palpable crepitus, indicating the presence of rib fractures. Alternatively, there may be signs of a penetrating injury. Anterior chest wounds medial to the nipples, or posterior wounds medial to the scapulae, should raise the suspicion of great vessel, hilar or cardiac injury. The classic signs of a haemothorax are decreased chest expansion, dullness to percussion and reduced breath sounds on the affected side. Tracheal deviation away from the affected side may occur with massive haemothorax. The difference in key clinical findings between a haemothorax and pneumothoraces is summarised in Table 11.2.

In the erect patient (usually those with a penetrating injury), the classic x-ray appearance of a fluid level with a meniscus is as seen in Figure 11.2. Although

Table 11.2 Differentiating signs of chest injuries.

	Look for chest movement	Listen for breath sounds	Feel for tracheal deviation	Percussion	Patient shocked?
Tension pneumothorax	Decreased on affected side	Absent on affected side	Deviated away	Hyper-resonant	Yes
Massive haemothorax	Decreased on affected side	Absent on affected side	Deviated away	Stony, dull	Yes
Simple pneumothorax	May be normal	Absent on affected side	Central	Hyper-resonant	No

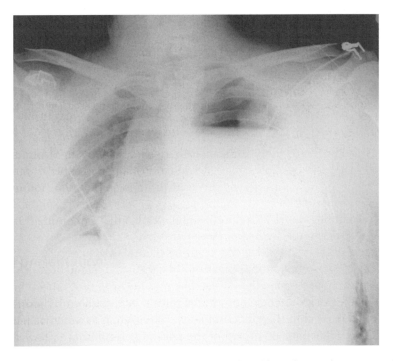

Figure 11.2 Erect chest x-ray of left haemothorax. Reproduced from the Royal Lancaster Infirmary Image Library, compiled by Dr Ray McGlone.

the erect film is more sensitive, it takes approximately 400–500 ml of blood to obliterate the costo-phrenic angle on a chest radiograph. In the supine position (usually blunt trauma patients with suspected spinal injury), no fluid level is visible because the blood lies posterior to the lung and is spread out over the whole hemithorax. The chest x-ray shows a diffuse opacification or 'ground glass' appearance on the affected side, through which lung markings can still be seen in Figure 11.3. It is sometimes difficult to differentiate a unilateral haemothorax from an anterior pneumothorax on the opposite side.

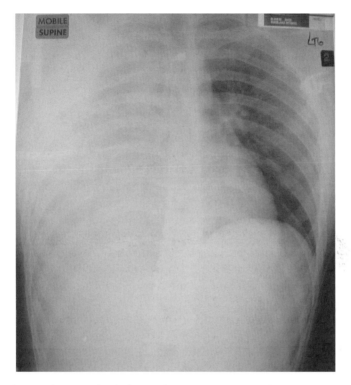

Figure 11.3 Supine chest ray of right haemothorax.

Immediate management

A massive haemothorax will cause both respiratory and circulatory problems. Respiratory compromise is the result of direct compression of the lung by the large amount of blood within the chest cavity. Chest drain insertion on the affected side allows the blood to be drained and the lung to re-expand. Circulatory effects are due first to contained blood loss within the chest. However, on inserting a chest drain, any containment of continuing haemorrhage will be lost and the patient may suddenly decompensate. Therefore, before placing a drain for haemothorax, good intravenous access should be secured (two large-bore cannulae) with cross-matching arranged and resuscitation fluids immediately available. Significant immediate drainage or ongoing blood loss into a chest drain necessitating transfusion may require urgent thoracotomy, and therefore needs prompt surgical review.

Cardiac tamponade

The heart muscle, or myocardium, is enclosed in a fibrous non-elastic sheath called the pericardium. Cardiac tamponade occurs when, as a result of an injury, blood accumulates within this sac as a pericardial effusion. External compression of the ventricles by this abnormal collection reduces the degree to which they can fill and hence the amount of blood which is ejected with each systolic contraction (stroke volume). Initial compensation by means of increased heart rate may maintain adequate cardiac output but, as the effusion expands, cardiac output will fall and the patient becomes shocked.

Causes

Tamponade is most often associated with penetrating injuries to the mediastinum or following cardiac surgery, central line insertion and cardiac catherisation. However, cardiac tamponade can also occur following severe blunt and penetrating chest injuries, in which case the outlook is extremely bleak.

Clinical presentation

The diagnosis of cardiac tamponade can be easily missed as the clinical signs are hard to elicit and the time course of presentation may vary. The pericardial effusion will expand at a rate dependent on the underlying structures injured: hence a ventricular laceration will present more rapidly than pericardial vessel injury. Some patients may present in traumatic cardiac arrest, where cardiac tamponade is a potentially reversible cause of pulseless electrical activity.

Some patients may report sharp, stabbing chest pain that radiates to the neck, shoulder, back or abdomen and is aggravated by deep breathing or coughing. A history of recent cardiac surgery greatly increases the chances of tamponade, but for those presenting in cardiac arrest, previous history may be difficult to acquire and the diagnosis will rely on clinical examination. The clinician should suspect cardiac tamponade in shocked patients who do not respond to volume resuscitation, particularly with penetrating chest injuries.

With a large pericardial effusion, the patient will be shocked and tachycardic and may be hypotensive (see also Chapter 8). The neck veins may be distended, but this is not seen if the patient is hypovolaemic from blood loss, and neck veins are usually obscured by rigid cervical collars in blunt trauma. The heart sounds may be muffled, though this is very difficult to appreciate in a noisy environment.

Immediate management

In the presence of circulatory compromise, intravenous fluids should be administered. Fluid resuscitation will improve cardiac filling, and temporarily improve cardiac output. However, a compressing, traumatic, pericardial effusion will need to be drained by pericardiocentesis.

On chest x-ray the heart may have a globular shape, and a 12-lead electrocardiograph (ECG) may show low *electrical alternans* which is characterised by alternating levels of voltage in P waves, QRS complexes, and T waves. Ultrasound examination, sometimes undertaken during 'FAST' scanning (focused assessment sonography in trauma), will confirm a pericardial effusion.

Cardiac contusion

Cardiac contusion most commonly occurs following blunt trauma to the front of the chest. The injury usually involves the ventricle, and this can have similar manifestations to a myocardial infarction. The damaged area of heart may become a focus for arrhythmias, or ventricular function may be impaired resulting in heart failure and hypotension.

Causes

Cardiac contusion typically occurs in an RTC, when the chest of a car driver involved in a head-on collision strikes the steering wheel. However, any cause of significant blunt chest trauma has the potential to cause cardiac contusion. There may be an associated sternal fracture or other evidence of anterior chest wall injury.

Clinical presentation

Cardiac contusion can be very difficult to diagnose clinically. The patient may complain of chest pain suggesting cardiac ischaemia (see Chapter 6) or anterior musculoskeletal chest pain as a result of an associated chest wall injury (see Chapter 13). There may also be dyspnoea. In severe cardiac contusion, hypotension and arrhythmias occur, with a risk of cardiac arrest. Cardiovascular examination rarely detects any abnormality aside from changes in pulse and blood pressure.

Immediate management

The best way of diagnosing cardiac contusion remains uncertain, and 12-lead ECG, cardiac enzymes and echocardiography (looking for ventricular wall motion abnormalities) all have a role. ECG abnormalities are variable and include ST changes, multiple premature ventricular extrasystoles, unexplained sinus tachycardia, atrial fibrillation and bundle branch block (usually right) (Kaye and O'Sullivan 2002).

   Treatment is supportive with close monitoring of blood pressure and cardiac rhythm. Inotropes may be used to treat hypotension that does not respond to fluid loading, and arrhythmias are managed as they occur according to Advanced Life Support protocols (Resuscitation Council (UK) 2005). Prophylactic antiarrhythmics are not routinely administered. Opioids form the mainstay of analgesia.

Great vessel injury

Traumatic rupture of the thoracic aorta is the most common cause of immediate death following a motor vehicle collision or a fall from a height. The anatomy of the thoracic aorta is such that it is fixed at specific points (the aortic valve, thoracic vertebrae and ligamentum arteriosum just distal to the subclavian artery). The aortic arch (between the aortic valve and subclavian artery) is mobile. During rapid deceleration, the arch is free to move creating a shearing force at its fixed points and leading to rupture. Complete rupture is rapidly fatal, but if the rupture is partial or the haematoma is contained within the mediastinum, patients may survive the initial impact. Specific signs are frequently absent, but the patient may complain of back or interscapular pain. Because the haematoma is contained, there is no ongoing haemorrhage and therefore no evidence of hypovolaemia unless other injuries cause significant bleeding. Abnormal chest x-ray findings may be present, but are easily overlooked. These include a widened mediastinum, deviation of the trachea and/or oesophagus to the right, and left haemothorax. Clinical staff should have a high suspicion of great vessel injury if there is a history of sudden deceleration such as a fall from a height or high speed RTC. The diagnostic investigations of choice are CT scanning or contrast angiography, and the treatment is definitive repair by a cardiothoracic surgeon.

Oesophageal injury

This is a rare injury that is frequently overlooked; however, untreated it can lead to mediastinitis and death.

Causes

Oesophageal injury is most common in penetrating trauma, but can also occur following a severe blow to the upper abdomen, by forceful expulsion of gastric contents into the oesophagus.

Clinical presentation

Oesophageal injury is difficult to diagnose. The history may provide a clue to the vigilant practitioner, as may the persistence of constant, unexplained chest pain, which may radiate to the neck. Dyspnoea is relatively common, as is epigastric pain. Dysphagia or unexplained pyrexia and systemic illness in the days following chest trauma suggest oesophageal injury. Oesophageal rupture can give rise to surgical emphysema in the neck and/or reduced breath sounds on the side of the injury, but these are relatively rare and the clinical examination is frequently unhelpful.

Immediate management

Any suspicion of oesophageal injury requires investigation by a contrast imaging study as leakage of gastric contents into the mediastinum causes mediastinitis and has a significant mortality. On chest x-ray there may be air in the mediastinum, a pleural effusion on the affected side or subcutaneous emphysema. Early surgical referral is required.

Diaphragmatic rupture or laceration

This injury occurs when the abdominal contents herniate into the chest through a tear or laceration in the diaphragm. Because the liver lies adjacent to the diaphragm on the right side, this injury is more commonly seen on the left.

Causes

Diaphragmatic rupture occurs following significant blunt trauma to the abdomen, which suddenly and substantially raises the patient's intra-abdominal pressure. Penetrating wounds to the chest can also lacerate the diaphragm, which rises as high as the 5th rib during expiration.

Clinical presentation

Diaphragmatic rupture or laceration follows significant trauma, and there will almost certainly be other injuries. The patient may complain of chest pain, abdominal pain or respiratory distress. On examination there may be abdominal tenderness with absent breath sounds, dull percussion or even bowel sounds on the affected side of the chest.

Injury to the diaphragm allows free communication between the chest and abdominal cavities. As a result, bleeding below the diaphragm (e.g. from a ruptured spleen) can be mistaken for a haemothorax because blood will be lost via a chest drain. Similarly, bowel or bowel contents may enter the chest, compromising respiration and predisposing to infection. There is a risk that herniated bowel will become incarcerated and obstructed, particularly if the hole in the diaphragm is relatively small. This can occur soon after injury or many months or years later, and may be the first indication of a previously overlooked diaphragmatic injury.

Immediate management

Significant herniation should be obvious on chest x-ray, although the insertion of a radio-opaque nasogastric tube can help identify the stomach above the level of the diaphragm. Diaphragmatic laceration occurring during penetrating trauma may be small, uncomplicated and overlooked in the initial stages. The treatment is open surgical repair.

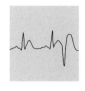

Initial investigations in the patient with chest pain due to trauma

The initial management of a patient with significant chest trauma always includes the administration of high flow oxygen and the application of monitoring, to include as a minimum:

- Continuous cardiac monitoring
- Continuous pulse oximetry

- Non-invasive blood pressure measurement
- Respiratory rate measurement

Vital signs should be regularly assessed and analgesia (usually opioids) provided at the first opportunity.

Once immediately life-threatening conditions have been identified and treated and the patient has been resuscitated, initial investigations are performed. These should include a chest x-ray, blood tests and an ECG.

Chest x-ray

The plain antero-posterior chest radiograph remains the standard first investigation in chest trauma. The indications and techniques are slightly different for blunt and penetrating trauma. All trauma patients should have a portable chest x-ray performed in the resuscitation area (see Figure 11.4). The discussion on physical examination above highlights the unreliability of clinical signs in this situation. The chest x-ray is a rapid screening tool that will identify significant chest injuries requiring intervention.

Blunt injuries

Chest x-rays in blunt trauma patients are taken in the supine position, since unstable spinal injuries may be present. Chest films should be slightly overpen-

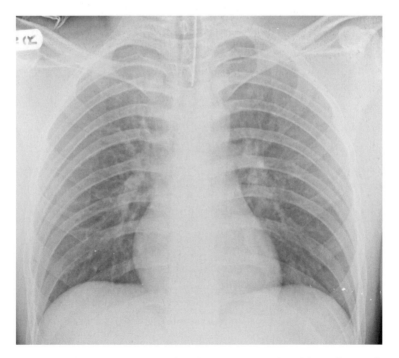

Figure 11.4 Supine chest x-ray in an intubated patient. Reproduced from the Royal Lancaster Infirmary Image Library, compiled by Dr Ray McGlone.

etrated to allow improved imaging of the thoracic spine, paraspinal lines and aortic outline.

Penetrating injuries

Patients with a penetrating wound that may have entered the thoracic cavity should have a chest x-ray (see Figure 11.5, which illustrates a dagger penetrating the chest wall). In practice, this means all patients with stab wounds between the neck and the umbilicus (front or back). For gunshot wounds, all patients with wounds between the neck and the pelvis/buttock area should have a chest film. This is especially true if the bullet track is unclear, or if there is a missing bullet or an odd number of entry/exit wounds. If possible, depending on the mechanism of injury and possibility of spinal injury, the chest x-ray in penetrating trauma should be taken with the patient sitting upright. This will increase the sensitivity for detecting a small haemothorax, pneumothorax or diaphragmatic injury.

Blood tests

The laboratory tests required may include full blood count, clotting screen, urea, creatinine, electrolytes, amylase, liver function and cross-match. In combined

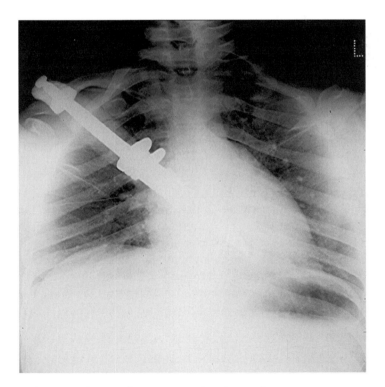

Figure 11.5 Chest x-ray showing dagger penetrating chest wall.

chest and abdominal trauma, amylase and liver function are crude markers of pancreatic and liver injury.

Part of the full blood count profile is the haemoglobin concentration. This will fall with significant haemorrhage, but there may be a considerable time delay between blood loss and changes in haemoglobin concentration. This is because the haemoglobin falls as a result of blood dilution, either by physiological compensation (renal reabsorption of fluid) or blood replacement by intravenous fluids. A normal haemoglobin in the early stages of trauma is to be expected, and does not rule out significant external or internal haemorrhage.

Troponin has been recognised as a potential marker of blunt cardiac injury and contusion. However, whilst a normal troponin taken 4–6 hours after the event appears to rule out significant blunt cardiac injury, the prognostic significance of a raised troponin in this context is currently unclear (Sybrandy et al. 2003).

Blood gases are very useful in assessing chest injuries. Arterial concentrations of oxygen and carbon dioxide permit assessment of the adequacy of ventilation, particularly with serial testing. Modern blood gas analysers often give values for haemoglobin and lactate, which can be helpful in assessing tissue perfusion and shock.

Electrocardiogram

The 12-lead electrocardiogram can be helpful in assessing a patient's previous cardiac status and may show abnormal changes in myocardial contusion (for example: bundle branch block, atrial fibrillation supraventricular tachycardia, ventricular tachycardia, fibrillation: Foot 2005) or cardiac tamponade.

Ultrasound

'FAST' (focused assessment sonography in trauma) ultrasound scanning is an initial screening investigation. It involves assessing four regions of the chest and abdomen, including the pericardium, for abnormal fluid collections (usually blood) and is invaluable in confirming a possible diagnosis of cardiac tamponade (ACSCT 2004). Its great advantage is that, with the use of small and portable machines, it is readily available at the bedside, potentially negating the need to transfer unstable patients to distant areas for specialised imaging.

Formal echocardiography may demonstrate wall motion abnormalities or pericardial effusion following blunt cardiac trauma, and also allows assessment of cardiac function, the heart valves and great vessels.

Computed tomography

Computed tomography (CT) provides detailed imaging of the chest. As CT technology has developed, it has established itself as the best screening modality for chest injury. Because CT uses x-rays, bony injuries are readily identified and newer multi-detector machines now allow faster and more detailed scanning of the soft tissues. It is far more sensitive than plain chest x-ray for identifying pulmonary contusion and simple pneumothoraces. In fact, it can reveal minor abnormalities that are not clinically significant. 'Occult pneumothoraces' found on CT may sometimes be managed without chest drainage, even in the presence of positive pressure ventilation. CT is particularly useful in the diagnosis of blunt aortic injury, which is notoriously difficult to diagnose clinically or on chest x-ray. The sensitivity of modern scanners is reported to be 97–100% (Dyer et al. 2000).

CT scanning does, however, have one major disadvantage. Transfer of a potentially unstable patient to and from the radiology department, and monitoring during the scanning process, are practically difficult and potentially hazardous. Patient deterioration may be difficult to manage in a remote scanning suite, and the time taken to obtain CT scans may inappropriately delay life-saving surgery. Transfer to CT requires the same degree of preparation as inter-hospital transfer, with trained staff, monitoring and equipment immediately available.

Interpretation of a chest x-ray following trauma

The following is a broad overview of the systematic evaluation of a chest x-ray, which can be used to facilitate the identification of significant abnormalities. As an aid to memory, it follows an ABCDE pattern.

- **A**dequacy, date and exposure of film.
- **A**lignment: A partially lateral or rotated x-ray may be more difficult to inter-pret, leading to a missed diagnosis.
- **A**irway: The trachea should be centrally located between the clavicles.

- **B**reathing: In an adequately aligned film, the lung fields should appear equally black. Lighter areas represent fluid or blood. Darker areas suggest air (pneumothorax), which will be at the lung apices on an erect film and at the most anterior space on a supine film (refer to Figure 11.6).
- **B**ones and peripheral soft tissues: The ribs should be scrutinised individually along their entire length to look for rib fractures. The clavicles, thoracic ver-tebrae and humeri should be examined for obvious abnormalities.

- **C**ardiac border and mediastinum: The peripheral soft tissues should be scruti-nised for air trapped within them, suggesting subcutaneous (surgical) emphy-sema. The maximum width of the heart shadow is difficult to assess on trauma films, which are usually taken with the x-ray machine in front of the patient (i.e. AP: antero-posteriorly). An AP chest x-ray magnifies the heart because it lies closer to the x-ray source than in a standard PA (postero-anterior) x-ray. However, a heart shadow greater than 50% of the thoracic diameter, or globular in appearance, is probably abnormal and warrants further investigation.

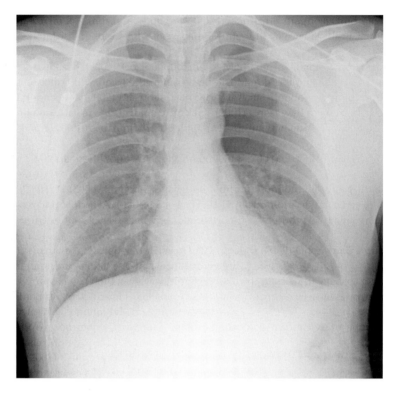

Figure 11.6 Erect antero-posterior inspiration chest x-ray of left-sided pneumothorax due to penetrating trauma. Reproduced from the Royal Lancaster Infirmary Image Library, compiled by Dr Ray McGlone.

The upper mediastinum should be relatively narrow, and mediastinal widening (greater than 8 cm at the level of the aortic arch), though again difficult to interpret on supine AP films, is suggestive of mediastinal or great vessel injury. If possible, sitting the patient up and repeating the chest x-ray will help to decide whether a mediastinum is truly widened, or whether this is due to the patient's position and the x-ray projection (Nagy 2000).

- **Diaphragm:** The diaphragm should be easily seen on both sides. The left diaphragm should be clearly visible behind the heart. Loss of diaphragm definition may be due to the accumulation of fluid or abnormal adjacent tissue (collapsed or consolidated lung).

- **Extras:** The position of lines, tracheal tubes, nasogastric tubes and chest drains needs to be checked, but x-rays should not be used as a substitute for clinical assessment or capnography in confirming correct tracheal tube placement.

Key learning points

- Chest injuries are common and occasionally life-threatening.
- The two types of injury mechanism (blunt or penetrating) require different approaches.
- Thorough and repeated clinical examination will elicit the majority of significant injuries.
- Life-threatening injuries include flail chest, tension pneumothorax, cardiac tamponade, open pneumothorax and massive haemothorax.
- The chest x-ray is the standard initial investigation, but requires knowledge and experience to interpret reliably.

References

Advanced Life Support Group (2005) *Advanced Paediatric Life Support – The Practical Approach, 4th edition*. London, BMJ Books.

American College of Surgeons Committee on Trauma (ACSCT) (2004) *Advanced Trauma Life Support for Doctors, Student Course Manual*, 7th edition. Chicago, American College of Surgeons.

Bersten A (2003) *Oh's Intensive Care Manual*, 5th edition. London, Butterworth Heinemann.

Bjerke HS (2002) Flail chest. eMedicine from webMD. Available at: http://www.emedicine.com/med/topic2813.htm (accessed 16th March 2006).

Britten S, Palmer SH (1996) Chest wall thickness may limit adequate drainage of tension pneumothorax by needle thoracocentesis. *Emergency Medicine Journal* **13**(6): 426–427.

Cohn SM (1997) Pulmonary contusion: review of the clinical entity. *Journal of Trauma* **42**(5): 973–979.

Demetriades D, Murray J, Charalambides K, Alo K, Velmahos G, Rhee P, Chan L (2004) Trauma fatalities: time and location of hospital deaths. *Journal of the American College of Surgeon* **198**(1): 20–26.

Dunitz M (2002) *Fundamental Principles and Practice of Anaesthesia*. London, Martin Dunitz.

Dyer DS, Moore EE, Ilke DN, McIntyre RC, Bernstein SM, Durham JD, Mestek MF, Heining MJ, Russ PD, Symonds DL, Honigman B, Kumpe DA, Roe EJ, Eule J Jr (2000) Thoracic aortic injury: how predictive is mechanism and is chest computed tomography a reliable screening tool? A prospective study of 1,561 patients. *Journal of Trauma* **48**(4): 673–682.

Foot L (2005) Exercise in EBM: cardiac contusion. *Critical Care and Resuscitation* **7**: 29–31.

Kaye P, O'Sullivan I (2002) Myocardial contusion: emergency investigation and diagnosis. *Emergency Medicine Journal* **19**: 8–10.

Leigh-Smith S, Harris T (2005) Tension pneumothorax – time for a re-think? *Emergency Medicine Journal* **22**: 8–16.

McRoberts R, McKechnie M, Leigh-Smith S (2005) Tension pneumothorax and the 'forbidden CXR'. *Emergency Medicine Journal* **22**: 597–598.

Nagy KK, Fabian T, Rodman G (2000) Guidelines for the diagnosis and management of blunt aortic injury. Chicago, EAST Trauma Practice Guidelines Committee. Available at: www.east.org/tpg/chap8.pdf (accessed 16th March 2006).

Resuscitation Council (UK) (2005) *Advanced Life Support Course Provider Manual,* 5th edition. London, Resuscitation Council.

Sybrandy KC, Cramer MJ, Burgersdijk C (2003) Diagnosing cardiac contusion: old wisdom and new insights. *Heart* **89**(5): 485–489.

World Report on Road Traffic Injury Prevention. Geneva, World Health Organization (2002) Available at: www.who/int/violence_injury_prevention (accessed 16th March 2006).

World Health Organization Department of Injuries and Violence Prevention (2000) *Injury – A Leading Cause of the Global Burden of Disease.* Geneva, World Health Organization. Available at: www.whqlibdoc.who.int/publications/2002 (accessed 16th March 2006).

Useful websites

http://www.trauma.org   Trauma.org is an independent, non-profit organization providing global education, information and communication resources for professionals in trauma and critical care.

http://www.alsg.org.uk   The Advanced Life Support Group exists to 'preserve life by providing training and education in life saving techniques'.

http://www.bestbets.org   The 'BestBETs' Best Evidence Topics for emergency medicine.

http://www.radquiz.com   Radquiz.com is a gateway to radiology teaching resources on the worldwide web.

http://www.library.nhs.uk/emergency   The Emergency Care Specialist Library of the National Library for Health is a unique resource aimed at supporting healthcare professionals by providing high quality information on all aspects of emergency healthcare.

http://www.chestnet.org/education   The American College of Chest Physicians Center of Excellence for Learning and Teaching is a practical source of information related to diseases of the chest.

Chapter 12

Assessing and managing the patient with chest pain due to oesophago-gastric disorders

Theresa M.D. Finlay and Jan Keenan

Aims

This chapter reviews oesophago-gastric causes of chest pain, and differentiates between these and other potential causes. Acute, severe chest pain associated with oesophago-gastric pathology is rare. Less severe but often troubling symptoms are far more common and can lead to presentation in general practice, the emergency department and chest pain clinics. For this reason, this chapter deals with acute presentations of oesophago-gastric related chest pain, which can present as medical or surgical emergencies, and separates these from subacute and chronic conditions. Whilst some patients may describe chest and epigastric pain in association with peptic ulceration, this seldom accounts for acute or initial presentation with chest pain. Therefore peptic ulcer disease is not considered here.

Learning outcomes

Having read this text and sought suitable practice experience it is anticipated that healthcare practitioners should be able to:

- Consider oesophago-gastric disorders as differential diagnoses in assessing the patient with chest pain.
- Include enquiry about oesophago-gastric symptoms and antacid use when taking a history from patients with chest pain.
- Appreciate the subtle differences in presenting symptoms between chest pain of cardiac, respiratory or oesophago-gastric origin.
- Discuss the immediate, medium- and long-term management of patients with confirmed oesophago-gastric causess of chest pain.
- Discuss the role of investigations in confirming the diagnosis of oesophago-gastric causes of chest pain.

OESOPHAGEAL RUPTURE

Background

Spontaneous oesophageal rupture was first described by Herman Boerhaave in 1724 in a patient who presented with repeated vomiting and retching, and who developed severe left-sided pleuritic pain and became increasingly toxic until his death three days later (Lemke and Jagminas 1999). Spontaneous barogenic perforation, or rupture, of an otherwise non-diseased oesophagus is therefore usually referred to in medical literature as Boerhaave's syndrome (Janjua 1997). Oesophageal rupture has also been described as a sequela of blunt trauma (Lomoschitz et al. 2001), and by Baric (2000) as a rare complication arising from postoperative nausea and vomiting. More common is iatrogenic traumatic perforation of the oesophagus following instrumentation for invasive procedures, or chest injury (Travis et al. 2005).

An intramural tear, or Mallory-Weiss tear, is a tear in the mucosa at the oesophago-gastric junction rather than a rupture perforating all the layers of the oesophagus. Mallory-Weiss tears are associated with forceful or prolonged vomiting due to a variety of causes such as alcohol-related vomiting, or the repeated forceful retching of 'morning sickness' during pregnancy, severe cases being referred to as 'hyperemesis gravidarum'.

Causes

Boerhaave's syndrome can follow forceful vomiting, often in conjunction with significant alcohol consumption when cricopharyngeal relaxation may fail as vomiting starts. This leads to a dramatically raised pressure in the oesophagus and subsequent rupture of the oesophageal wall. Intramural tears are also associated with vomiting but do not rupture the oesophagus. More commonly, instrumentation of the oesophagus or chest trauma results in smaller perforations of the oesophagus. Age, barotrauma, malignancy or infection may contribute to the risk of perforation (Mamun 1998).

Traumatic causes of oesophageal rupture

- Instrumentation of the oesophagus for:
  - Oesophago-gastro-duodenoscopy (OGD)
  - Oesophageal dilatation for achalasia or benign stricture
  - Oesophageal stenting for malignant stricture
  - Laser therapy for oesophageal carcinoma
  - Treatment of oesophageal varices
- Oesophageal surgery
- Penetrating foreign body
- Ingestion of caustic material

Pathophysiology

The oesophagus is a muscular tube beginning at the pharynx and ending at the stomach. It lies close to the trachea, the great vessels and the left atrium of the heart. The walls of the oesophagus reflect the general organisation of the intestinal wall, and are formed from outside to inside by:

- Adventitia
- Longitudinal muscle
- Circular muscle
- Submucosa
- Muscularis mucosa
- Mucosa and epithelium

The muscle in the upper third of the oesophagus is striated, with smooth muscle in the lower two-thirds. Peristalsis conveys food down the oesophagus and comprises a co-ordinated wave of contraction behind a bolus of food, with relaxation ahead of it, propelling the bolus downward (Keshav 2004).

Following forceful vomiting the oesophageal wall can rupture longitudinally. A retrospective study of 14 cases of Boerhaave's syndrome found that all tears were found in the longitudinal axis of the oesophagus, ranging from 0.6 to 8.9 cm in length, suggesting that the longitudinal muscle layer was disrupted (Lemke and Jagminas 1999). Perforation of the oesophagus allows direct contamination of the mediastinum by gastric contents, leading to acute mediastinitis. Once the mediastinal pleura is disrupted, further negative pressure exerted by respiratory effort promotes further emptying of the gastric contents into the mediastinum and pleural space, rapidly creating hydropneumothorax and pneumomediastinum. Perforation of the oesophagus following blunt trauma most commonly occurs in the cervical region as a result of direct force to the neck or laceration by fracture fragments (Lomoschitz et al. 2001). The cause of the injury is uncertain, though the mechanism may be similar to Boerhaave's syndrome if sudden high oesophageal intraluminal pressure is generated at the time of injury.

The extent and type of traumatic rupture will relate to the nature of the instrument, type of force or foreign body causing penetration of the oesophageal wall. Mallory-Weiss syndrome arises when only the inner, mucosal layer of the lower oesophagus is torn following forceful vomiting. The tear develops close to the oesophago-gastric junction, and the syndrome is characterised by initial bouts of vomiting without haematemesis, which develops later (Travis et al. 2005).

Clinical presentation

Traditionally, if Boerhaave's syndrome was suspected, the presence of a triad of symptoms that included vomiting followed by chest pain and subcutaneous emphysema confirmed the diagnosis (Lemke and Jagminas 1999). However, the same authors contest this often-quoted presentation on the basis that the literature is replete with case studies and small case series which contradict these findings. In their review, they argue that up to 25% of patients do not present with prior vomiting, 75% may present with abdominal pain and 63% with chest pain. Additionally some may present with back pain. Subcutaneous emphysema was reported in only 8–30% of cases and this appeared to develop over time from the onset of symptoms and may therefore be a late sign. Boerhaave's syndrome should be regarded as a rare condition in which patients may present with one or a combination of sudden onset of chest, abdominal or back pain, and in around 75% of cases this will be preceded by forceful vomiting. In addition to chest, back and abdominal pain, patients will develop respiratory distress and are likely to experience odynophagia (painful swallowing) and/or dysphagia.

Clinical findings also include shock and abdominal tenderness or rigidity (Baric 2000). Overwhelming sepsis will develop in those not treated promptly; the risk of mortality after 48 hours rises above 50%, although Schattner et al. (2005) argue that most patients do well with prompt diagnosis and adequate treatment. As studies and reviews have highlighted, acute oesophageal rupture is difficult to diagnose not least because it is often omitted in differential diagnoses for chest pain (Travis et al. 2005). Relying on the triad of symptoms described above is unlikely to help the clinician arrive at the rapid diagnosis necessary to reduce mortality, as patients seldom present with vomiting followed by chest pain and emphysema (Baric 2000).

In patients who present with iatrogenic intramural rupture following instrumentation, the clinical presentation will be a gradual or sudden onset of chest and/or epigastric pain (with or without haematemesis). Onset follows investigation involving instrumentation of the oesophagus, surgery, ingestion of a foreign body, or rarely, ingestion of a caustic substance. Patients with a Mallory-Weiss tear present with chest pain and haematemesis ranging from mild to severe. Because the mucosa of the oesophagus is disrupted rather than the muscular wall, they are not usually shocked unless haematemesis is excessive.

History taking

Onset of symptoms will depend on the underlying pathology. Boerhaave's syndrome is acute and there is sudden onset associated with vomiting in 75% of cases. Pain will start in the back, chest or upper abdomen but may involve all three, and may begin with a history of retrosternal pain progressing to excruciating and become more widespread (see Figure 12.1). Presentation will usually be fairly early and will be prompted by pain, dyspnoea, shock, distress, collapse, vomiting and/or haematemesis (Lemke and Jagminas 1999). Pain will be intractable and not relieved by movement, and there may be little relief from opiate analgesia. Associated dysphagia or odynophagia will usually be present. Whilst Boerhaave's syndrome is associated with an otherwise normal oesophagus, Baric (2000) points out that 10% of patients who have oesophageal rupture have pre-existing conditions such as hiatus hernia, oesophagitis or diverticulosis, although this may be unknown at the point of presentation.

Patients with iatrogenic oesophageal tear will also present with chest and/or upper abdominal discomfort, along with odynophagia and dysphagia. Pain is less acute. The patient is unlikely to be shocked or distressed and will have a history of instrumentation in the preceding 24–48 hours. A patient with a Mallory-Weiss tear will describe a history of vomiting which provoked chest

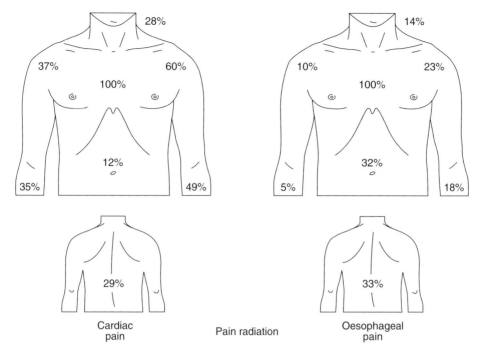

Cardiac pain

Pain radiation

Oesophageal pain

Figure 12.1 Comparison of pain radiation between oesophageal and cardiac. Reproduced with permission from Logan et al. (2002).

pain and, later, haematemesis. There may be a history which reflects the underlying cause of the vomiting, for example alcohol intoxication or pregnancy. In women of reproductive age, reviewing the reproductive system and establishing menstrual history may be relevant where vomiting is otherwise unexplained.

Clinical examination

An initial survey of the patient with Boerhaave's syndrome reveals shock, manifested by tachypnoea, tachycardia, hypotension, poor peripheral perfusion and peripheral cyanosis. The patient may be cold, clammy and grey, with a varying degree of respiratory distress. Heart sounds will usually be normal unless there is coexisting heart failure, which may be evidenced by raised jugular venous pressure and/or abnormal heart sounds. Auscultation over the lung fields will reveal reduced or absent breath sounds and there will be dullness to percussion over pleural effusions and hyper-resonance over any pneumothorax. Abdominal examination may be difficult if the patient is in pain. There may be tenderness over the epigastrum, rigidity and guarding of the abdomen with pain on examination which would indicate peritonitis if a lower oesophageal tear is leaking into the abdominal cavity. In some patients there will be subcutaneous emphysema that collects around the upper chest wall and neck, although this tends to develop a few hours after the onset of symptoms. Other clinical signs will be dependent on concomitant pathology causing vomiting or requiring instrumentation for investigation or treatment, such as carcinoma of the oesophagus. Examination of the abdomen may reveal indications of liver disease characterised by an enlarged liver span, a firm, non-tender liver edge, and spider naevi on the abdomen. Patients with portal hypertension may have enlarged veins and/or ascites.

Initial investigations

A range of traditional investigations will usually be performed in the patient with chest pain suggestive of an oesophageal rupture. Of these the electrocardiogram is helpful in ruling out evidence of myocardial ischaemia/infarction: see differential diagnosis section. Specific investigations are discussed below

Radiography

Studies and reviews largely support the view that the simplest and most valuable diagnostic test is an upright chest x-ray which reveals pneumomediastinum, effusion, hydropneumothorax, subcutaneous emphysema, basal consolidation or pneumothorax (Lemke and Jagminas 1999; Baric 2000). A water-soluble contrast (Gastrograffin) oesophagram is the test of choice to confirm the presence of the tear. A leak from the oesophagus will be evident if there is a long tear; the area of collection of fluid in the chest will vary anatomically dependent on its location. Upper oesophageal perforations tend to leak into the mediastinum, mid-oesophageal perforations leak into the mediastinum and right pleura, distal oesophageal perforations into the mediastinum, left pleural cavity or abdomen (Travis et al. 2005).

Imaging

Instrumentation perforations are small and not always evident on a contrast swallow, although if no leak is demonstrated a chest CT scan may be helpful. The advantage of CT is that it is widely available, fast, requires minimal patient co-operation, and allows evaluation of the pleura, mediastinum and aorta. On CT, extraluminal air is the most useful finding, reported in up to 92% of patients with rupture of the distal oesophagus (Lomoschitz et al. 2001).

Differential diagnosis

Boerhaave's syndrome is most likely to present with features that may be mistaken for myocardial infarction, dissecting aortic aneurysm, pulmonary embolism, perforated peptic ulcer or acute pancreatitis. Myocardial infarction can usually be excluded by the electrocardiogram (ECG), although patients with concomitant coronary heart disease (CHD) may present with ST segment changes on the ECG provoked by oesophageal rupture. Indeed Schattner et al. (2005) describe a case of oesophageal submucosal haemorrhage in a patient with known

CHD in which the only differentiating factors from myocardial infarction were odynophagia and dysphagia.

Dissecting aortic aneurysm tends to present similarly with pain radiating to the back (see Chapter 9) but there is unlikely to be accompanying dysphagia, and a CT scan would differentiate the diagnosis from an oesophageal tear or rupture. Pulmonary embolism manifests as acute chest pain but is not preceded by vomiting, although vomiting may follow the onset of pain (see Chapter 10). Equally, in pulmonary embolism, a chest radiograph is frequently normal and is in fact most useful in diagnosing other causes of acute chest pain. Perforated peptic ulcer gives rise to abdominal rather than chest signs, including a rigid, silent abdomen, and air under the diaphragm visualised on chest radiograph. In this instance signs may have been increasing in intensity for some time and vomiting tends to follow, rather than precede, the onset of symptoms.

Acute pancreatitis is characterised by severe abdominal pain that may radiate to the back, nausea and vomiting, distension and possibly fever. Diagnosis is confirmed by a serum amylase raised to a minimum of four times the normal value. In severe cases additional signs include Grey Turner's sign where there is bruising discoloration of the flanks due to extravasation of blood, and fat necrosis as pancreatic enzymes digest blood vessel walls. Cullen's sign is similar discoloration around the umbilicus (Long and Cheshire 2002).

Immediate management and interventions

For patients with Boerhaave's syndrome, resuscitation should be with intravenous fluid, intravenous analgesia (such as morphine) and early surgical involvement. The principles of management for spontaneous rupture of the oesophagus are fasting, oesophageal and gastric suction, antibiotics, and early surgical drainage and repair (Baric 2000). Recovery is dependent on early diagnosis and intervention. Late surgery may be unsuccessful in debriding damaged tissue because of digestion of tissues; surgery is therefore advocated within 24 hours of the onset of symptoms (Travis et al. 2005). Intravenous antibiotics (metronidazole and cefuroxime) should be commenced immediately a leak has been identified.

Small tears with no contrast leak such as Mallory-Weiss tears or tears following instrumentation are usually managed conservatively. Nasogastric suction and drainage are advocated for three days along with intravenous fluid and antibiotics, as for ruptured oesophagus (Baric 2000). Surgery may be indicated if there is persistent fever or pneumothorax after 48 hours.

Further investigations

Further investigation is dictated by the patient's condition. Repeat chest radiograph is indicated to observe for changes consistent with a leak into the mediastinum, or for signs of pneumothorax if respiratory distress occurs or fever persists in patients with small tears. Any underlying pathology may also be identified and appropriate referral made.

Medium- to long-term management plan

Investigation, counselling and appropriate referrals in respect of alcohol use are indicated for those in whom the episode was related to vomiting associated with alcohol consumption. Similar plans are required for those whose vomiting is associated with eating disorders, whilst patients with hyperemesis gravidarum should be referred for management by obstetricians.

Key learning points

- Oesophageal rupture, whether severe such as Boerhaave's syndrome or as a result of Mallory-Weiss tear, is rare and often overlooked as a differential diagnosis for chest pain.
- A 'classic triad' of symptoms, namely vomiting followed by chest pain and subcutaneous emphysema, present simultaneously in very few cases.
- Check for odynophagia and/or dysphagia
- Consider history of instrumentation of the oesophagus or vomiting prior to symptom onset.
- Look for fluid or pleural air on CXR.
- Fever, shock and respiratory distress may emerge later.

OESOPHAGEAL MOTILITY DISORDERS

Background

Oesophageal motility disorders are extremely common and comprise any condition whose symptoms are suspected of being oesophageal in origin, especially dysphagia and chest pain (Richter 2001). Approximately 10% of the population seek medical advice for typical symptoms of gastro-oesophageal reflux such as heartburn, epigastric or retrosternal discomfort and regurgitation, although the British Society of Gastroenterology (BSG) suggest that this may represent only 25% of those who regularly experience these symptoms (BSG 2005). Dyspeptic symptoms account for approximately 4% of general practice consultations per year (Baird 2005), and anecdotal evidence suggests that oesophageal disorders cause the discomfort which drives a significant proportion of patients to be referred to rapid access chest pain clinics.

Diffuse oesophageal spasm is a potential cause of intermittent chest pain and/or dysphagia (Barham et al. 1997). Considerably less prevalent than gastro-oesophageal reflux, oesophageal motility disorders such as diffuse oesophageal spasm and achalasia may cause distressing symptoms such as dysphagia and chest pain, and can only be diagnosed and categorised accurately by oesophageal function studies, including manometry and pH testing. Achalasia, defined as 'failure to relax', is the most recognised motor disorder of the oesophagus and the only primary motility disorder with an established pathology (Richter 2001).

Pathophysiology

Abnormal oesophageal contractions can be responsible for causing severe chest pain that is commonly mistaken for cardiac pain. Patients present with severe central chest pain as the oesophagus contracts abnormally. However, it is often not possible to directly associate patients' symptoms with abnormal motility although pain and altered motility may both be experienced (Barham et al. 1997; Tobin and Pope 1998).

Whilst no structural abnormality is demonstrable in patients with oesophageal spasm, symptoms are thought to be caused by abnormal contractions of the oesophageal muscularis. Causes for this are not known although association with gastro-oesophageal reflux disease, irritable bowel syndrome and stress are thought to contribute (Richter 2001; Travis et al. 2005). Following a study involving 390 patients, Barham et al. (1997) proposed that the chest pain experienced in hypertensive (or 'nutcracker') oesophagus was due to repeated high amplitude, peristaltic contractions. However, symptomatic diffuse oesophageal spasm (corkscrew oesophagus) was related to high amplitude, simultaneous, non-peristaltic contractions of more than 15 seconds' duration over 10 cm or more of the oesophagus. Richter (2001) suggests that diffuse oesophageal spasm is not necessarily associated with high pressure contractions; rather that normal peristalsis is interrupted by simultaneous contractions that may have multiple peaks. However, he does indicate that those patients who experience chest pain are likely to experience contractions at higher pressures than those who experience dysphagia, whose oesophageal contraction pressures are lower.

In achalasia there is increased lower oesophageal sphincter pressure and decreased or absent peristalsis in the body of the oesophagus due to degeneration of the myenteric plexus, the reasons for which are not known (Travis et al. 2005).

Causes

Aetiology of abnormal oesophageal motility in the absence of any lesion is not clearly understood, and consensus is lacking (Tobin and Pope 1998). In some patients it is thought to be associated with symptoms of irritable bowel syndrome or abnormal neurological nociception in the viscera, possibly influenced by psychological factors, hence its relationship to stress (Bennett 2000). Richter (2001) suggests that myenteric plexus degeneration in achalasia may be due to hereditary, degenerative, autoimmune and infectious causes.

Clinical presentation

Oesophageal motility disorders account for many patients referred with oesophageal symptoms that present with chest pain. The chest pain experienced may mimic cardiac pain, and may be provoked or exacerbated by stress and associated with intermittent dysphagia to liquids and solids. However, a persistent ache between severe episodes usually distinguishes it from angina. Severe pain associated with oesophageal spasm may be accompanied by a vagal response, along with grey skin, pallor and sweating with or without nausea and/or vomiting. Oesophageal spasm tends to be worse in the recumbent position. It characteristically persists for up to 20–30 minutes at a time and may leave the patient with a persistent ache in the centre of the chest for some time following a severe attack, although, to further distinguish this from angina, activity does not tend to exacerbate the discomfort (Travis et al. 2005).

Chest pain experienced by those with achalasia can be severe. Dysphagia to liquids and solids will be progressive with concomitant weight loss. The characteristics of oesophageal-related chest pain may be insufficient to distinguish it from a cardiac cause, and it is believed that the similarity in presentation in terms of the pain itself can be explained by the convergence of afferent signals from the heart and oesophagus to the same dorsal neurons of the spinal cord (Van Meigham et al. 2004). The patient may complain of moderate to severe, crushing, central chest pain. Unlike angina, the onset of symptoms tends to be unpredictable and in this sense the history tends to rule angina in or out, rather than suggesting oesophago-gastric causes of chest pain *per se.*

History taking

A careful history is the most helpful source of information for diagnosis; it may reveal progressive attempts which have helped in the first instance but have failed to relieve their symptoms over time. Selective use of questioning may confirm a history of intermittent dysphagia to both solids and liquids, and worsening pain lasting for over 30 minutes that is exacerbated by dietary factors or lying in a specific position and unlikely to be induced by physical activity. Additionally, patients presenting with oesophago-gastric symptoms may report self-medicating with over-the-counter antacid preparations to relieve their symptoms. These findings may signal a gastric disturbance, and if patients describe having recent episodes of gastro-intestinal blood loss, the individual should be referred to specialists for urgent investigations.

Clinical examination

On examination, there are often no clinical signs to support a diagnosis of oesophageal dysmotility; rather findings may rule out other causes for the symptoms. In an acute episode of pain, the patient may be in distress, with pallor, sweating and nausea. Further abdominal examination is unlikely to be remarkable.

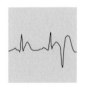

Initial investigations

Barium swallow often reveals a normal oesophageal contour as symptoms often cannot be elicited 'to order'. However, disruption of peristalsis and the characteristic 'corkscrew' appearance of the oesophagus can be demonstrated in diffuse oesophageal spasm (Figure 12.2). Oesophago-gastro-duodenoscopy (OGD) should be undertaken to rule out the presence of a lesion or oesophagitis.

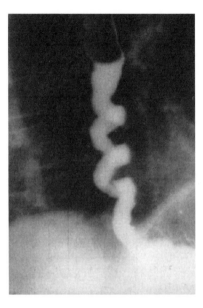

Figure 12.2 Barium swallow showing diffuse oesophageal spasm with a typical 'corkscrew' deformity. Reproduced with permission from Travis et al. (2005).

Oesophageal manometry measures intraluminal and sphincter pressures, and the pH in the lower oesophagus. Manometry is used to ascertain whether oesophageal peristaltic and sphincter pressures are normal, and to elicit the oesophageal pH as acid reflux may be associated with similar symptoms (Richter 2001; Travis et al. 2005). Testing may be conducted at a single appointment in a clinical laboratory but is likely to miss intermittent abnormal oesophageal contractions. A higher yield of correlation of symptoms to physiological abnormality may be obtained with 24-hour ambulatory manometry in which oesophageal pressures and pH are measured and linked to a patient record of normal daily activity and symptoms experienced (Barham et al. 1997). However, negative findings do not necessarily rule out a positive diagnosis (Tobin and Pope 1998; Richter 2001; Travis et al. 2005).

Differential diagnosis

If the pain is to be distinguished from ischaemic-type chest pain, then the characteristics of acute coronary syndromes, including the electrocardiographic and cardiac enzyme markers, need to be ruled out (see Chapter 6). Unless there is good reason to suspect cardiac pain, then a oesophago-gastric cause should be considered.

Medium- to long-term management plan

Proton pump inhibitors (PPIs) should be used initially as abnormal motility may be provoked by acid reflux (Travis et al. 2005). Reassurance that symptoms are not cardiac-related is important, particularly as pharmacological management for oesophageal spasm employs drugs also used in patients with angina, including nitrates and calcium channel blockers (Tobin and Pope 1998; Richter 2001). Small doses of tricyclics (imipramine, amitriptyline) can be useful, whereas botulinum toxin, dilatation and finally oesophago-myotomy are reserved for very severe cases (Tobin and Pope 1998; Richter 2001). In achalasia, balloon dilatation is indicated for dysphagia. Post-procedure chest radiograph after the procedure (before resuming oral intake) is required to exclude perforation.

Key learning points

- Oesophageal motility disorders can cause patients to present with severe central chest pain almost indistinguishable from cardiac pain.
- Often associated with dysphagia, the pain is likely to radiate to the back rather than the arms, while cardiac pain will radiate more frequently to arms than to the back (Bennett 2002).

GASTRO-OESPHAGEAL REFLUX DISEASE

Background

Gastro-oesophageal reflux disease (GORD) is a significant problem in adult Western populations. Jones (2004) reports that about 40% of the United States population experience acid reflux on a monthly basis. With detrimental effects on sufferers' quality of life, the socio-economic burden of this disease in the West is significant (Jones 2004). It is a more important cause of angina-like pain than oesophageal motility disorders (Van Meigham et al. 2004), and its importance lies not only in the frequency of symptoms in the population, but also in its potential for the development of complications such as stricture and Barrett's columnar-lined oesophagus, which is a pre-malignant condition.

Pathophysiology

Reflux of gastric contents through the lower oesophageal sphincter into the lower oesophagus exposes unprotected mucosa to corrosive material containing acid (pH < 4), pepsin and sometimes bile. Oesophagitis can result following damage to the mucosa, while repeated exposure may result in chronic symptoms including retrosternal chest pain and dysphagia. Acid reflux into the oesophagus can trigger myocardial ischaemia and ECG changes in patients with concomitant coronary artery disease (Van Meigham et al. 2004), which gives rise to difficulty both in diagnosing the condition and differentially managing symptoms.

The term GORD (known as GERD in North America) is given to those in whom there is a risk of complications or impaired quality of life due to gastro-oesophageal reflux (Jalal and Heatley 2000). Symptoms include:

- Heartburn related to meals, position and sometimes exercise
- Reflux of stomach contents into the mouth

- Dysphagia
- Chest pain related to position or exercise
- Asthma (often experienced at night only)
- Laryngitis (hoarseness)

GORD is often associated with hiatus hernia or other functional gastrointestinal problems such as irritable bowel syndrome, although they are not diagnostic criteria for GORD (Jalal and Heatley 2000; Travis et al. 2005). Patients may have asymptomatic or 'silent' reflux with significant damage to the mucosa, or alternatively describe severe symptoms but have no oesophagitis on investigation (Jalal and Heatley 2000; Jones 2004).

Complications relate to altered histology as a result of exposure of the oesophageal mucosa to gastric contents and include oesophagitis, peptic stricture, Barrett's oesophagus in which histological changes result in columnar lined lower oesophagus, and adenocarcinoma of the oesophagus. Both GORD and Barrett's oesophagus are known to be risk factors for the development of adenocarcinoma of the oesophagus, and this in spite of effective treatment (Jones 2004).

Clinical presentation

The patient presents with pain or chest discomfort which may be upper or lower retrosternal pain, frequently described as burning. There may be accompanying epigastric discomfort with radiation to the upper back, shoulders, neck or arms. Duration is variable, unlike angina in which there is usually predictable relief within a few minutes. Antacids may provide relief although persistent symptoms may have only mild or short-lived relief with over-the-counter antacid preparations.

History taking

In such patients, there is likely to be a history of heartburn or symptoms suggestive of acid reflux. The symptoms may have a relationship to dietary intake, occurring more frequently before or after food. There may be a relationship to exercise, including sexual activity, and symptoms may be provoked by position and also while straining which mimics angina (Travis et al. 2005). Given that pain may be provoked by exercise and on bending forward, it is important to assess whether symptoms are provoked by carrying out usual daily activities, for example in the course of working life. In patients with oesophagitis, oesophageal dysmotility or a peptic stricture in the oesophagus, there may additionally be intermittent dysphagia.

Clinical examination

The clinical examination in patients presenting with GORD is essentially normal though there may be residual chest or epigastric discomfort. Palpation of the epigastrum may reveal tenderness though there is unlikely to be reproducible discomfort in the chest on palpation.

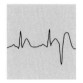

Initial investigations

The ECG in patients presenting with chest pain is usually normal but may not be so if there is co-existing coronary disease. Exercise tolerance testing in this group of patients may be sufficient to rule out the presence of coronary disease, although equivocal results are common, particularly where symptoms are provoked on exercise without concomitant ECG changes.

Differential diagnosis

Both cardiac and oesophageal disease may produce similar chest pain, and the two entities frequently coexist, creating confusion for the clinician. The documentation of ECG abnormalities is an important finding as it makes the diagnosis of an oesophageal disorder unlikely. Of patients with chest pain, normal exercise ECG and normal angiography, 20–40% have an oesophageal disorder. The pain may be severe, wake patients from sleep, or occur during emotional stress.

Patients presenting with chest pain who have GORD are more likely to indicate the pain stroking their hand down the sternum as opposed to those with cardiac pain who will hold a tightly clenched fist to the sternum (Bickley and Szilagyi 2003). The duration and type of pain and the provoking or relieving factors may help to differentiate the diagnosis. Oesophageal reflux and diffuse oesophageal spasm most commonly mimic angina.

It is important in the first instance to identify risk factors for an organic pathway. Guidelines indicate that age over 45 years at first presentation with unexplained and recent onset dyspepsia alone should be further investigated, along with those with a family history of early onset gastric cancer (age <50 years), those with persistent symptoms, previous peptic ulcer disease, unexplained weight loss, evidence of gastrointestinal bleeding, dysphagia, persistent vomiting, or upper abdominal mass (Scottish Intercollegiate Guidelines Network 2003; NICE 2004).

Immediate management and interventions

Proton pump inhibitors are recommended in the first instance for 1–2 months (NICE 2004). If the symptoms abate during treatment, and they will do so gradually, this is sufficient to confirm the presence of GORD. Provided that cardiac pain has been ruled out, then the patient should be reassured that their symptoms do not have a cardiac origin.

Further investigations

Angiography may be indicated for persistent chest discomfort with cardiac features. However, between 10 and 50% of patients with anginal pain are found to have normal coronary arteries. An oesophageal cause of non-cardiac chest pain is found in 60% of cases, and ECG abnormalities may be found in these patients, which highlights that changes in T wave morphology and ST segment morphology, both of which are manifestations of coronary disease, may be misleading (Van Meigham et al. 2004).

Oesophago-gastro-endoscopy (OGD) is indicated for a first presentation if the patient is >45 years or has alarming symptoms including dysphagia and/or weight loss. Those with chronic, severe symptoms related to reflux should also have OGD (Jalal and Heatley 2000) and, in both cases, evaluation of oesophagitis or diagnosis of Barrett's oesophagus can be made if present (Jones 2004; Travis et al. 2005).

In patients with unusual symptoms 24-hour ambulatory manometry to measure the pH in the lower oesophagus is indicated. Previously, 24-hour pH testing was considered to be the gold standard to confirm GORD, but it has been shown to lack sensitivity or specificity, with many symptomatic patients having normal acid exposure times (Tobin and Pope 1998).

Medium- to long-term management plan

Therapy for GORD is aimed at symptom relief and improving quality of life. There is a hierarchy of approaches to treatment (Figure 12.3), which may be followed in a step-up or step-down approach. Most favour a step-down approach, the rationale being to achieve healing of oesophagitis and then maintenance on the lowest possible interventional level or dose of medication (Jalal and Heatley 2000; Jones 2004; Travis et al. 2005).

Step up	Therapeutic intervention	Step down
	High dose PPI (e.g. Lanzoprazole 30 mg od/bd)	
	Low dose PPI (e.g. Lanzoprazole 15 mg od/bd)	
	H₂ receptor antagonist (e.g. Ranitidine) and/or prokinetic (e.g. Domperidone)	
	Antacids (e.g. Maalox) and alginates (e.g. Gaviscon Advance)	
	Lifestyle modifications • lose weight • stop smoking • low fat diet • reduce alcohol and caffeine intake • reduce citrus and chocolate intake • avoid eating within 4 hours of bedtime • raise the head of the bed	

Figure 12.3 Hierarchical treatment approaches for gastro-oesophageal reflux disease (Jalal and Heatley 2000; NICE 2004).

Given the significant economic impact of either suffering or being treated for GORD, there is a balance to be struck between symptom relief and costly drug treatments. Proton pump inhibitors have been shown to be the most effective treatment for healing oesophagitis and for symptom control in endoscopy-negative GORD. NICE guidelines (2004) recommend that patients should be treated until symptoms remit and should then be prescribed the lowest dose of PPI possible. In addition, it is advocated that patients be facilitated to manage their therapy independently, using treatment on an 'as required' basis.

Key learning points

- Early presentation of GORD is difficult to distinguish from angina.
- The presence of dysphagia may offer the clinician insight into whether GORD may be the cause of the symptoms.
- Response to PPI therapy is indicative of a positive diagnosis for GORD.

References

Baird A (2005) The management of gastro-oesophageal reflux in primary care. *Nurse Prescribing* **3**(5): 184–187.

Barham CP, Gotley DC, Fowler A, Mills A, Alderson D (1997) Diffuse oesophageal spasm: diagnosis by ambulatory 24-hour manometry. *Gut* **41**: 151–155.

Baric A (2000) Oesophageal rupture in a patient with postoperative nausea and vomiting. *Anaesthesia and Intensive Care* **28**: 325–327.

Bennett JR (2000) Clinical history taking. In Adam A, Mason RC, Owen WJ (Eds) *Practical Management of Oesophageal Disease*, pp. 1–12. Oxford, Isis Medical Media.

Bennett J (2002) Oesophagus: atypical chest pain and motility disorders. In Logan RPH, Harris A, Misiewicz JJ, Baron JH (Eds) *ABC of the Upper Gastrointestinal Tract*, pp. 791–794. London, BMJ Books.

Bickley LS, Szilagyi PG (2003) *Bates' Guide to Physical Examination and History Taking*, 8th edition. Philadelphia, Lippincott Williams & Wilkins.

British Society of Gastroenterology (2005) *Guidelines for Oesophageal Manometry and pH Monitoring*. www.bsg.org.uk/pdfworddocs/oespman.pdf.

Jalal PK, Heatley RV (2000) Medical treatment of gastro-oesophageal reflux disease. *Hospital Medicine* **61**(7): 478–482.

Janjua KJ (1997) Boerhaave's syndrome. *Postgraduate Medical Journal* **73**: 265–270.

Jones MP (2004) Acid suppression in gastro-oesophageal reflux disease: Why? How? How much and when? In Mayberry J (Ed.) *Gastroenterology Update*. Abingdon, Radcliffe Publishing.

Keshav S (2004) *The Gastro-intestinal System at a Glance*. Oxford, Blackwell Publishing.

Lemke T, Jagminas L (1999) Spontaneous oesophageal rupture: a frequently missed diagnosis. *The American Surgeon* **65**: 449–452.

Logan RPH, Harris A, Misiewicz JJ, Baron JH (Eds) (2002) *ABC of the Upper Gastrointestinal Tract*. London, BMJ Books.

Lomoschitz FM, Linnau KF, Mann FA (2001) Pneumomediastinum without pneumothorax caused by esophageal rupture. *American Journal of Radiology* **177**: 1416.

Long MS, Cheshire E (2002) *Mosby's Crash Course: the Gastrointestinal System*. London, Mosby.

Mamun M (1998) Spontaneous oesophageal perforation: long known but still not easy to diagnose. *Hospital Medicine* **58**: 968–969.

National Institute for Clinical Excellence (2004) *Clinical Guideline 17; Management of Dyspepsia in Adults in Primary Care*. NICE, London.

Richter JE (2001) Oesophageal motility disorders. *The Lancet* **358**: 823–828.

Schattner A, Binder Y, Melzer E (2005) An elderly man with excruciating retrosternal pain and dysphagia. *Canadian Medical Association Journal* **172**: 1556.

Scottish Intercollegiate Guideline Network (SIGN) (2003) *Dyspepsia: Quick Reference Guide*. SIGN Executive, Royal College of Physicians Edinburgh. www.sign.ac.uk.

Tobin RW, Pope CE II (1998) Disorders of swallowing and chest pain. In Phillips SF, Wingate DL (Eds) *Functional Disorders of the Gut*, pp. 177–195. London, Churchill Livingstone.

Travis SPL, Ahmad T, Collier J, Steinhart AH (2005) *Gastroenterology: Pocket Consultant*. Oxford, Blackwell Publishing.

Van Meigham C, Sabbe M, Knockaert D (2004) The clinical value of the ECG in non-cardiac conditions. *Chest* **125**(4): 1561–1576.

Useful websites

http://gut.bmjjournals.com
http://bnf.org.uk
http://bsg.org.uk
http://www.nice.org.uk
http://www.surgical-tutor.org.uk/system/abdomen
http://www.medicine.ucsd.edu/clinicalmed/introduction.htm

Chapter 13

Assessing and managing the patient with musculoskeletal chest pain

Rebecca Hoskins

Aims

Musculoskeletal chest pain tends to be used as a collective term for chest pain caused by soft tissue injury and is not thought to be cardiac in origin. This chapter aims to encourage the reader to identify specific musculoskeletal causes in patients presenting with chest pain. It will also outline specific treatment strategies and management plans for the identified complaints. The differentiation of a musculoskeletal origin rather than a cardiac cause of chest pain in the patient presenting with chest discomfort lies in taking a comprehensive history coupled with an accurate examination of the patient. A cardiac cause of chest pain should always be thought of and ruled out by careful examination and appropriate investigation if necessary.

Learning outcomes

While this chapter gives an outline of the more common conditions and presentations of musculoskeletal causes of chest pain, theory must be augmented by development of practical clinical examination and diagnostic reasoning skills (under the supervision of a mentor if appropriate). By the end of this chapter the reader should be able to:

- Identify causes and presenting features of musculoskeletal chest pain.
- Understand the pathophysiology of musculosketetal causes of chest pain including those due to trauma, inflammation, infection and cancer.
- Differentiate between various musculoskeletal causes for chest pain.
- Identity the key findings in the clinical examination of a patient presenting with musculoskeletal chest pain.

There are a vast variety of conditions that may give rise to chest pain with an underlying musculoskeletal cause which, with appropriate history taking, examination and investigation will enable a more accurate diagnosis and subsequent treatment plan for the patient.

Studies examining the prevalence of non-cardiac chest pain are rare. Wise (1994) suggests that musculoskeletal chest wall pain syndromes account for between 10 and 15% of cases of adults presenting with chest pain in the emergency setting, and as a group account for about 15–20% of patients who have had chest pain but whose coronary angiograms were normal.

This chapter will concentrate on non-life-threatening injuries, as conditions caused by major trauma are covered elsewhere. Musculoskeletal conditions can be separated into those caused by minor trauma and those caused by an inflammatory disease.

MINOR TRAUMA: RIB INJURY, INTERCOSTAL MUSCLE STRAIN AND RIB FRACTURE

Background

Injury to the ribs or chest wall is thought to be the commonest thoracic injury with which patients present to an emergency department (Wardrope and English 1998). There have been no significant studies carried out to quantify the incidence.

Causes

The majority of patients will present with so-called minor injuries to the chest resulting from blunt injury such as that acquired from a direct contact sport, e.g. rugby. Some patients may present following a low speed road traffic collision (RTC) or a fall from a height or on to an object such as the side of the bath. Others may have been the victim of a physical assault. Occasionally patients may present with a pathological rib fracture caused by very minor trauma because of their co-existing disease, for example a 'cough fracture'.

Pathophysiology

The bony skeleton of the chest is comprised of 12 thoracic vertebrae, the ribs, costal cartilages and the sternum. The bony cage of the ribs, clavicles, sternum, scapulae and vertebrae provides protection for the heart, lungs and great vessels, the liver, spleen and upper abdominal organs. It is important to remember that the abdomen reaches to the level of the nipple on inspiration (see Figure 13.1). The intercostal vessels run close to the underside of the ribs. Tears in these vessels can result in a significant haemothorax.

Rib fractures or intercostal muscle strain can compromise effective ventilation because pain from rib injuries and/or a fracture can result in hypoventilation and subsequent atelectasis and pneumonia. Multiple contiguous rib fractures can result in a flail chest (see Chapter 11). Rib fractures occur most often between the 4th and 10th ribs (Peavey 2003). Subcutaneous emphysema or crepitus may be present. Fractures that separate the sternum from costal cartilage are not evident on an x-ray.

It is important to be aware that older patients may present with rib fractures or even a flail segment after a minor fall due to reduced compliance within the thoracic cage, which reduces the ability of the thorax to withstand blunt trauma

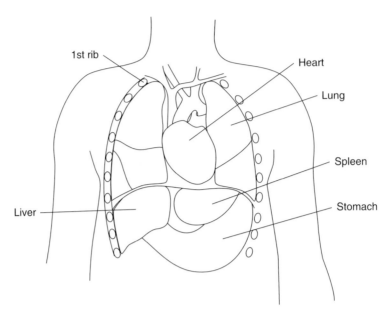

Figure 13.1 Normal position of organs in the thorax.

(Greaves and Johnson 2002). There also tends to be a rise in the incidence of osteopenia in older patients, contributing to an increased risk of fractures following minor trauma (Lee et al. 1990). Whether the fall was caused by tripping up or as a consequence of a loss of consciousness needs further investigation (National Institute for Clinical Excellence (NICE) 2004).

Clinical presentation

It is usual for the patient to present several days after the initial injury because of worsening pain which may be preventing the individual from carrying out their usual activities of daily living. The patient may complain of pain on inspiration as well as dyspnoea (Greaves and Johnson 2002). They may also have restricted movement in the ipsilateral upper limb. The patient may describe the pain as sharp and localised to a specific area (such as the xiphoid, lower ribs or midsternum). Conversely, some patients may describe the pain as diffuse and poorly localised. Most chest wall pain is positional and exacerbated by deep breathing, turning, or arm movement.

History taking

A detailed history of the mechanism of the original injury can provide useful information in predicting the injury pattern to be found on clinical examination. It is relevant to ask about coexisting respiratory disease as this may influence the subsequent management of such patients. Those with decreased pulmonary function from asthma or chronic obstructive pulmonary disease also require careful assessment because vital capacity is already decreased (Cox and Roper 2005). It is also important to discover whether the patient is a smoker and to elicit how many cigarettes are smoked a day as this can put the patient at greater risk of developing a subsequent lower respiratory tract infection.

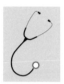

Clinical examination

In addition to general information regarding clinical examination of patients presenting with chest pain (see Chapter 4), specific information relating to musculoskeletal presentations is also required regarding cervical spine and respiratory systems.

The cervical spine of the patient should be examined in order to discount a concurrent injury caused by the same incident. Palpation of each cervical vertebra down to the cervicothoracic junction should be carried out. Any bony pain elicited points to a positive finding and the patient should be placed in c-spine precautions. A negative examination of the c-spine and the absence of distracting injury or pain in a patient who is fully alert, with no head injury and who is not intoxicated by alcohol or drugs, allows the range of movement of the c-spine to be carried out thus:

- Rotation to left and right
- Flexion and extension
- Lateral flexion to left and right (Moulton and Yates 2006)

If there are no associated abnormal neurological findings, then an injury in the patient's c-spine may be ruled out (Wardrope et al. 2004). It is important to measure the patient's vital signs, especially an accurate respiratory rate to identify any increased work of breathing. The chest should be examined for any signs of bruising, wounds, deformity, swelling or emphysema (Westaby and Odell 1999). The position of the trachea should be noted (see Figure 4.7).

When examining the chest, there may be asymmetrical chest movement because of splinting of the muscles of respiration. This can be assessed by placing the examiner's hands together with thumbs lightly touching on the patient's chest wall. When the patient takes a breath in, the examiner's thumbs should move symmetrically apart (refer to Figure 13.2). Determine the exact site of tenderness, and test for pain by compressing or springing the chest laterally and anteriorly–posteriorly at sites away from the area of the blow. Pain on compression indicates a clinical fracture (Purcell 2003).

Palpation of subcutaneous emphysema or crepitus is an abnormal finding and indicates a possible rib fracture or injury to the respiratory tract. In a study by Liman et al. (2003), 75% of patients presenting with subcutaneous emphysema had an associated haemothorax and/or pneumothorax. While subcutaneous emphysema is self-limiting, it is essential to identify and treat the underlying cause.

The anterior and posterior chest wall should be gently percussed to assess for resonance. Hyper-resonance indicates the presence of a pneumothorax. Next, the

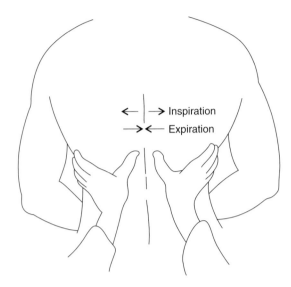

→ Inspiration
→← Expiration

Figure 13.2 Technique for assessing bilateral chest expansion.

anterior and posterior lung fields should be auscultated to ascertain that equal air entry is present and that no added sounds exist. Decreased air entry may indicate the presence of a pneumothorax. Finally, if there is an injury to the lower chest wall, an examination of the patient's abdomen is indicated (Douglas et al. 2005). Fracture of the left lower ribs is associated with splenic injuries, while fracture of the right lower ribs may indicate an injury to the liver. Injury of the floating ribs (ribs 11 and 12) is associated with renal injuries.

Initial investigations

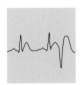

If the blow to the chest has been minor, the patient is well, displaying no abnormal signs on clinical examination with no previous respiratory problems, then no further investigation is indicated. However, a relatively low threshold for requesting a chest x-ray is indicated in the majority of patients presenting with a chest wall injury. The chest x-ray should be examined carefully in order to exclude any signs of a pneumothorax. Rib fractures can be difficult to see on x-ray, and suspicion of a simple rib fracture with no associated abnormal clinical findings is not an indication for requesting a chest film (Raby et al. 2005). Injury to the posterior lower thorax may indicate a renal injury, and the patient's urine should be tested in order to rule out the presence of blood.

Differential diagnosis

Associated abdominal trauma should be ruled out by clinical examination and further investigation if necessary. Injuries to the acromioclavicular and sternoclavicular joint should also be considered and a detailed clinical examination carried out. Major injuries, such as a pneumothorax, haemothorax, aortic arch injury, and cardiac injury, should also be ruled out during clinical examination, although the mechanism of injury and physical examination should exclude the possibility of major trauma (Westaby and Odell 1999).

Immediate management and interventions

Treatment for most rib injuries and fractures is analgesia and simple chest physiotherapy in the form of deep breathing exercises. Non-steroidal anti-inflammatory drugs such as Diclofenac are effective in relieving pain (Barkin et al. 1998). Coughing and deep breathing are used to prevent complications, including pneumonia or atelectasis.

Further investigations

A chest x-ray is indicated if multiple rib fractures are suspected from the clinical examination, or if a pneumothorax or haemothorax is suspected. It is helpful to be aware that only 70% of rib fractures are identified on plain chest films. The presence of more than two rib fractures is a marker of severe injury, and associated injuries should be sought and ruled out (Lee et al. 1990).

Medium- to long-term management plan

The patient can be discharged from hospital if only a single rib fracture is suspected and there are no clinical findings to suggest underlying injury which compromises effective ventilation. The patient should be discharged with adequate analgesia, such as Diclofenac 50 mg three times a day if there are no contraindications (Moulton and Yates 2006). Additional analgesia such as codeine may also be required. The patient will need specific education as to the importance of deep breathing exercises and splinting their chest wall with a pillow when coughing. Specific advice on when to seek further help should also be given, preferably in written form including:

- If the patient becomes acutely short of breath (indicating a possible pneumothorax)
- If they develop haemoptysis
- If they become unwell with a pyrexia and purulent sputum
- If their pain is not controlled despite taking prescribed analgesia (Greaves and Johnson 2002)

There are specific groups of patients who may be assessed as being at high risk of developing a chest infection as a consequence of a chest wall injury. For example, elderly patients with coexisting disease may need to be referred for admission or to a discharge planning team in order to monitor for signs of deterioration, and to ensure that adequate analgesia and aggressive chest physiotherapy are provided (Liman et al. 2003).

INFLAMMATORY CONDITIONS: COSTOCHONDRITIS

Background

Costochondritis is common cause of chest pain in children and adolescents that is seen in the emergency department setting. According to Garry and Myones (2005) costochondritis occurs mainly in patients aged 10–35 years; Disla et al. (1994) claim that this condition is higher in women.

Causes

Although it is thought that most cases of costochondritis are idiopathic, the cause and aetiology are not well defined (Tough 2004). However, direct trauma to cos-tochondral cartilage and aggressive exercise involving the upper torso or cough-ing that result in repetitive stretching, twisting and strain at the costochondral junction are main culprits for costochondritis (Garry and Myones 2005). Costo-chondritis may occur with viral respiratory infections because inflammation leads to excessive coughing and straining. Bacterial or fungal infections of these joints occur uncommonly, usually in patients who are intravenous drug users and in those who have had breast or thoracic surgery. It is thought that following surgery the cartilage can become more prone to infection because of the reduced blood flow in the region that has been operated on (Tough 2004).

Pathophysiology

Costochondritis is an inflammatory process of one or more costochondral or costosternal joints that causes localised pain and tenderness in the anterior chest wall (Isenberg et al. 2004). The exact pathophysiology of cartilage and capsular movement is unknown because costochondritis does not warrant surgical inter-vention or tissue biopsy (Garry and Myones 2005). It is thought that the cartilage involved in costochondritis is either inflamed or torn, and either condition leads to inflammation with subsequent stimulation of pain receptors. Any of the seven costochondral junctions may be affected, and more than one site is affected in 90% of cases (see Figure 13.3). The most commonly affected sites are those between the second and fifth costochondral junctions (Smith and Wordsworth 2005), but there is no local swelling (Freeston et al. 2004).

Tietze syndrome has some similarities to costochondritis, although they are distinct conditions. Tietze syndrome is twice as frequent in men as in women and approximately a third of all patients are in the third decade of life (Smith and Wordsworth 2005). Typically, there is swelling over affected joints and the syndrome usually comes on abruptly, with chest pain radiating to the arms or shoulder and lasting several weeks.

Clinical presentation

The onset of pain tends to be subtle and develop over several days or weeks, often following a chest infection, injury or activities which involve stretching or

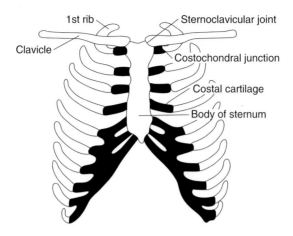

Figure 13.3 Location of costochondral joints.

twisting the upper rib cage. The pain is sharp and stabbing, and is found over the anterior chest wall; it is usually unilateral but can be bilateral. The pain often radiates to the chest, upper abdomen and back, and can be exacerbated by coughing, sneezing, deep inspiration and movement of the upper limbs. The pain is reproducible on compressing the affected costochondral junctions (Garry and Myones 2005).

History taking

Asking the patient about any recent upper respiratory infection, episodes of repeated chest trauma or sporting activities is important, as these may be a precursor to an episode of costochondritis. The mechanism and onset of chest pain are a vital part of history. A history of a recent viral infection, however, may suggest pericarditis (Chapter 8). Furthermore, because of the age group and associated causes, social and family history are relevant, and sensitive exploration of home circumstances is essential to exclude drug, aerosol and alcohol misuse and the possibility of physical abuse.

Clinical examination

A full respiratory, abdominal and cardiac assessment should be undertaken in order to exclude other serious pathology. Inspection for symmetrical chest movements is essential to exclude rib injury or chest trauma, whereas auscultation of lungs, heart and abdomen should confirm no abnormalities. With costochondritis, there is no noticeable swelling. However, in Tietze syndrome, swelling at the second and third costochondral junctions may be present. In costochondritis, pain is reproducible usually over the fourth to sixth costochondral junctions and over the second to third costochondral junctions in Tietze syndrome (Garry and Myones 2005). In

Tietze syndrome there is frequently radiation of pain to arms and shoulders as well. Percussion of the anterior and posterior chest wall should reveal equal resonance. Pulmonary auscultation in costochondritis or Tietze syndrome should reveal equal air entry with no added sounds.

Initial investigations

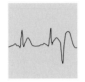

A chest x-ray is only indicated if pneumonia, chest trauma or other pathologies are suspected. A 12-lead electrocardiogram (ECG) is only indicated in order to rule out a cardiac cause of chest pain, as are blood tests (see Chapter 6). There is no specific investigation used to confirm the diagnosis; however, where an infection is suspected, microbiological findings should identify underlying cause. In Tietze syndrome biochemical markers of inflammation such as C-reactive Protein (CRP) or erythrocyte sedimentation rate (ESR) will be raised, demonstrating an inflammatory response (Isenberg et al. 2004).

Differential diagnosis

In middle-aged patients, Tietze syndrome and costochondritis may be confused with ischaemic chest pain initially and it is essential to rule out a cardiac cause (Freeston et al. 2004). However, patients aged 21 years or younger presenting with chest pain pose specific problems. In addition to excluding serious pathology, Garry and Myones (2005) suggest that staff consider muscle strain, stress fractures, gynaecomastia, dysrhythmias, oesophagitis, pneumothorax, pneumonia, viral pericarditis, viral myocarditis, asthma, physical abuse and child neglect as differential diagnoses. Other alternative diagnoses are detailed below.

Herpes zoster (shingles)

Shingles results from the reactivation of the varicella zoster virus (VZV) in individuals who have been previously exposed to it in the form of chickenpox. Shingles never occurs as a primary presentation as it results from reactivation of latent VZV in the dorsal root or cranial nerve ganglia. The patient may experience a prodromal phase of tingling or pain, which is followed by the eruption of blisters in the distribution pattern of one or more dermatomes (see Chapter 15 for a detailed account).

Fibromyalgia (chronic widespread pain/chest wall tenderness)

A patient may present with diffuse muscle and joint pain including severe discomfort in the chest wall. Chest pain associated with fibromyalgia is described as widespread and unremitting, with aching discomfort, and it occurs most commonly in around 11% of women, who may also have normal coronary angiograms (Ho et al. 2001). A typical feature of fibromyalgia is tender trigger points such as in the arm or shoulder. Chronic fatigue syndrome, irritable bowel syndrome, anxiety, depression and sleep disorders are common (Isenberg et al. 2004). Diagnosis is based on eliminating other possible conditions such as rheumatoid disease, as well as on identifying at least 11 of 18 tender points in both sides of the body, above and below the waist, and axial skeletal pain for at least three months (Wolfe et al. 1990).

Polymyalgia rheumatica (syndrome)

Polymyalgia rheumatica is described as a large vessel vasculitis classified as a rheumatic disease. It is accompanied by widespread severe musculoskeletal pain and specific tender points all over the body. There is a sudden onset of symptoms with severe pain and stiffness in shoulders, neck, hips and lumbar spine. The patient often describes the symptoms as being worse in the morning, usually resolving after several hours (Wolfe et al. 1990). Polymyalgia rheumatica is seen in patients over 50 years old, who describe accompanying systemic symptoms of fatigue, fever, weight loss, depression and occasionally night sweats. Appropriate investigations to support preliminary diagnosis from clinical history and examination include the following.

- ESR and/or CRP will be raised.
- Serum alkaline phosphatase and glutamyltranspeptidase may be raised as markers of the acute phase.
- Full blood count, anaemia will often be present (mild normochromic or normocytic).

Treatment of the condition is with corticosteroids. The disease process usually settles after 12–36 months in 75% of patients, although the remaining 25% of patients will require long-term low-dose corticosteriods (Kumar and Clark 2005).

Ankylosing spondylitis

This is an inflammatory disorder affecting approximately 1.4% of the general population. It is more commonly found in men, with a ratio of 3:1 male to female. It tends to affect young adults aged between 15 and 30 years old. (Dawes et al. 1988). There is lymphocyte and plasma cell infiltration and local erosion of bone at the attachments of the ligaments. This heals with new bone (syndesmophyte) formation. The patient may present with the clinical signs and symptoms of costochondritis due to involvement of the costochondral junction with inflammation causing anterior chest pain and reduced chest expansion; however, the pain is more diffuse.

The key to differentiation of diagnoses is the associated symptoms and classical points in the clinical history. Episodes of inflammation of the sacroiliac joints may be the first symptoms reported by the patient. Pain in the buttocks, low back pain and stiffness, typically worse in the morning, are relieved by exercise. According to Wolfe et al. (1990) the diagnosis is often missed because the patient is asymptomatic between episodes of pain, and abnormalities on x-ray are absent in the early stages of the disease process. Lumbar lordosis during spinal flexion is an early sign, which is important not to miss. Uveitis (inflammation of eyes) is also associated with this disease, so a whole systems approach to examination is important. Referral to a rheumatologist is appropriate in order that active management of the condition can be instigated before syndesmophytes form.

Sternalis syndrome

This is a rarely described condition in which localised tenderness is found directly over the body of the sternum or overlying sternalis muscle with palpation causing pain radiation bilaterally (Pace 1975). This syndrome is generally self-limited, and less likely to cause persistent pain than costochondritis (Chambers et al. 1999). Xiphoidalgia is another relatively rare syndrome that is characterised by localised discomfort and tenderness over the xiphoid process of the sternum with no associated history of trauma.

Bone tumours

Tumours of the chest wall may be malignant or benign and, if malignant, primary or metastatic. Other sources of malignancy found in the chest wall may be from a tumour originating in the bronchus or breast. Tumours may be found in the sternum, ribs or diaphragm. Primary tumours in the chest account for about 8% of all bone tumours (Kumar and Clark 2005). The most common malignancy in the chest wall is chondrosarcoma, which is a malignancy of cartilage cells, accounting for about 10% of primary bone malignancies, occurring most often on the pelvis, ribs, shoulder girdle and humerus. Patients present complaining of bone pain or a pathological fracture, and on examination a localised swelling may be found over the site of the chondrosarcoma. There is a 2:1 ratio of affected males to females, with a peak incidence between the ages of 30 and 40 years old (Wise et al. 1992).

It is important also to consider that chest wall pain may be referred from another part of the body, such as the cervical spine and the thoracic spine. Other problems that should be considered if a cause for musculoskeletal chest pain cannot be found are referred pain from cervical spondylitis, and nerve entrapment syndrome such as thoracic outlet syndrome.

Immediate management and interventions

Management of chest wall pain with nonsteroidal anti-inflammatory analgesics (NSAIDs) such as Diclofenac 50 mg TDS and codeine are the mainstay of treatment (Greaves and Johnson 1999). If NSAIDs are contraindicated, then paracetamol and codeine may be used (Greaves and Johnson 2002). If there is an underlying infective cause, the patient should be admitted for a course of intravenous antibiotics. Additionally, the patient with costochondritis should be advised to limit strenuous physical movements and avoid exercise until such time as these activities may be performed without aggravating chest pain (Garry and Myones 2005). Many adult patients may have multiple readmissions and investigations for chest pain. Early referral to rheumatology specialists is recommended to reduce delays to diagnosis and institute appropriate management therapies (Freeston et al. 2004).

Further investigations

Normally costochondritis is benign and resolves without further intervention, and does not require additional investigations.

Medium- to long-term management plan

After one year, about half of patients may still have discomfort; approximately one-third report continued tenderness with palpation (Wise 1994). Isenberg et al. (2004) suggest that local injection of steroids can be helpful, particularly when combined with sulfasalazine (Freeston et al. 2004). Patients and parents should be reassured that the cause of chest pain is not indicative of malignancy or other chronic pathology.

Key learning points

> The key to accurate diagnosis and differentiation of musculoskeletal causes of chest pain is effective history-taking skills and accurate clinical examination of the patient.
> - The aetiology of musculoskeletal chest pain may be acute and chronic conditions without specific limitations on age.
> - It is imperative to adopt a whole systems approach to clinical examination and diagnostic reasoning in order to provide the answer to the underlying cause of musculoskeletal chest pain.
> - A cardiac or pulmonary cause for chest wall pain should always be sought and ruled out first.
> - Pain which is reproducible on palpation is usually due to a musculoskeletal cause.

References

Barkin R, Rosen P, Hockberger R (1998) *Emergency Medicine, Concepts and Clinical Practice.* Mosby, St Louis.

Chambers J, Bass C, Mayou R (1999) Non-cardiac chest pain: assessment and management. *Heart* **82**: 656.

Cox N, Roper T (2005) *Clinical Skills.* Oxford, Oxford University Press.

Dawes PT, Sheeran TP, Hothersall TE (1988) Chest pain – a common feature of ankylosing spondylitis. *Postgraduate Medical Journal* **64**: 27.

Disla E, Rhim HR, Reddy A, Karten I, Taranta A (1994) Costochondritis. A prospective analysis in an emergency department setting. *Archives of Internal Medicine* **154**(21): 2466–2469.

Douglas G, Nicol F, Robertson C (2005) *Macleod's Clinical Examination*, 11th edition. London, Churchill Livingstone.

Freeston J, Karim Z, Lindsay K, Gough A (2004) Can early diagnosis and management of costochondritis reduce acute chest pain admission? *Journal of Rheumatology* **31**(11): 2269–2271.

Garry JP, Myones B (2005) Costochondritis. e-Medicine available from http://www.emedicine.com/PED/topic487.htm (accessed 3rd March 2006).

Greaves I, Johnson G (2002) *Practical Emergency Medicine*. London, Arnold.

Ho M, Walker S, McGarry F, Pringle S, Pullar T (2001) Chest wall tenderness is unhelpful in the diagnosis of recurrent chest pain. *QJM: An International Journal of Medicine* **94**: 267–270.

Isenberg D, Maddison P, Woo P, Glass D, Breedveld F (2004) *Oxford Textbook of Rheumatology*. Oxford, Oxford University Press.

Kumar P, Clark M (2005) *Clinical Medicine*, 6th edition. London, Elsevier Saunders.

Lee RB, Bass SM, Morris JA, MacKenzie E (1990) Three or more rib fractures as an indicator for transfer to a level 1 center. A population-based study. *Journal of Trauma* **30**(6): 689–694.

Liman ST, Kuzucu A, Tastepe AI, Ulasan GN, Topcu S (2003) Chest injury due to blunt trauma. *European Journal of Cardiothoracic Surgery* **23**: 374–378.

Moulton C, Yates D (2006) *Emergency Medicine*. Oxford, Blackwell Science.

National Institute for Clinical Excellence (2004) *Falls: The Assessment and Prevention of Falls in Older People*. London, NICE.

Pace JB (1975) Commonly overlooked pain syndromes responsive to simple therapy. *Postgraduate Medicine* **58**: 107.

Peavey A (2003) Thoracic trauma. In Peavey A, Newberry L (Eds) *Sheehy's Emergency Nursing, Principles and Practice*, p. 278. St Louis, Mosby.

Purcell D (2003) *Minor Injuries: A Clinical Guide for Rurses*. London, Churchill Livingstone.

Raby N, Berman L, deLacey G (2005) *Accident and Emergency Radiology – A Survival Guide*. London, Elsevier Saunders.

Smith R, Wordsworth P (2005) *Clinical and Biochemical Disorders of the Skeleton*. Oxford, Oxford University press.

Tough J (2004) Assessment and treatment of chest pain. *Nursing Standard* **18**(37): 45–53.

Wardrope J, English B (1998) *Musculo-skeletal Problems in Emergency Medicine*. Oxford, Oxford University Press.

Wardrope J, Ravichandran G, Locker T (2004) Risk assessment for spinal injury after trauma. *British Medical Journal* **328**: 721–723.

Westaby S, Odell J (1999) *Cardiothoracic Trauma*. London, Arnold.

Wise CM (1994) Chest wall syndromes. *Current Opinion in Rheumatology* **66**: 197–202.

Wise CM, Semble EL, Dalton CB (1992) Musculoskeletal chest wall syndromes in patients with noncardiac chest pain: a study of 100 patients. *Archives of Physical and Medical Rehabilitation* **73**: 147.

Wolfe F, Smythe HA, Yunus MB, Bennett RM, Bombardier C, Goldenberg DL (1990) The American College of Rheumatology 1990 criteria for the classification of fibromyalgia. Report of the Multicenter Criteria Committee. *Arthritis and Rheumatism* **33**(2): 160–172.

Useful websites

www.eboncall.co.uk
www.arc.org.uk

Chapter 14

Assessing and managing the patient with pulmonary chest pain

Jenny Tagney and Sarah Green

Introduction

This chapter focuses on the assessment and management of chest pain that results from pulmonary and respiratory causes. These disorders were identified as the most common reason for visiting a general practitioner (GP) or presenting to an emergency department in the United Kingdom (British Thoracic Society 2001b). Incidence and mortality rates can vary considerably around the world and not all pulmonary or respiratory conditions give rise to chest pain. However, the prevalence of these conditions means that numerous healthcare professionals may encounter patients whose chest pain is associated with a pulmonary or respiratory cause.

Aim

This chapter aims to identify characteristics, incidence, investigation, diagnosis, treatment and management of a selection of acute pulmonary and respiratory conditions that can cause chest pain.

Learning outcomes

Through reading this chapter and undertaking any necessary clinical practice with appropriate supervision, the reader should be able to:

- Identify selected respiratory and pulmonary conditions that cause chest pain.
- List identifying characteristics of different types of pulmonary chest pain.
- Identify relevant risk factors for developing specific respiratory illnesses.
- Discuss associated features that may accompany pulmonary chest pain.
- Discuss differential diagnoses in pulmonary chest pain.
- Identify prognostic indicators to aid severity assessment in community acquired pneumonia (CAP).
- Gain an overview of preferred tests and investigations used to confirm suspected diagnosis in the conditions discussed.

Background

Chest pain attributed to pulmonary causes (including pneumonia, pleuritic disease and lung cancer) accounts for approximately 20% of patients presenting in primary care settings and 12% of those presenting in emergency departments in Europe (Cayley 2005). A variety of disorders affecting the lower respiratory tract and lungs may be associated with chest pain. These may be acute (infection, spontaneous injury), progressive (malignancy) and chronic (chronic obstructive pulmonary diseases – COPD), although the latter rarely cause chest pain (National Institute for Clinical Excellence 2004). Many of these patients also exhibit associated symptoms, particularly shortness of breath or breathlessness, which can be a feature of other disease presentations as identified in previous chapters (6, 7, 10). According to the British Thoracic Society (2001b), respiratory illnesses are the cause of one in four deaths in the United Kingdom, with more people dying from respiratory disease than from coronary heart disease (CHD) or non-respiratory cancer.

This chapter will focus on selected acute pulmonary/respiratory conditions where chest pain occurs as one of the key presenting features. The selection is by no means exhaustive but intended to guide the reader towards a likely diagnosis by a thorough assessment of symptoms and signs.

PNEUMONIA

Pneumonias are typically classified as being either community-acquired or hospital-acquired (nosocomial) (Chesnutt and Prendergast 2006). As the latter often occurs as a complication associated with another condition or following other interventional procedures, this chapter will focus on community-acquired pneumonia.

Prospective population studies in Finland, the UK and North America have suggested the incidence of CAP to be between 5 and 11 cases per 1000 (BTS 2001a). It is estimated that over 66,000 people died from pneumonia in the UK in 1999 (BTS 2001a) and it is the sixth leading cause of death in the United States of America (Chesnutt and Prendergast 2006). Approximately 250,000 adults are affected by CAP in the UK annually. Of these, 83,000 are admitted to hospital (33.3%) and those over 65 account for approximately 67% of this figure (Guest and Morris 1997). The British Thoracic Society developed guidelines for the diagnosis and management of CAP (BTS 2001a) and, although these guidelines were updated in 2004, epidemiology figures remain unchanged (BTS 2004).

Pathophysiology

Pneumonia may be defined as an inflammation of the lungs, most frequently caused by bacterial infection (Holgate and Frew 2002). In health, pulmonary defence mechanisms (such as the cough reflex and mucociliary clearance systems) prevent the development of lower respiratory tract infections following aspiration of infected oropharyngeal secretions or inhalation of airborne pathogens

(Chesnutt and Prendergast 2006). CAP occurs when there is a defect in one or more of the normal host defence mechanisms, or when a very large infectious inoculum or highly virulent pathogen overwhelms the host (Chesnutt and Prendergast 2006). Bacteria typically enter the lung with inhalation, though they can reach the lung through the bloodstream if other parts of the body are infected. This invasion triggers release of neutrophils and cytokines, leading to a general activation of the immune system resulting in the fever, chills and fatigue common in CAP. The neutrophils, bacteria and fluid leaked from surrounding blood vessels fill the alveoli and result in impaired oxygen transportation and increased secretions (Light 1999).

Pathogens associated with CAP and their specific clinical features are outlined in Table 14.1, from BTS guidelines (BTS 2001a). In the UK, the most common pathogen responsible for CAP is *Streptococcus pneumoniae*, also known as pneumococcal pneumonia (Farrant 2003) and this is often precipitated by a viral infection with influenza or parainfluenza (Holgate and Frew 2002).

Clinical presentation

As identified in Table 14.1, the clinical presentation will depend to a certain extent on the infecting pathogen but is also affected by the age and immune state of individual patients plus the presence of comorbidities such as chronic obstructive pulmonary disease (BTS 2001a; Holgate and Frew 2002). Patients may present with a cough, which may be productive or non-productive; rapid, shallow breathing; pleuritic chest pain (sharp, localised, respirophasic) or dull chest discomfort and may be pyrexial or hypothermic (Duke et al. 2000; Chesnutt and Prendergast 2006). Older patients are less likely to be pyrexial and may present with non-specific or apparently unrelated symptoms such as a fall or

Table 14.1 Clinical features of specific pathogens associated with CAP. Reproduced with permission from BTS (2001).

Streptococcus pneumoniae
- Increasing age, comorbidity, acute onset, high fever and pleuritic chest pain

Bacteraemic *Streptococcus pneumoniae*
- Female sex, excess alcohol, diabetes mellitus, chronic obstructive pulmonary disease, dry cough

Legionella pneumophila
- Younger patients, smokers, absence of comorbidity, diarrhoea, neurological symptoms, more severe infection, evidence of multisystem involvement (e.g. abnormal liver function tests, elevated serum creatine kinase)

Mycoplasma pneumoniae
- Younger patients, prior antibiotics, less multisystem involvement

Chlamydia pneumoniae
- Longer duration of symptoms before hospital admission, headache

Coxiella burnetii
- Male sex, dry cough, high fever

confusion. They require particularly careful assessment as their mortality risk from pneumonia is high (BTS 2001; Farrant 2003; Chesnutt and Prendergast 2006).

Diffuse pneumonia (bronchopneumonia) is common, particularly as part of a terminal illness. Patients with conditions such as cancer or a dense stroke may be unable to cough up retained secretions, which leads to consolidation within the lungs (Holgate and Frew 2002).

History taking

In addition to recording duration of current symptoms and confirming whether the patient has had a recent viral illness, information regarding altered mental state, loss of appetite and night sweats may be helpful in assisting diagnosis. Evidence of precipitating risk factors such as cigarette smoking, alcohol excess, bronchiectasis (e.g. in cystic fibrosis), previous episodes of pneumonia or diminished immunity may assist in clarifying a clinical picture (Almirall et al. 1999; Holgate and Frew 2002). As elderly patients may present in a confused state with atypical symptoms and are likely to have at least one coexisting illness, their assessment may be more challenging. History of chest injury, particularly in the elderly, is an important feature as pain may have inhibited normal breathing and coughing, thus allowing build-up of secretions leading to increased susceptibility to infection.

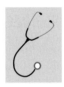

Physical examination

On presentation the patient may appear pale or flushed depending on the presence or absence of fever. Respiratory rate may be increased, with shallow, painful breaths, and observation of chest movements may reveal that the affected side of the chest moves less (if unilateral pneumonia). A raised respiratory rate of >30 per minute is associated with poor outcomes (Holgate and Frew 2002). Palpation of the chest may reveal increased vibration during speech (tactile fremitus), whereas dulled resonance may be evident during chest percussion (particularly if a parapneumonic pleural effusion is present) and basal crackles and/or a pleural rub on the affected side may be heard on auscultation of breath sounds (Holgate and Frew 2002). The presence of bronchial breath sounds heard over the periphery of the lung (as opposed to over the suprasternal notch) is abnormal and implies pulmonary consolidation (Chesnutt and Prendergast 2006).

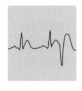

Initial investigations

The BTS (2004) stresses that diagnosis by history and assessment of clinical signs alone is unreliable. The following tests and investigations are recommended for confirming the clinically suspected diagnosis:

- Chest x-ray
- Full blood count
- Urea, electrolytes and liver function tests
- C-reactive protein (CRP) when locally available
- Oxygenation assessment. Those with SaO2 of <92% on pulse oximetry proceed to arterial blood gas measurement
- Blood cultures (not necessary in patients with no comorbid illness or severity factors – see 'assessing severity')
- Sputum cultures for *all* with severe CAP and those patients classified as non-severe who are able to expectorate purulent sputum and have not received prior antibiotic therapy

Specific microbiological tests will be guided by the severity of CAP plus clinical factors such as age, comorbid illness plus epidemiological factors and previous antibiotic therapy (BTS 2004). In those assessed as having severe CAP, a full range of microbiological tests should be performed including blood cultures, sputum cultures, and urine tests for pneumococcal and legionella urine antigen.

Predictive models for assessing severity

Because the recommended treatment of CAP varies according to severity, the updated BTS guidelines have incorporated a six-point scoring tool to guide severity assessment, called the CURB-65 (Lim et al. 2003 cited in BTS 2004). This was developed and tested prospectively on patients from New Zealand, the UK and the Netherlands and is summarised below:

C = confusion	suggest using Abbreviated Mental Test to gain an idea of the severity of the illness
U = urea	a level above 7 mmmol/litre may indicate presence of infection
R = respiratory rate	rates of 30 breaths or more per minute indicates severe disease
B = blood pressure	a blood pressure of below 90 mmHg systolic or 60 mmHg diastolic indicates severe disease

Age ≥ 65

Patients can be individually stratified according to increasing risk of mortality or need for intensive care unit admission. Those scoring 0 or 1 are at low risk of death and classed as having non-severe CAP. They may be considered suitable for home treatment, depending on the social context. Those scoring 2 are at increased risk of death but are still classed as having non-severe CAP. However, hospital assessment and admission should be considered, if only for short-stay treatment. Patients with CURB-65 scores of 3 or more are classed as having severe CAP and are at high risk of death. They require urgent hospitalisation and may require admission to ITU.

The Pneumonia Patient Outcomes Research Team (PORT) have also devised a more complex tool for prognostic risk assessment in patients with CAP used in the USA. Please see Chesnutt and Prendergast (2006) for further details.

Differential diagnosis

The presence of chest pain and breathlessness or shortness of breath can also be features of acute coronary syndromes (ACS), particularly in women (Chapters 6 and 7), and pulmonary embolism (Chapter 10), and can be associated with chest trauma (Chapter 11). Congestive heart failure may also be present and exacerbated by the acute condition, particularly in the elderly, which may be a confounding factor. Other non-cardiac differential diagnoses that should be considered include: upper respiratory tract infections, lung cancer, pulmonary vasculitis, pulmonary thromboembolic disease and atelectasis. The clinical history, specific features and tests, including chest x-ray and ECG interpretation, will assist in clarifying diagnosis but special caution should be taken in assessing elderly patients due to their increased risk and atypical presentations (Farrant 2003).

Immediate management

Non-severe CAP, home management

For those patients assessed as having mild, non-severe CAP (CURB-65 score of 0 or 1), management may continue in the community. They should be advised to rest, to avoid smoking and, especially when febrile, to drink plenty of fluids to maintain adequate hydration. Analgesia such as paracetamol and non-steroidal anti-inflammatory medication may be required to relieve pleuritic chest pain, which is important in order to ensure that patients are able to cough up any secretions. If, however, the cough is non-productive and distressing, suppressants such as simple linctus may be prescribed (Holgate and Frew 2002). Maintaining a good nutritional state is associated with better outcomes, so nutritional supplements may be considered, particularly in the elderly, to avoid any deficit (BTS 2001a).

Hypoxia is common due to inadequate ventilation, which can lead to tachypnoea, dyspnoea, altered mental state and increased chest discomfort. However, it may be non-specific and may be difficult to detect in the early stages (BTS 2001a). Pulse oximetry is used increasingly within primary care to assess arterial oxygen saturation (SaO_2) when reviewing patients at home. However, whilst supporting increased use of pulse oximetry, the BTS guidelines also recommend appropriate training in its use and in interpreting results, as patients with poor peripheral perfusion, jaundice and pigmented skin can exhibit potentially false low readings (BTS 2001a, 2004).

Treatment strategies and specific choice of antibiotic therapy vary globally, and the contentious issue seems to revolve around specific versus empiric treatments (BTS 2004; Chesnutt and Prendergast 2006). The BTS make their empiric recommendations based on the large body of epidemiological evidence to suggest that the majority of patients with CAP in the UK are infected with *Streptococcus pneumoniae*. Empiric treatments are therefore aimed at this pathogen initially but may be changed if the patient fails to respond, or subsequent microbiological tests indicate that alternative treatments may be more appropriate. See Table 14.2 for a summary.

Table 14.2 Preferred and alternative empirical treatment for CAP. Reproduced with permission from BTS (2004).

	Preferred	Alternative*
Home treated – not severe	Amoxicillin 500 mg – 1 g tds po	Erythromycin 500 mg qds po *or* clarithromycin 500 mg bd po
Hospital treated – not severe	Amoxicillin 500 mg – 1 g tds po *plus* erythromycin 500 mg qds po	Fluoroquinolone with some enhanced pneumococcal activity, e.g. moxifloxacin (for doses see BNF 2006) *or* levofloxacin 500 mg od po
● If intravenous treatment needed:	Ampicillin 500 mg qds iv *or* benzylpenicillin 1.2 g qds iv *plus* erythromycin 500 mg qds iv *or* clarithromycin 500 mg bd iv	Levofloxacin 500 mg od iv *(moxifloxacin not licensed for iv use in UK at time of guidance)*
Hospital treated, severe	Co-amoxiclav 1.2 g tds *or* cefuroxime 1 g tds *or* ceftriaxone 2 g od *(all iv) plus* erythromycin 500 mg qds iv *or* clarithromycin 500 mg bd iv *(with or without rifampicin 600 mg od or bd iv)*	Fluoroquinolone with some enhanced pneumococcal activity, e.g. levofloxacin 500 mg bd iv *plus* benzylpenicillin 1.2 g qds iv

*Alternative is provided for those intolerant of or hypersensitive to the preferred regimen, or where there are local concerns over *Clostridium difficile* associated diarrhoea.
bd = Twice daily; iv = intravenous; po = oral; qds = four times per day; tds = three times per day.

Patients who fail to improve after 48 hours should be considered for hospital admission.

Non-severe CAP, hospital management

All the above principles still apply to this group but they will additionally benefit from high-flow oxygen therapy of 35% if SaO_2 < 92%, unless complicated by COPD. Patients with pre-existing COPD may have carbon dioxide retention, therefore high-concentration oxygen can reduce hypoxic drive and increase ventilation/perfusion mismatching (BTS 2001a). Lower starting concentrations of continuous O_2 (24–28%) should be used first, up-titrating in accordance with serial arterial blood gas measurements, keeping PaO_2 > 6.65 kPa and pH < 7.26 as per COPD management guidelines (BTS 2001a).

Severe CAP, hospital management +/– ITU

For those with severe CAP (CURB-65 score of 3 or above), hospitalisation is mandatory and consideration for high dependency or intensive care unit admission may be necessary along with intravenous antibiotics, pain relief, fluid resuscitation and either invasive or non-invasive ventilatory (NIV) support. Persistent PaO_2 < 8 kPa +/– $PaCO_2$ ≥6 kPa on arterial blood gas measurement (see Table 14.3

Table 14.3 Normal arterial blood gas values (normal ranges).

H⁺	35–45 mmol/l	pH 7.35–7.45
PO_2	10–13.3 kPa	(75–100 mmHg)
PCO_2	4.8–6.1 kPa	(36–46 mmHg)
Base deficit	+/–2.5	
Plasma HCO_3^-	22–26 mmol/l	
O_2 saturation	95–100%	

for normal ranges) despite maximal oxygen administration, progressive hypercapnia and exhaustion, severe acidosis (pH < 7.26, base excess < –8), shock or depressed consciousness are all indications for HDU/ITU admission with ventilatory and cardiovascular support. The BTS note that, whilst patients treated with NIV may initially improve, there is over 50% failure rate. Therefore, close monitoring is recommended, particularly in those aged over 40 years or those with an initial respiratory rate of >38 (BTS 2004). Additional nutritional support should also be considered, either via enteral (nasogastric, gastrostomy, jejunostomy) or parenteral (peripheral or via central venous route) feeding (BTS 2001a); Kumar and Clark 2002).

Medium- to long-term management plan

Failure to improve or respond to antibiotic treatment should prompt further investigations/tests for more unusual pathogens plus other underlying pathology, and treatment altered accordingly. Holgate and Frew (2002) suggest the overall mortality for patients admitted to hospital with CAP is approximately 5% and the most common reason cited for death is not receiving appropriate antibiotics of sufficient doses. However, in severe CAP, mortality rates are nearer 50%.

Once patients are being considered for discharge, it is important to ensure that this is not attempted too soon. One study from North America demonstrated that 20% of patients in hospital with CAP were discharged despite having one or more 'unstable' factor present within the previous 24 hours. These included temperature > 37.8°C, heart rate > 100 beats per minute, respiratory rate > 24 breaths per minute, systolic blood pressure < 90 mmHg and oxygen saturation <90% amongst others. Of those discharged with two or more of these features, 46% died or were readmitted within 30 days. In contrast, only 11% of those with no such features died or were readmitted (Halm et al. 2002). Therefore, patients should be reviewed 24 hours prior to planned discharge and should remain in hospital if unstable features are present (BTS 2004).

Longer term strategies for prevention

There is still some debate as to the effectiveness of vaccination against pneumococcal pneumonia, although there is acknowledgement of some benefit in 'at risk' groups such as those over 65 years (Willcox 2003). Within England, all those aged over 65 are entitled to pneumococcal vaccination and it is currently offered at the same time as the influenza vaccine, also thought to assist in reducing incidence of severe influenza leading to pneumonia (Willcox 2003). The BTS point to an expected new conjugate pneumococcal vaccine to help improve reduction in disease prevalence (BTS 2004).

PLEURISY

Pleurisy or pleuritis is the term used to describe the pain arising from any inflammation of the pleura (Holgate and Frew 2002; Chesnutt and Prendergast 2006) . Localized inflammation produces the typically described sharp, localised chest or thoracic pain, worse on deep inspiration, coughing, sneezing and sometimes when twisting or bending movements are made (Holgate and Frew 2002; Chesnutt and Prendergast 2006). There may be referred pain. For example, if the diaphragmatic area of the pleura is inflamed, shoulder pain may be the presenting symptom.

Causes

In young, otherwise healthy individuals, the cause is usually a viral respiratory infection or pneumonia. Pleurisy also occurs with pulmonary infarct, carcinoma and, more rarely, in rheumatoid arthritis and systemic lupus erythematosus (Holgate and Frew 2002). Simple rib fracture can induce severe pleuritis (Chesnutt and Prendergast 2006).

Treatment

This mostly consists of treating the underlying cause (see also pneumonia above, and pleural effusion below) and controlling pain with analgesia and nonsteroidal anti-inflammatory medications.

PLEURAL EFFUSION

A pleural effusion is an abnormal collection of fluid in the pleural space signifying a variety of underlying mechanisms and diseases (Hayes 2001; Maskell and Butland 2003). Pleural effusions are a common problem and the patient's symptoms and any coexisting illness will determine the prognosis (Allibone 2006). The British Thoracic Society issued guidelines for the diagnosis and management of both unilateral (Maskell and Butland 2003) and malignant (Antunes et al. 2003) pleural effusions.

Causes

Up to 57% of patients with bacterial pneumonia also develop a pleural effusion – so-called 'parapneumonic effusion'. Pleural effusions can also arise as a result of other pathology including other infections, malignancy, or inflammatory

Table 14.4 Drugs reported to cause pleural effusions (rarely). Reproducted with permission from Maskell and Butland 2003.

Over 100 reported cases globally
- Amiodorone
- Nitrofurantoin
- Phenytoin
- Methotrexate

20–100 reported cases globally
- Carbamazepine
- Procainamide
- Propylthiouracil
- Penicillamine
- Recombinant human granulocyte-colony stimulating factor (G-CSF)
- Cyclophosphamide
- Bromocriptine

Table 14.5 Causes of pleural effusions. (Maskell and Butland 2003: Allibone 2006).

	Transudates	Exudates
Common	Left ventricular failure Liver cirrhosis Hypoalbuminaemia Peritoneal dialysis	Malignancy Parapneumonic effusions Other infections
Less common	Hypothyroidism Nephrotic syndrome Mitral stenosis Pulmonary embolism	Pulmonary infarction Rheumatoid arthritis Autoimmune diseases Benign asbestos effusion Pancreatitis Post-myocardial infarction syndrome
Rare	Constrictive pericarditis Urinothorax Superior vena cava obstruction	Drugs (see Table 14.2) Fungal infections Sarcoidosis Oesophageal perforation

processes (Davies et al. 2003; Allibone 2006). Rarely, pleural effusions may also be caused by certain medications (see Table 14.4). Classification of the type of effusion is dictated by the causative mechanism, explained below and listed in Table 14.5.

Pathophysiology

The pleura are the serous, semi-transparent, elastic membranes covering the lung parenchyma, mediastinum, diaphragm and rib cage. They are made up of two layers – the visceral and parietal pleura, which are in close contact, giving rise to a potential rather than actual space (Allibone 2006). Pleural effusions are classified as transudates or exudates and arise from a variety of causes (see Table 14.5). A transudative pleural effusion occurs when there is an altered balance of hydrostatic pressures influencing formation and absorption of pleural fluid such that fluid accumulates. An exudative pleural effusion develops when the permeability of the pleural surface and/or local capillaries is altered (Maskell and Butland 2003), usually due to disease of the pleura (Allibone 2006).

Clinical presentation

Patients will often present with dyspnoea, dry cough and features associated with the underlying disease (e.g. cardiac failure or pneumonia) and complain of persistent pleuritic chest pain or chest discomfort described as a heavy sensation (Allibone 2006; Chesnutt and Prendergast 2006). However, some patients may be asymptomatic and the effusion is discovered on routine chest x-ray (Sahn and Heffner 2003). Patients with existing cardiopulmonary disease are likely to be more symptomatic than those without. In symptomatic patients, pleuritic pain is present in approximately 75% of those subsequently found to have pleural effusion and pulmonary embolism (Maskell and Butland 2003). Additionally, patients may present with weight loss and lethargy if there is underlying malignancy.

History taking

Severity of symptoms may influence when patients present to healthcare professionals and relates to the specific pathology involved. Severity also influences whether patients present in primary care or emergency departments. Delayed presentation of patients with pneumonia adds to the likelihood of developing a parapneumonic pleural effusion (Light 2001). Information regarding general health, recent infections, appetite, diet, weight gain or loss, investigations or treatments for other conditions will give important clues regarding potentially altered physiology. Detailed medication history (start dates, doses, recent changes) should also be sought as, although uncommon, some have been reported as causing pleural effusions (see Table 14.4). Combined with careful evaluation of physical signs and symptoms, such information will guide practitioners in assessing the likelihood and type of pleural effusion.

Physical examination

General examination should assess for signs of cardiopulmonary disease (see Chapter 4) and signs of rheumatoid arthritis or other disease processes implicated in pathophysiological processes contributing to formation of pleural effusions (see Table 14.5). Specific physical findings will depend on the size of the effusion, underlying pathology and severity of symptoms, and are usually absent in small effusions (Chesnutt and Prendergast 2006). In larger effusions, the respiratory rate is often increased and breathing may be altered due to pleuritic pain associated with inspiration. Percussion of the chest may indicate dullness on the affected side in larger effusions, while pulmonary auscultation may reveal diminished or absent breath sounds over the effusion. If the effusion is causing compressive atelectasis, bronchial breath sounds and egophony (increased resonance of voice sounds) may be heard just over the effusion (Chesnutt and Prendergast 2006). If there is atelectasis and reduced expansion, oxygen saturation may be reduced, particularly if there is underlying cardiopulmonary disease.

Differential diagnosis

Specific clinical presentation and underlying disease mechanisms greatly influence symptoms but differential diagnoses can include malignant mesothelioma, pneumonia and pulmonary embolus (Allibone 2006).

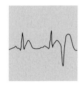

Initial investigations

Other than confirmatory chest x-ray, investigations will depend on the suspected cause of the pleural effusion, based on clinical presentation and underlying pathology. For example, pleural aspiration is not recommended in the context of bilateral effusions in a clinical setting strongly suggestive of a pleural transudate (e.g. left ventricular failure), unless there are atypical features or there is no response to other therapy (e.g. intravenous diuretics) (Maskell and Butland 2003).

Radiography

Chest x-ray will confirm the presence, position and approximate volume of a suspected pleural effusion and will assist in evaluating the aetiology (transudate or exudate) plus the presence of any diagnostic abnormalities above the fluid levels or in the opposite lung (Allibone 2006). Pleural fluid characteristically shows up as a dense, white shadow with a concave upper edge or fluid level (Bourke 2003). Ideally, a posterior–anterior, upright chest x-ray will be performed as much of this diagnostic information is lost if the patient is supine (as may be the case in patients in intensive care settings), causing the fluid to layer out posteriorly (Allibone 2006).

Ultrasound

This is more accurate than plain x-ray for estimating fluid volume and can aid identification of appropriate location if thoracocentesis or biopsy is planned. It is also helpful in distinguishing pleural fluid from pleural thickening and identifying whether the fluid is loculated (trapped in pockets) (Bourke 2003).

Computerised tomography (CT) scan

This investigation is most helpful in differentiating between benign and malignant tumours and evaluating the underlying lung parenchyma, and can assist in identifying the most appropriate site for pleural biopsy (Maskell and Butland 2003). However, ultrasound is the investigation of choice in identifying the presence or absence of pleural fluid (Allibone 2006).

Pleural aspiration and pleural fluid analysis

When there is no clinically apparent cause for a new pleural effusion, diagnostic thoracocentesis should be performed to remove a sample of the fluid gathered in the pleural space for further evaluation (Maskell and Butland 2003). The gross appearance of pleural fluid may be illuminating, purulent fluid signifying empyema (Chesnutt and Prendergast 2006) and bloodstained fluid indicating malignancy, pulmonary infarction or severe inflammation (Allibone 2006). Colour and odour should be noted and samples analysed for:

- Protein
- Lactate dehydrogenase (LDH)
- pH
- Gram stain
- Cytology
- Microbiological culture

Identification of exudative or transudative pleural fluid is achieved through tests comparing protein and LDH levels (see Maskell and Butland 2003). The normal pH of pleural fluid is slightly alkaline (around 7.64). A low pH signifies an exudate and may be associated with malignancy, tuberculosis or rheumatoid arthritis (Hayes 2001). A pH less than 7.2 suggests empyema (Allibone 2006).

Gram staining and microbiological culture of pleuritic fluid is of diagnostic value if infection is suspected. Stains for acid-fast organisms are necessary if TB is suspected (Buchanan and Neville 2004).

Cytologic evaluation of pleural fluid is recommended in all exudative effusions and in any patients suspected of underlying malignancy (Chesnutt and Prendergast 2006). Sixty percent of malignant cases will be diagnosed with the first sample (Maskell and Butland 2003). However, negative results in highly clinically suggestive cases should be repeated and followed up by pleural biopsy if necessary (Maskell and Butland 2003; Chesnutt and Prendergast 2006).

Immediate management

Transudates

Treatment is aimed at the underlying condition and, in 90% of cases, this will be congestive heart failure where the mainstay of treatment is often administration of intravenous diuretics. Therapeutic thoracocentesis is rarely indicated for relief of breathlessness (Allibone 2006; Chesnutt and Prendergast 2006). Administration of oxygen and analgesia plus anti-inflammatory medication to relieve any pleuritic pain may also be indicated. If the heart failure is treated successfully, effusions usually resolve in less than a month (Cohen and Sahn 2001).

Exudates

In contrast, only selected exudate effusions are likely to resolve following treatment of the underlying cause, e.g. drug-induced or secondary to collagen vascular disease (Cohen and Sahn 2001). Empyema requires prompt treatment with appropriate antibiotics and insertion of a chest drain (Allibone 2006). Malignant effusions are often large and patients may require therapeutic thoracocentesis for relief of breathlessness (Antunes et al. 2003). However, further treatment will depend on prognosis from the underlying disease, the primary tumour and its response to systemic treatment and lung re-expansion following removal of pleural fluid. Choices may include thoracic surgery or intercostal tube drainage and pleurodesis (Antunes et al. 2003), although palliative care options should also be considered.

SPONTANEOUS PNEUMOTHORAX

Pneumothorax is an accumulation of air in the pleural cavity and can be classed as spontaneous (primary or secondary) or traumatic (Chesnutt and Prendergast 2006). Primary spontaneous pneumothorax occurs in the absence of underlying lung disease and affects mainly tall, slim males aged between 10 and 30 years (Chesnutt and Prendergast 2006), with a reported global incidence of approximately 18–32/100,000 per year (Henry et al. 2003). The male-to-female ratio is estimated as 6:1 (Holgate and Frew 2002), with an approximate incidence of 1.2–6/100,000 in women (Henry et al. 2003). Secondary spontaneous pneumothorax occurs as a complication of pre-existing pulmonary disease, the most common being chronic obstructive pulmonary disease (COPD) with bronchial asthma, carcinoma, severe pulmonary fibrosis with cyst formation, cystic fibrosis and tuberculosis being rarer causes (Holgate and Frew 2002; Chesnutt and Prendergast 2006).

Pathophysiology

It is thought that sub-pleural blebs or bullae (cyst or blister type structures) play a significant role in the pathogenesis of primary spontaneous pneumothorax as they are found in up to 90% of cases at thoracoscopy or thoracotomy and in up to 80% of cases on CT scanning of the thorax (Henry et al. 2003). Primary spontaneous pneumothorax is thought to be caused by the rupture of these pleural blebs or bullae. The precise aetiology is uncertain, although they may be associated with congenital defects in the connective tissue of the alveolar walls (Holgate and Frew 2002) and there is increased incidence in tall, slim people (Henry et al. 2003). Those who smoke have an increased risk (Henry et al. 2003) and there may be a family history of spontaneous pneumothorax (Chesnutt and Prendergast 2006).

In a small percentage of cases (2–5%), haemothorax may complicate spontaneous pneumothoraces but anecdotal reports suggest that non-traumatic haemopneumothoraces may also occur spontaneously, with bleeding most commonly resulting from a tear in the visceral pleura or rupture of a vascilated bulla (Hart et al. 2002).

Clinical presentation

The onset of chest pain in spontaneous pneumothorax is usually sudden, pleuritic and unilateral and can be mild to severe on the affected side. In most patients, it is accompanied by progressively increasing dyspnoea (Chesnutt and Prendergast 2006). Initially, symptoms begin at rest and in some mild cases can resolve within 24 hours, even if the pneumothorax persists, in previously healthy individuals. In general, clinical symptoms associated with secondary pneumothoraces are worse than those related to primary pneumothoraces (Henry et al. 2003) and patients may present with life-threatening respiratory failure if underlying COPD or asthma is present (Chesnutt and Prendergast 2006). However, severity of symptoms is not a reliable indicator of pneumothorax size (Henry et al. 2003).

Often, patients with primary pneumothoraces do not seek immediate medical advice, with up to 46% waiting two or more days with symptoms (Henry et al. 2003). This is an important feature because the occurrence of re-expansion pulmonary oedema after re-inflation may be related to length of time the lung has been collapsed (Henry et al. 2003).

History taking

Ascertaining time of onset of symptoms is important as it can indicate the potential clinical path and potential recovery problems (see previous paragraph).

Age, general health status, smoking and family history of spontaneous pneumothorax are important elements to determine in addition to any previous personal history of spontaneous pneumothorax. The risk of recurrence of primary pneumothorax is 54% within 4 years (Henry et al. 2003). Although there are no known precipitating events for either primary or secondary pneumothorax, in those with a known history of pulmonary disease it is important to establish whether they have had a recent acute infection or a decrease in respiratory function as this may inform treatment plans.

Location, nature and severity of any chest discomfort and dyspnoea must be established and monitored as increases may indicate enlargement of the pneumothorax (Holgate and Frew 2002).

Physical examination

If the patient is a tall, slim, young, cigarette-smoking male with suggestive symptoms as described above, a high degree of clinical suspicion is indicated for the possibility of primary spontaneous pneumothorax. The patient may have a mild tachycardia (rates of 100–110) and may be tachypnoeic, and signs of unequal chest movement may be evident.

Palpation of the chest at the suprasternal notch will identify any mediastinal or tracheal deviation. Tension pneumothorax should be suspected if this is accompanied by marked tachycardia and hypotension (Chesnutt and Prendergast 2006). Chest percussion may reveal an area of hyper-resonance over the affected side (Chesnutt and Prendergast 2006). In patients with a pneumothorax, breath sounds heard during chest auscultation may be reduced or absent on the affected side (Holgate and Frew 2002). If the pneumothorax is small (less than 15% of a hemithorax), other than mild tachycardia, physical findings may be unimpressive.

Initial investigations

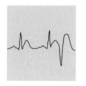

Clinical history and physical examination are often sufficient to suggest the presence of a pneumothorax, although gauging the size in this way is unreliable (Henry et al. 2003).

Chest radiograph

A plain chest x-ray is the diagnostic tool of choice in both primary and secondary pneumothoraces. If a pneumothorax is suspected but not confirmed by a standard posterior–anterior (PA) x-ray, lateral views may add additional information in up to 14% of cases (Henry et al. 2003). In patients suspected of diffuse bullous lung disease, CT scanning will differentiate between emphysematous bullae and pneumothoraces, saving the patient from an unnecessary and potentially dangerous aspiration (Henry et al. 2003).

Electrocardiograph (ECG)

This test may prove unhelpful as left-sided primary pneumothorax may produce left axis deviation and precordial ECG changes, which may be misinterpreted as acute myocardial infarction.

Laboratory tests

Arterial blood gas measurements are frequently abnormal, revealing hypoxaemia PO_2 (<8 kPa) and acute respiratory alkalosis (pH > 7.46) in most patients, which may be worse in patients with underlying pulmonary disease (Henry et al. 2003; Chesnutt and Prendergast 2006).

Pulmonary function tests are weakly sensitive to detection of a pneumothorax and are not recommended (Henry et al. 2003).

Differential diagnosis

Occasionally, a pneumothorax may mimic myocardial infarction (see above), pulmonary embolisation or pneumonia (Chesnutt and Prendergast 2006).

Targeted history, clinical examination and results of relevant tests are required to clarify the diagnosis as detailed above.

Immediate management and interventions

This will depend on the size and severity of the pneumothorax and the nature of any underlying disease. If the primary pneumothorax is small (<2 cm on PA chest x-ray) and closed and there is no significant breathlessness, no immediate intervention is indicated (Henry et al. 2003). Patients with a primary pneumothorax in this category do not require admission to hospital but should be considered for early discharge and early out-patient follow-up, with clear guidance regarding what to do if they experience increased breathlessness before their appointment (Henry et al. 2003). Many pneumothoraces resolve spontaneously as air is absorbed from the pleural space, and supplementary oxygenation can increase the rate of reabsorption (Chesnutt and Prendergast 2006).

Secondary pneumothoraces are also treated according to size but 'small' is classified as 1 cm or less, equivalent to 15% of the hemithorax. If patients experience minimal symptoms, admission to hospital for observation and monitoring of any change in condition is recommended (Henry et al. 2003).

Patients with primary or secondary pneumothoraces of 2 cm or greater, as confirmed by PA chest film, and those experiencing breathlessness or chest discomfort require active treatment. Severe breathlessness in patients with a small primary pneumothorax may herald tension pneumothorax (Henry et al. 2003). Supplemental, high flow (10 litres/min) oxygen should be administered as this may help to reduce the total pressure of gases in the pleural capillaries by reducing the partial pressure of nitrogen (Henry et al. 2003).

Simple aspiration is recommended by the BTS for all primary pneumothoraces requiring intervention (dictated by size of pneumothorax and severity of symptoms). It can be considered in minimally breathless patients with small secondary pneumothoraces as an initial treatment strategy but is more likely to fail in this group (Henry et al. 2003). Repeat aspiration is considered reasonable in primary pneumothorax but secondary cases should progress to tube drainage where simple aspiration fails.

Tube or catheter drainage and connection to underwater sealed systems is recommended in patients with larger pneumothoraces, tension pneumothorax or severe symptoms (Henry et al. 2003; Chesnutt and Prendergast 2006).

Medium- to long-term management

Where patients experience recurrent pneumothoraces, treatment options are similar to those for pleural effusions and include pleurodesis, transaxillary minithoractomy, video assisted thoracoscopic surgery (VATS) or thoracic surgery such as open thoracotomy and pleurectomy (Henry et al. 2003).

Key learning points

- Community acquired pneumonia (CAP) is treated at home or in hospital according to severity assessment.
- Specific clinical features of CAP are associated with the specific causative pathogen.
- People over 65 with CAP may present with non-specific symptoms and are at higher risk of poor outcomes.
- Pleurisy or pleuritis is the term given to describe pain arising from inflammation of the pleura and may be due to a variety of mechanisms.
- Pleural effusions are classed as transudates or exudates.
- If initial pleural aspiration test for cytology is negative, one further sample should be checked followed by pleural biopsy in clinically suspicious cases.
- Tall, slim, young, cigarette-smoking males presenting with acute onset, unilateral, pleuritic chest pain should generate high levels of clinical suspicion for spontaneous primary pneumothorax.

References and useful websites

Allibone L (2006) Assessment and management of patients with pleural effusions. *Nursing Standard* **20**(22): 55–64.

Almirall J, Bolibar I, Balanzo X, Gonzalez CA (1999) Risk factors for community acquired pneumonia in adults: a population-based case-control study. *European Respiratory Journal* **13**: 349.

Antunes G, Neville E, Duffy J, Ali N *on behalf of the BTS Pleural Disease Group* (2003) British Thoracic Society Guidelines for the management of malignant pleural effusions. *Thorax* **58**(Suppl. II): ii29–ii38.

Bourke SJ (2003) *Lecture Notes on Respiratory Medicine*, 6th edition. Oxford Blackwell Publishing.

British National Formulary (2006) Antibiotic therapy, respiratory system. www.bnf.org/bnf/bnf/current/102037.htm.

British Thoracic Society (2001a) Guidelines for the management of adults with community acquired pneumonia (CAP). *Thorax* **56**(Suppl. IV). Also available via www.brit-thoracic.org/guidelines (accessed 16th May 2006).

British Thoracic Society (2001b) *The Burden of Lung Disease. A Statistics Report from the BTS.* www.brit-thoracic.org (accessed 28th April 2006).

British Thoracic Society (2004) Guidelines for the management of community acquired pneumonia (CAP) in adults – 2004 update. www.brit-thoracic.org/guidelines (accessed 16th May 2006).

Buchanan DR, Neville E (2004) *Thoracoscopy for Physicians: A Practical Guide.* Arnold, London.

Cayley WE (2005) Diagnosing the cause of chest pain. *American Family Physician* **72**(10): 2012–2021. www.aafp.org/afp (accessed 15th March 2006).

Chesnutt M, Prendergast TJ (2006) Lung. In: Tierney LM Jr, McPhee SJ, Papadakis MA *Current Medical Diagnosis and Treatment*, 45th edition, pp. 9218–9311. New York, Lange Medical Books.

Cohen M, Sahn SA (2001) Resolution of pleural effusions. *Chest,* **119**(5): 1547–1562.

Davies CWH, Gleeson FV, Davies RJ (2003) British Thoracic Society guidelines for the management of pleural infection. *Thorax* **58**(Suppl II): 18–28.

Duke JR, Good JT, Hudson LD, Hyers TM, Iseman MD, Mergenthaler DD, Murray JF, Petty TL, Rollins DR (2000) Frontline Assessment of Common Pulmonary Presentations. National Lung Health Education Programme. The Snowdrift Pulmonary Foundation, Denver. www.nlhep.org (accessed 28th April 2006).

Farrant A (2003) Better than a cure. *Nursing Standard.* **18**(3): 18–19.

Guest JF, Morris A (1997) Community acquired pneumonia: the annual cost to the National Health Service in the UK. *European Respiratory Journal* **10**(7): 1530–1534.

Halm EA, Fine MJ, Kapoor WN (2002) Instability on hospital discharge and the risk of adverse outcomes in patients with pneumonia. *Archives of Internal Medicine.* **162**: 1278–1284.

Hart SR, Willis C, Thorn A, Barfoot L (2002) Spontaneous haemopneumothorax: are guidelines overdue? *Emergency Medical Journal* **19**: 273–274.

Hayes DD (2001) Stemming the tide of pleural effusions. *Nursing Management* **32**(10): 30–34.

Henry M, Arnold T, Harvey J *on behalf of the BTS Pleural Disease Group* (2003) British Thoracic Society guidelines for the management of spontaneous pneumothorax. *Thorax* **58**(Suppl. II): ii39–ii52. www.brit-thoracic.org/guidelines (accessed 10th May 2006).

Holgate ST, Frew A (2002) Respiratory disease. In Kumar P, Clark M *Clinical Medicine*, 5th edition. Oxford, WB Saunders.

Kumar P, Clark M (Eds) (2002) *Clinical Medicine*, 5th edition, Oxford, WB Saunders.

Light RB (1999) Pulmonary pathophysiology of pneumococcal pneumonia. *Seminars in Respiratory Infection* **14**(3): 218–226.

Light RW (2001) *Pleural Diseases*, 4th edition. Philadelphia, Lippincott Williams and Wilkins.

Lim WS, van der Eerden MM et al. (2003) Defining community acquired pneumonia severity on presentation to hospital: an international derivation and validation study. *Thorax* **58**: 377–382, cited in British Thoracic Society Guidelines (2004) www.brit-thoracic.org/guidelines.

Maskell NA, Butland RJA *on behalf of the BTS Pleural Disease Group* (2003) British Thoracic Society Guidelines for the investigation of a unilateral pleural effusion in adults. *Thorax* **58**(Suppl. II): ii8–ii17.

National Institute for Clinical Excellence (2004) Chronic obstructive pulmonary disease. Management of chronic obstructive pulmonary disease in adults in primary and secondary care. Clinical guideline 12 developed by the National Collaborating Centre for Chronic Conditions. www.nice.org.uk/CG012NICEguideline (accessed 12th May 2006).

Sahn S, Heffner J (2003) Pleural fluid analysis. Cited in Light RW, Lee G (Eds) *Textbook of Pleural Diseases* pp. 191–210. London, Arnold.

Willcox A (2003) Ready for vaccination. *Nursing Standard* **18**(3): 19.

Chapter 15

Assessing and managing the patient with chest pain due to cardiac syndrome X, cocaine misuse and herpes zoster

John W. Albarran and Helen Cox

Introduction

In addition to the more common causes of chest pain, there are other subtle presentations that lead health professionals to suspect that the presenting symptoms of a patient relate to conditions other than coronary heart disease. While chest pain induced by cardiac syndrome X, recreational use of cocaine or herpes zoster has been considered unusual or even rare, the incidence and detection level seem to be on the increase. Exploring these conditions will help to advance the knowledge and skills of health staff in assessing for differential diagnoses.

Aim

The aim of this chapter is to specifically review how symptoms chest pain manifest in cardiac syndrome X, recreational use of cocaine and herpes zoster, and how these differ from other cardiac and non-cardiac conditions. In addition, other aspects of clinical presentation, as well as assessment and management priorities, will be discussed in detail.

Learning outcomes

Following the completion of this chapter, the reader will have:

- An understanding of the rates of morbidity and mortality associated with cardiac syndrome X, cocaine misuse and herpes zoster.
- An appreciation of the underlying causes and pathophysiology of cardiac syndrome X, misuse of cocaine and herpes zoster.
- An ability to assess and distinguish the unique characteristics of chest pain and related symptoms linked with cardiac syndrome X, misuse of cocaine and herpes zoster.
- Awareness of specific clinical investigations for establishing a differential diagnosis.
- An appreciation of the acute and long-term treatment for individuals diagnosed with cardiac syndrome X, misuse of cocaine and herpes zoster.

CARDIAC SYNDROME X

Background

The term 'cardiac syndrome X' (cardiac SX) was first coined in 1973 but controversy remains over the lack of a universal definition. Currently it is accepted that the syndrome encompasses a triad of symptoms including:

- The presence of exertional angina-like chest pain
- Exercise-induced ST segment depression
- Angiographically normal coronary arteries

Additionally, an absence of spontaneous or provoked coronary artery spasm and cardiac or systemic diseases that may be linked with microvascular dysfunction are integral to the overall definition (Crea and Lanza 2004; Kaski et al. 2004; Pasqui et al. 2005).

In recent years, the incidence of the syndrome has increased due to wider acceptance of this diagnosis. Cardiac SX affects both genders, although 60–70% of those who are diagnosed with this syndrome tend to be women, the majority of whom are post-menopausal (Maseri 2004).

Despite an excellent prognosis of low mortality rates and a decreased risk of cardiovascular events compared with patients with coronary heart disease (CHD), patients with cardiac syndrome X have a poor quality of life (Kaski et al. 2004). This is often due to persistent and worsening angina-like symptoms (Crea and Lanza 2004). High rates of psychiatric morbidity are particularly common in around 30% of patients with cardiac SX. Evidence of psychological morbidity in the form of poor health and general anxiety, as well as depression, have also been identified in 30% of women with cardiac SX (Asbury et al. 2004). Reasons for anxiety and depression may include:

- Inadequate reassurance about the limiting effects of the symptoms
- Doubts over the diagnosis
- Failure of traditional treatments to improve quality of life
- Recurrent episodes of chest pain (Crea and Lanza 2004; Kaski et al. 2004)

Gurjinder et al. (2001) add that when angiography does not confirm evidence of CHD or other aetiology, rather than being reassured, patients' anxiety levels may worsen and further contribute to their chronic chest pain. These factors may impact negatively on the health, social and economic status of patients.

Causes

The exact causes of cardiac syndrome X remain a mystery. Smoking, oestrogen deficiency and high cholesterol may contribute to the pathogenesis of cardiac SX, although their specific role remains elusive (Kaski 2004). Patients excluded from the diagnosis of cardiac SX are those in whom angina is known to be caused by left ventricular hypertrophy, hypertension, diabetes mellitus and epicardial coronary artery spasm (Kaski et al. 2004).

Pathophysiology

Several competing theories have been proposed to explain cardiac SX. These relate to either ischaemic or non-ischaemic mechanisms (Schwartz and Bourassa 2001; Kaski et al. 2004).

Ischaemic mechanisms

Coronary microvascular dysfunction

Abnormalities in coronary blood flow caused by microvascular endothelial dysfunction are speculated to be highly significant. In health, the endothelium is responsible for local regulation of vascular tone and ventricular function. An intact endothelium maintains a balance through release of nitric oxide (NO), causing vessel dilatation, and the peptide endothelin 1 (ET-I), which initiates vasoconstriction. This balance can be affected by injury, damage or toxicity of the endothelium. For example, raised levels of C–reactive protein, monocyte chemotactic protein-1 and structural vessel damage can impair the functioning of the endothelium and coronary flow reserve, altering the bio-availability of NO and ET-1 (Desideri et al. 2000; On et al. 2005; Pasqui et al. 2005). Interestingly, a lower basal NO/ET-1 ratio has also been observed in cardiac SX patients, supporting the premise that abnormalities in the levels of NO and ET-I are integral to the pathogenesis of this syndrome (Kaski et al. 2004). It is, however, questionable whether the degree of microvascular dysfunction can cause cardiac ischaemia (Crea 2003). In addition to the known factors leading to endothelial dysfunction, smoking, lipids, obesity, diabetes mellitus and oestrogen deficiency may be responsible for precipitating these effects (Kaski et al. 2004).

Oestrogen deficiency

Oestrogen deficiency occurring in post-menopausal women has been implicated as having a pathogenic role in this syndrome (Kaski 2002). Indeed, post-menopausal women comprise 70% of patients who are eventually diagnosed with cardiac SX. In such individuals, the administration of exogenous oestrogen has been demonstrated to decrease episodes of chest pain (Crea and Lanza 2004; Kaski et al. 2004). Improvements in frequency and duration of pain were attributed to the endothelial mediated vasodilatory properties of oestrogens.

Myocardial ischaemia

Myocardial ischaemia has also been implicated in the pathogenesis of cardiac SX. However, there are a number of reasons why the role of myocardial ischaemia has been rejected. These are linked to: the good prognosis, a limited response to nitrates, the presence of normal findings during stress echocardiography, and lack of objective markers of ischaemia in these patients (Crea 2003; Kaski 2004).

Non-ischaemic mechanisms

Abnormal pain perception

According to Valeriani et al. (2005) enhanced pain sensitivity is a feature of patients with cardiac SX but the reasons for this remain unclear (Lanza and Crea 2002). Increased chest pain perception, induced by either mechanical or pharmacological means, has been shown to be proportionately higher in patients with cardiac SX (Kaski et al. 2004). Alterations in potassium and adenosine ionic pumps appear to be one explanation for heightened chest pain perception in these patients. The abnormal reaction of the central nervous system in responding to specific afferent stimuli has likewise been considered to influence the level of pain perceptions. It is hypothesised that the 'thalamic gate' which regulates the response to such stimuli may be ineffective in cardiac SX patients, therefore allowing a stream of afferent heart signals to reach and activate the cortex causing increased pain perception (Rosen et al. 2002). Crea and Lanza (2004), however, argue that cardiac rather than cortical abnormalities are central to this debate.

Autonomic nervous system imbalance

This theory suggests that cardiac SX patients have an imbalance in autonomic system responses, which account for changes in endothelial functioning, pain sensitivity and other cardiovascular findings (Kaski et al. 2004). This hypothesis is underdeveloped and remains questionable. To date there is no consensus over the exact mechanisms behind the chest pain experienced in cardiac syndrome X.

Clinical presentation

The majority of people admitted or referred to out-patient clinics with chest pain attributed to cardiac SX are post-menopausal women. The nature of the pain, pattern of location, precipitating factors and electrocardiographic ST segment depression characteristics make it almost impossible to differentiate from CHD (Kaski et al. 2004). In these patients chest pain can be provoked by physical activity whilst others may have symptoms at rest. The pain can be long in duration; however, response to nitrates is ineffective (Crea and Lanza 2004). As with women with a history of CHD, patients with cardiac SX may also present with increased dyspnoea on exertion.

History taking

As the primary symptom is chest pain, the focus of history taking should be to rule out evidence of cardiac ischaemia, specifically an acute myocardial infarction. Careful history taking should help to eliminate other plausible causes which may explain the symptoms, for example vasospastic angina. Some patients may deny or minimise the significance of their symptoms, therefore consulting family members and friends is also vital. Since over half of women with underlying CHD present with a vague and unspecific history of symptoms (see Chapter 7), it is important to have a high level of suspicion for either an acute coronary event or cardiac syndrome X, particularly if the patient is post-menopausal. If chest pain occurs at rest but without a positive response to sublingual nitrates, the possibility of cardiac SX should be considered.

Clinical examination

There may be no unusual or abnormal findings in the physical examination of patients with cardiac SX. Physical signs may only be present if the patient has hypertension, or is diabetic or overweight. The systematic and comprehensive approach described in Chapter 4 that includes the gender-specific issues outlined in Chapter 7 remains applicable.

High levels of anxiety, depression, panic disorder, hostility, paranoia and neuroticism have been identified in patients with cardiac SX, which in part may be attributed to the lack of a firm diagnosis (Asbury and Collins 2005). Additionally, fears of a recurrence of cardiac pain may fuel anxiety, resulting in greater disability and concern over cardiovascular health. Health professionals need to recognise and respond appropriately by referring patients to relevant specialists.

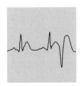

Initial investigations

Initial investigations must include those that apply to the patient presenting with acute chest pain suspicions of CHD (see Chapter 6).

Exercise testing

A positive exercise stress test is of limited value as it is potentially misleading, particularly in the absence of other investigations. It should be noted that ST segment elevation is rare in patients with this syndrome.

Echocardiograms

The approach to cardiac syndrome X is a 'rule out' process, where the presence of normal coronary angiograms forms the basis for the diagnosis. However, reliance on coronary angiography as a diagnostic criterion may be of limited value, since it offers little information on early atherosclerotic changes within the arterial walls (Kaski et al. 2004). Nevertheless, it will exclude angiographically significant stenoses and therefore the findings can assist in treatment decisions. Testing patients with angina at rest with intravenous ergonovine is helpful in excluding occlusive coronary artery spasm (Crea and Lanza 2004). Angina-induced symptoms and ST segment changes, provoked by pharmacological or physical techniques and assessed through echocardiography (stress echo), may be more helpful in excluding angina and epicardial coronary stenoses. Instead this investigation may positively suggest a microvascular origin to the symptoms.

Differential diagnosis

The spectrum of causes precipitating an onset of chest pain is varied, because cardiac syndrome X mimics the symptoms of CHD, although cases of the former tend to be of younger age and mainly women (Mirza 2005). Diagnosing patients with cardiac SX poses a unique challenge, although the following causes of chest pain must be eliminated as possible diagnoses:

- Coronary heart disease
- Prinzmetal angina
- Cardiomyopathy
- Oesophageal spasm
- Costochondritis
- Fibromyalgia

Immediate management and interventions

Due to its similarities to myocardial ischaemia, cardiac syndrome X is a challenge and represents a 'diagnostic and therapeutic riddle' (Kaski 2004: 568). The management of cardiac SX is as complex as the pathophysiology which defines this syndrome. In the immediate stages symptom control is important; however, to date the value of many medications used in CHD is far from proven in patients with cardiac SX.

- Beta-blockers have been reported to have some modest benefit in reducing anginal symptoms and exercise test findings if given as a monotherapy. Beta-blockers should be considered first-line therapy unless contraindicated. Imipramine has been found to decrease anginal attacks in patients with chest pain and normal coronary arteries because it decreases pain transmission to visceral tissues (Crea and Lanza 2004). However, because of its undesirable side effects it may impair patients' quality of life.
- Trials of nitrates have demonstrated that they may only be effective in around 50% of patients with cardiac SX. As such they have limited use in the acute setting (Crea and Lanza 2004; Kaski et al. 2004). However, the contribution of long-acting nitrates remains controversial owing to the lack of large and well controlled studies.
- Angiotensin converting enzyme inhibitors (ACE) have been considered as useful due to their ability to affect coronary vasomotor tone by interfering with sympathetic activity. Recent findings suggest that, in those with cardiac SX, enalapril improves microvascular function by provoking NO availability (Crea and Lanza 2004; Kaski et al. 2004).

- Oestrogen administration also improves pain relief and coronary dilatation in patients with cardiac SX by manipulating endothelial behaviour. However, the increased risk of cardiovascular disease and breast cancer identified in a number of clinical trials (Hulley et al. 1998; Herrington et al. 2000) has limited the use of hormone replacement therapy in individuals where a clear relationship exists between oestrogen deficiency and the syndrome (Kaski et al. 2004).
- Statin use seems to be beneficial in reducing cholesterol levels, increasing exercise tolerance and improving systemic blood flow by enhancing the effects of endothelial vasodilator functioning (Kayilcioglu et al. 2003; Fabian et al. 2004). The aggressive use of lipid lowering therapies is recommended (Kaski 2004).
- Aminophylline derivatives have been shown to have positive effects on symptom and exercise test results, although these are not well tolerated. Administration of oral or intravenous aminophylline-based drugs blocks the effects of adenosine which trigger anginal pain in cardiac SX patients (Crea and Lanza 2004).

Medium- to long-term management plan

The aggressive management of risk factors is one key element of the long-term treatment plan. However, because of the debilitating nature of this condition and the recurrence of chest pain, many patients may develop emotional problems or have unresolved concerns which need to be managed. This may be achieved by a follow-up appointment after their cardiac clinic to explore conceptions of illness (Gurjinder et al. 2001) and by referral to specialist services (Kaski et al. 2004; Asbury and Collins 2005).

- Stress reduction, relaxation therapy, transcendental meditation and cognitive behavioural therapy are interventions which in cardiac SX patients produce significant improvements in symptom severity, frequency of pain attacks and decreased psychological morbidity (Asbury and Collins 2005), although some patients may also benefit from anti-depressants or mild sedation.
- Physical tolerance is normally impaired in cardiac SX patients. Regular exercise can increase physical capacity and improve pain thresholds. Whilst cardiac SX patients may not be routinely offered cardiac rehabilitation, the philosophy of exercise and appropriate support mechanisms are important factors optimising feelings of well-being.
- Transcutaneous electrical nerve stimulation (TENS) and spinal cord stimulation may be a viable alternative method of pain control (Kaski 2004).

COCAINE MISUSE

Background

In the past 5000 years, cocaine has been widely used for recreational and medicinal purposes (Erwin and Deliargyris 2002). It is one of the most common illicit drugs used, and owing to its adverse effects on the central nervous and cardio-vascular systems it causes the majority of drug-related deaths. Cocaine-related deaths from overdose are rare; most occur following prolonged misuse as a result of adverse molecular, cellular and tissue derangements (Karch 2005). Men aged 18 to 45 years comprise the highest known user group, although estimates suggest that 11% of the population in the United Kingdom have experimented with this drug at some point in their life (Egred and Davis 2005). Cocaine abuse is also more prevalent amongst unemployed and unskilled workers. Within Europe, the UK tops the league for cocaine use with the number of misuse offences rising from 1500 in 1994 to 8000 in 2004 (Sadler 2006). Estimates in the United States suggest that 25 million Americans have experimented at least once with cocaine, 3.7 million have used it in the past seven months, and the number of regular users now exceeds 1.5 million (Erwin and Deliargyris 2002; Kloner and Rezkalla 2003; Jones and Weir 2005). Consequently, the number of patients presenting to emergency departments (ED) with cardiac complications linked to cocaine misuse has risen. A recent report suggests that half of patients aged less than 40 years who were admitted with chest pain to one London ED during Friday and Saturday nights had cocaine within their circulation (Sadler 2006). Trends suggest that levels of misuse are increasing due to reduced costs, wider availability and misconceptions among the young about the low risks associated with such drugs. This may account for the current rise in health problems among this group (Lange and Hillis 2001). The immediate and pro-found euphoric effects explain cocaine's appeal and its addictive potential.

Routes and onset of effects

Cocaine can be smoked, inhaled nasally or injected intravenously, all of which produce powerful euphoric effects. In addition, because it is absorbed by mucus membranes, it may be applied to the genitalia. Typically, there is a rapid onset of action of 3 to 5 minutes with effects lasting for about an hour (Lange and Hillis 2001). Depending on the route, its onset of action, peak effect and duration of action will vary. Inhalation of cocaine has the shortest onset, peak effect and longest duration of action, intravenous and intranasal routes have between 20–90 minute duration of action, whereas the effects when taken orally can last for up to 3 hours. If cocaine is mixed with alcohol, it creates the compound cocaethyl-ene, which significantly increases the risk of death (Egred and Davies 2005).

Pharmacology

Cocaine is an alkaloid extract prepared from the leaves of the *Erythroxylon coca* plant (Lange and Hillis 2001), which has been used in medicine for over 150 years for its anaesthetic and analgesic properties. There are two forms of cocaine:

• Cocaine hydrochloride is made by dissolving the drug in hydrochloric acid which forms a water-soluble white powder, crystals or granules that will decompose when heated. Cocaine in this form may be prepared for administration via sublingual, intra-vaginal or rectal routes.

● Freebase or crack cocaine is manufactured by mixing cocaine hydrochloride with baking soda and water. This from of 'pure' cocaine is regarded as one of the most potent and addictive illicit drugs available (Erwin and Deliargyris 2002; Egred and Davis 2005).

Cocaine has two mechanisms of action. Initially, it works by inhibiting cellular sodium transport by blocking fast sodium channels resulting in membrane stabilisation and a local anaesthetic effect. As such, it is not too dissimilar to Class I anti-arrhythmic agents. The secondary action is a noticeable increase of catecholamine activity at the synaptic level, prompting marked sympathetic activation. This process is achieved by the augmented release and blocked reuptake of adrenaline, noradrenaline and dopamine (Erwin and Deliargyris 2002). It is the rapid and steep increase of these catecholamines which is responsible for the stimulation of α- and β-receptor sites that leads to a series of clinical manifestations.

The combined reactions to catecholamine release in the cardiovascular system include increased myocardial workload and oxygen consumption, coronary artery vasoconstriction, increased heart rate, vascular resistance and an elevated systolic blood pressure. In patients with pre-existing coronary heart disease (CHD), vasoconstriction is more likely to occur in stenotic regions and therefore magnifies their risks for myocardial ischaemia. Cocaine can also stimulate increased platelet aggregation and potentiate thromboxane production which may precipitate thrombus formation (Mittleman et al. 1999; Erwin and Deliargyris 2002). Long-term cocaine use has been linked with intimal hyperplasia and endothelial dysfunction which collectively may accelerate the early onset of atherosclerosis (Erwin and Deliargyris 2002; Karch 2005).

Clinical presentation

Since cocaine has immediate effects, users tend to present early with a sudden onset of chest pain. Most patients are male, smoke tobacco and have an average age of 38 years (Mittlemann et al. 1999; Weber et al. 2003). However, cocaine misuse is also common in women, the elderly and ethnic minority groups (Wasilow-Mueller and Erickson 2001; Weber et al. 2003; McGrath et al. 2005). Chest pain after cocaine-use occurs in 50–57% of patients and is often associated with episodes of dizziness (Egred and Davis 2005). Additionally, 56% may present with dyspnoea, 32% may report clammy sensations and 28% nausea (Erwin and Deliargyris 2002). Around half have had previous episodes of chest pain, described as sharp in nature and radiating to the shoulders. Despite these observations, the incidence of cocaine-induced non-fatal myocardial infarction (MI) is small, ranging between 6 and 30% (Qureshi et al. 2001; Carley et al. 2003; Weber et al. 2003). The risk for MI is highest in the first hours after cocaine intake, although patients remain vulnerable for adverse cardiac events for up to 12 hours. Importantly, there is no clear relationship between the dose of cocaine and the incidence of adverse cardiac events. Indeed myocardial complications can be induced among first-time and long-term users alike (Karch 2005).

Regardless of administration route, significant cardiac disorders associated with cocaine intoxication include: myocardial ischaemia, ventricular dysrhythmias and congestive heart failure. However, to accurately diagnose cocaine-induced myocardial infarction is problematic, partly because of interpretation difficulties with the electrocardiogram (ECG) (Egred and Davis 2005). Additionally, some patients who have used cocaine may present with unexplained syncope or rhythm disturbances but because they have no definitive ECG or radiographic abnormalities are at risk of being misdiagnosed (Nallamothu et al. 2001). History taking and clinical examination are therefore essential to diagnosis.

The major changes triggered from regular use of cocaine involve:

- Cardiac dysrhythmias: these are short-lived, occur mainly in the first 6 hours post cocaine use and may involve asystole, ventricular fibrillation, bradycardias, tachycardias and torsade des pointes
- Dilated cardiomyopathy, which is caused by a combination of myofibril destruction, interstitial fibrosis and wall dilatation, in addition to the sustained effects of circulating catecholamines
- Left ventricular hypertrophy
- Myocarditis: this commonly occurs in 20–30% of cocaine users
- Cerebrovascular events
- Aortic dissection, commonly seen with use of crack cocaine

Although the above list relates to the cardiovascular system, drug abuse has a number of negative consequences for the social and general health of individuals, resulting in sexually transmitted diseases, mental health disorders, engagement in criminal activities and unplanned pregnancies.

History taking

Most authors suggest that male patients presenting with chest pain, who smoke and are under the age 40 years, should be suspected of misusing cocaine and therefore should be questioned about their drug habits (Erwin and Deliargyris 2002; Egred and Davis 2005). This needs to be done after careful consideration involving evaluation of signs and symptoms as well data from clinical examination and history taking. Karch (2005) adds that blood screening for cocaine toxicity is unreliable; in such circumstances disclosure of cocaine usage is most valuable. However, there is reticence and reluctance among health professionals to question suspected patients during examination (Hollander et al. 1998). Conversely, patients may be reluctant to admit using illegal substances for fear of prosecution, and may therefore need to be reassured that any disclosures regarding drug misuse will remain confidential.

Table 15.1 CAGE questionnaire: screening for alcohol or drug misuse. Adapted from Ewing (1984).

1. Have you ever felt you should **Cut down** on your drinking or drug use?
2. Have people **Annoyed** you by criticising or complaining about your drinking or drug use?
3. Have you ever felt bad or **Guilty** about your drinking or drug use?
4. Have you ever had a drink or drug in the morning (**Eye opener**) to steady your nerves?

Additional question
5. Do you use any drugs apart from those prescribed by your physician?

Screening tools, for example the CAGE questionnaire for adults (see Table 15.1) and Community Reinforcement and Family Training (CRAFT) for adolescents comprise a series of questions designed to ascertain clinical warning signs of drug misuse that could be integrated into history taking in suspected individuals where no immediate explanation can be attributed to their chest pain symptom (Kaye 2004; McGrath et al. 2005). However, some patients may arrive in A&E departments in an unconscious state and this delays diagnosis (Attaran et al. 2005). Other areas that should be explored entail history of misuse, such as frequency, quantity and usual pattern of use. The social history should be directed at examining relationships, social networks, housing situation and evidence of substance misuse within the patient's family.

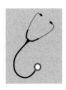

Clinical examination

A detailed clinical examination of the patient may highlight the tell-tale signs of cocaine abuse. The presence of physical changes may depend on how cocaine was administered and whether the patient is a habitual user. To avoid arousing suspicion some patients may attempt to disguise their mode of ingestion by refusing to have a physical examination or to cooperate with staff.

- Specific physical signs may include new venepuncture sites, track marks, nasal irritation, nasal septum damage, unexplained bruising, enamel erosion of the front teeth from wiping residue across the mouth, and callus formation on thumbs due to lighter overuse (see Figure 15.1). Other effects identified may be increased temperature, unexplained weight loss, seizures and damage to some mucous membranes, for example of the vagina and anus.
- Generally patients with cocaine intoxication may exhibit anxiety with feelings of paranoia, hyperactivity, agitated behaviour and changes in personality (Bonomo and Proimos 2005). Others may have persecutory delusions, auditory and visual hallucinations and aggression that could well be confused with psychiatric disorders.

Bonomo and Proimos (2005) add that physical examination should include assessing for evidence of drug withdrawal, which may also include sweating, cramps, rhinorrhea and dilated pupils.

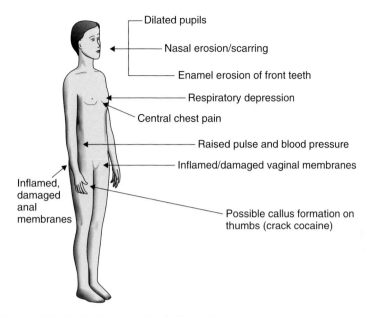

Figure 15.1   Possible physical examination findings of cocaine users.

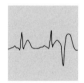

Initial investigations

As with other causes of chest pain, specific clinical investigations may help with the differential diagnosis, although occasionally they may cloud or confuse the situation.

Electrocardiogram

Up to 70% of patients with a history of cocaine misuse and recent onset of chest pain have abnormal or non-specific ECG changes for the diagnosis of MI (Erwin and Deliargyris 2002). Within the patient population there is also a high incidence of early repolarisation and left ventricular hypertrophy, making the ECG difficult to interpret (Kloner and Rezkalla 2003; Egred and Davis 2005). Some patients may even have ST elevation but without MI, thus stress testing may be indicated unless serum troponin levels suggest otherwise (Weber et al. 2003).

If an MI does occur, this is most likely to involve the anterior surface due to occlusion of the left anterior descending artery. This is the most frequently affected vessel among cocaine users (Egred and Davis 2005; Karch 2005). In those who develop ventricular hypertrophy, QT prolongation/dispersion is a potential complication which may cause torsade des pointes. QTc changes may also be present due to changes in cardiac automaticity generated from cocaine use (Karch 2005). The development of torsade des pointes is a rare form of ventricular tachycardia that is described as polymorphic because there is wide beat-to-beat variation in the QRS morphology, alternating every 5–20 beats along the baseline (Albarran 2005).

Radiology

A chest x-ray in these patients may not reveal any significant abnormalities unless aortic dissection or pericardial bleeding have developed secondary to regular intake of cocaine.

Laboratory tests

Serum CK MB level is an unreliable marker for myocardial injury in these patients, as it may be elevated due to muscle injury vasomotor activity or unusually as a result of rhabdomyolosis (Erwin and Deliagyris 2002; McCann et al. 2002). Troponin I and T assays are more sensitive and specific for detecting those with evolving changes and who progress to MI (see Chapter 6). In patients suspected of substance misuse, urine testing may be an effective way of screening for the presence or absence of cocaine metabolites and other drugs taken in recent days (Bonomo and Proimos 2005).

Differential diagnosis

Patients who present with specific demographics that include young age, male gender and minimal evidence of coronary heart disease risks, need to be carefully assessed. As noted in previously, a history of sudden chest pain in those below the age of 40 years can be attributed to a number of causes, making differential diagnosis a challenge. Cocaine use needs to be discriminated against the following:

- Acute coronary syndromes
- Acute myocardial infarction
- Aortic dissection
- Cardiomyopathy
- Brady/tachyarrhythmias
- Myocardial ischaemia
- Acute pericarditis/myocarditis
- Sudden cardiac death

Immediate management and interventions

This largely depends on the condition of the patient, and whether there is a risk of respiratory arrest. In bradypnoeic patients, naloxone should be administered intravenously and in those with evidence of ventricular dysrhythmias, intravenous lignocaine or amioderone should be administered (Attaran et al. 2005). Immediate care should encompass oxygen therapy, continuous ST segment monitoring (Weber et al. 2003) and access to resuscitation equipment. Additionally, the recommended first-line management approach for cocaine-intoxicated patients who have ECG changes includes the following:

- Aspirin should be considered for its anti-platelet properties in preventing thrombus formation. Heparin should be added to maintain anti-thrombotic state.

- Benzodiazepines are recommended as primary therapy for patients with hypertension, tachycardia and/or anxiety because of their effects in reducing cardiovascular and central nervous system toxicity (Jones and Weir 2005).
- Nitroglycerine IV or sublingually has cardiac and systemic effects on vascular tone, reversing the vasoconstrictive effects of cocaine and easing chest pain symptoms. As such, nitrates are beneficial in this group of patients (Jones and Weir 2005).
- In the acute stage blood pressure control poses difficulties because the administration of beta-blockers may augment existing vasoconstriction and therefore should be avoided (Egred and Davis 2005; Jones and Weir 2005). Intravenous calcium channel blockers, such as verapamil and α-blockade with phentolamine are recommended as second-line treatment options, as both decrease the rise in mean arterial pressure triggered by cocaine (Braunwald et al. 2002; Erwin and Deliargyris 2002; Attaran et al. 2005; Egred and Davis 2005).
- The use of thrombolytics remains controversial as the hypertensive effects of cocaine misuse increase the risk of intracranial haemorrhage. Thrombolytics should only be administered if there are signs and symptoms of an evolving MI, when initial interventions have been ineffective. Primary angioplasty may be an option for patients with a high systolic blood pressure and where thrombolysis is contraindicated.

Further investigations

The findings of one study indicate that patients with cocaine-associated chest pain who do not have evidence of ischaemia during an initial 12-hour observation period, have a low risk for MI in the first 30 days and therefore may be safely discharged after this time (Weber et al. 2003).

Medium- to long-term management plan

Cocaine dependence is a relapsing, chronic disorder and the long-term implication is the acceleration of atherosclerosis. Referral to a drug rehabilitation unit or to a residential drug withdrawal programme may be appropriate when supported by counselling and cognitive behaviour therapy (Hollander 1995; Bonomo and Proimos 2005). Pharmacological alternatives include the drug Disulfiram, which also appears to be effective in reducing cocaine abuse. Clinical trials of other drugs including Baclofen, Topiramate, Modafinil and Naltrexone have produced some encouraging results but further studies are needed to validate preliminary findings (Vocci and Elkashef 2005).

HERPES ZOSTER

Background

Herpes zoster is an acute infectious disease caused by the varicella zoster virus (shingles), which is spread by secretions from the respiratory tract (Reisz et al. 1998; Lovitt 2003). The incidence of herpes zoster increases with advancing age, for example 80% of cases involve those older than 20 years and up to half of people over 85 years of age become infected with this virus (Johnson and Dworkin 2003; Melton 2005). Within the population, the incidence rises from 1/1000 person years in children to 12/1000 person years in those aged 65 years or older (Melton 2005). Despite these figures, the incidence of herpes zoster has, however, fallen dramatically, particularly since the advent of mass vaccination (Moon and Hospenthal 2006). There is minimal difference between the genders, although it is 25% more prevalent among Caucasians despite exposure to chicken-pox (Melton 2005). Mortality is low, although immunocompromised patients who develop herpes zoster are at greater risk of death.

Causes

People with reduced cell immunity are at greatest risk of herpes zoster, although the exact mechanisms remain unclear (Johnson and Dworkin 2003; Melton 2005). Such people include those with HIV infections, individuals with certain forms of malignancy, transplant recipients receiving immunosuppressant therapy, and those being treated with either radiotherapy, chemotherapy, or high dose steroid therapy (Johnson and Dworkin 2003; Humphreys and Irving 2004). Trauma, including surgery, may also reactivate the varicella zoster virus (VZV), as can psychological stress and bacterial infections. Specifically, VZV can have serious implications for those with encephalitis and pneumonia. However, the most common complication in immunocompetent adult patients is *post-herpetic neuralgia*, which is characterised by pain that continues for months and even years (Melton 2005).

Pathophysiology

Most people infected with a primary varicella virus (Chicken-pox) carry the varicella zoster virus (VZV), but it may remain inactive for decades. This is due to the acquired cell-mediated immunity accumulated from the primary infection and by repeated storing by the immune system. The mechanism reactivating the VZ virus is unknown, but a deficiency in virus-specific immune response is considered significant (Lovitt 2003). Once the primary infection has been acquired, the virus journeys along sensory nerve fibres until it reaches the satellite cells of dorsal root ganglia where it becomes dormant or permanently inactive (Moon and Hospenthal 2006). Reactivation of dormant viruses in some individuals can cause inflammation of sensory nerves like the dorsal (thoracic) root and cranial nerve ganglia causing herpes zoster. Consequently, pain may be located across the chest and in parts of the face.

Herpes zoster begins with inflammation of the sensory ganglia and peripheral nerves resulting in hypersensitivity and abnormal sensations along the affected nerve (Harke et al. 2002). A vesicular rash in a single dermatome follows, leading to the development of skin lesions. In around half of all cases of herpes zoster the thoracic nerve root is involved (Fallon and Jaime 1997). In particular, T4 dermatomal distribution embraces the anterior chest wall and so patients will typically present with chest pain or distressing pain sensations across the chest

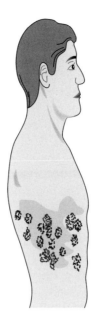

Figure 15.2 Distribution of herpes zoster rash across the trunk.

(Reisz et al. 1998). Because the affected nerve is situated in the trunk, a band-like rash with fluid-filled blisters across either the right or left of the chest/arm (see Figure 15.2) or in the abdomen will appear three to five days after pain sensations (Lovitt 2003; Moon and Hospenthal 2006).

Improvements in understanding have led to revised definitions of pain that persists beyond blister resolution, currently termed post-herpetic neuralgia, and a spectrum of symptoms that comprise:

- Acute herpetic neuralgia occurring within 30 days of the rash onset
- Sub-acute herpetic neuralgia exceeding the acute phase, but resolving within a 120-day timescale
- Post-herpetic neuralgia, which presents 120 days following rash onset; this is rare and affects between 10 and 15% of sufferers (Dubinsky et al. 2004; Jung et al. 2004).

Post-herpetic neuralgia occurs in approximately 10–15% of all patients with shingles but most commonly in those over 60 years of age. This may become chronic in those who experienced intense pain prior to and during the eruptive stage (Johnson and Dworkin 2003; Lovitt 2003; Jung et al. 2004).

Clinical presentation

In the pre-eruptive stage patients will initially complain of skin irritation and pain in the affected dermatome (Moon and Hospenthal 2006). In 50% of cases the infected nerve involves the dorsal root, therefore patients may report tightening, tearing, aching, tingling or itching sensations along one side of the chest.

Distribution of pain can extend to the upper limbs and abdominal regions. Complaints of malaise, headaches, fever and myalgia prior to the development of blisters are common and therefore during this phase there is the potential for misdiagnosis (Lovitt 2003; Melton 2005). The post-eruptive phase occurs three to five days or more after the onset of pain, when erythematous lesions appear and begin to erupt.

History taking

History taking is an important step in identifying the cause of virus reactivation. The virus may be the primary manifestation for a number of diseases, resulting in an immuno-deficient state.

Investigation into the underlying trigger is therefore essential (Humphreys and Irving 2004). Symptoms such as malaise, low-grade fever, headaches and fatigue may need to be carefully evaluated (Melton 2005). Moon and Hospenthal (2006) suggest that an immunocompromised status may be suggestive in patients younger than 50 years of age, therefore evidence of HIV needs to be assessed for and eliminated. Additionally, information concerning contact with infected adults or children may prove an important clue.

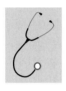

Clinical examination

On examination the patient may be tender over the thoracic region; regional lymph nodes may be enlarged and tender. This tenderness will be distributed along the affected dermatome(s) and manifests itself prior to the development of blisters which are usually distributed across one side of the trunk (Humphreys and Irving 2004). The blisters may become erythematous, vesicular, pustular and crusted over, reflecting the stage of the disease (Melton 2005; Moon and Hospenthal 2006). If viral reactivation affects the central nervous system, corneal ulcers, conjunctivitis, cranial and peripheral facial nerve palsies and confusion could be present during physical examination (Johnson and Dworkin 2003). Additionally, there may be evidence of muscular weakness, diaphragmatic wall paralysis and neurogenic bladder.

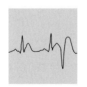

Initial investigations

In patients with herpes zoster the history and clinical findings should be sufficient to confirm the diagnosis. Electrocardiogram and chest x-ray should help eliminate other causes. Occasionally the presentation of herpes zoster can be atypical, and specific investigations may be required, especially for those who are immunosuppressed (Melton 2005). If the presence of a rash and its pattern suggest a clear diagnosis, virology studies must be performed. The virus may be detected in vesicle fluid by electron microscopy (Humphreys and Irving 2004). A Tzanck smear can also be obtained from the vesicular lesions but this will not discriminate between varicella zoster virus infections, for example herpes zoster and herpes simplex (Melton 2005). If available, modern tests such as direct immunofluorescence with fluorescein-tagged antibody (DFA) are preferred because of their higher specificity and sensitivity (Moon and Hospenthal 2006).

Differential diagnosis

Virology studies, history taking and clinical examination will help elucidate the diagnosis. However, chest pain associated with the herpes zoster virus may suggest a variety of differential diagnoses that may include:

- Pleurisy
- Myocardial infarction
- Cholecystitis
- Appendicitis
- Renal colic
- Varicella myocarditis (very rarely, Alter et al. 2001).

Immediate management and interventions

The initial aim of medical therapy in herpes zoster infections is to provide effective analgesia, relieve symptoms, shorten the clinical course of the disease, prevent complications, and decrease incidence of post-herpetic neuralgia and spread of infection (Melton 2005; Moon and Hospenthal 2006). As herpes zoster infections can be extremely painful, immediate treatment with either non-steroidal anti-inflammatory drugs or opiate-based analgesics may be used (Johnson and Dworkin 2003; Melton 2005). Additionally, recommended management includes the following:

- Topical therapy, such as calamine lotion and antipruritic creams, can be used to relieve itching sensations caused by the rash and blisters.
- Antiviral therapy appears to be most effective if administered within the first 72 hours of symptoms. Acyclovir, for example, may prevent post-herpetic neuralgia and reduce the duration and intensity of cutaneous symptoms (Dubinsky et al. 2004) by speeding up the healing of skin lesions (Johnson and Dworkin 2003).
- In those at risk for post-herpetic neuralgia, corticosteroids may be used with antiviral agents to accelerate resumption of quality of life to pre-infection levels.

Further investigation

Additional investigations are rare unless the patient presents with an atypical skin lesion, in which case biopsy may be indicated.

Medium- to long-term management plan

Around 20% of patients older than 50 years will suffer with some degree of persistent chest pain for up to six months following rash onset and treatment. Post-herpetic neuralgia must be considered as a continuum in the management of herpes zoster. Specific interventions such as ketamine gel and pregabalin have some therapeutic benefits (Lovitt 2003). Amitriptyline is also effective in decreasing the chronic pain symptoms of herpes zoster (Dubinsky et al. 2004). Likewise the anti-epileptic drug gabapentin and 5% lidocaine patches have been demonstrated to be effective alternative forms of pain relief but without unpleasant side effects (Johnson and Dworkin 2003; Dubinsky et al. 2004).

Key learning points

Cardiac syndrome X

- Cardiac syndrome X is characterised by a triad of symptoms including angina-like chest pain, exercise-induced ST segment depression and angiographically normal coronary arteries.
- Post-menopausal women are most at risk for this syndrome.
- Patients with cardiac SX are vulnerable to high levels of psychiatric and psychological morbidity.
- The causes of cardiac SX are not fully understood and are controversial.
- Symptom control and lipid lowering therapies are recommended for reducing anginal symptoms and their frequency and for improving health status.
- Prevention of psychiatric and psychological morbidity must be integral to ensure that the patient's quality of life is optimal.

Cocaine use

- Cocaine misuse occurs across a wide spectrum of society but is most common in men aged 18–45 years who are tobacco smokers.
- The main symptom of cocaine use is chest pain which may radiate to the left shoulder with a risk for adverse cardiac complications occurring within the first hour after intake.
- Focused questioning, use of specific assessment tools and clinical examination will help inform the differential diagnosis.
- Benzodiazepines, nitrates and aspirin are recommended first-line interventions.
- Rehabilitation options of behavioural modification and drug therapy should be considered for the long-term management and secondary prevention treatment.

Herpes zoster

- Herpes zoster is the reactivation of the virus that causes the childhood disease of chicken-pox, which has remained dormant in the body, with immunosuppressed or immunocompromised patients most at risk.
- If the affected dermatome is located within the chest, sharp and intense pain may be reported within a strip of the front or/and back of the chest and upper abdomen, usually occurring within 3–5 days before rash appears.
- Treatment with anti-viral medication is most effective when initiated within 3 days of symptom onset.
- Topical therapy and analgesia (with opiates) is essential to relieve symptoms of pain and skin itching.
- Chronic pain or post-herpetic neuralgia is more common in the elderly and may require a combination of therapies to facilitate control.

References

Albarran JW (2005) Monitoring and assessing cardiac rhythms. In Moule P, Albarran JW (Eds) *Practical Resuscitation: Recognising and Responding.* Oxford, Blackwell Publishing.

Alter P, Grimm W, Maisch B (2001) Varicella myocarditis in an adult. *Heart* **85**: e2.

Asbury E, Collins P (2005) Psychological factors associated with non-cardiac chest pain and cardiac syndrome X. *Herz* **30**: 55–60.

Asbury E, Creed F, Collins P (2004) Distinct psychological differences between women with coronary heart disease and cardiac syndrome X. *European Heart Journal* **25**: 1695–1701.

Attaran R, Ragavan D, Probst A (2005) Cocaine-related myocardial infarction: concomitant heroin use can cloud the picture. *European Journal of Emergency Medicine* **12**: 199–201.

Bonomo Y, Proimos J (2005) ABC of adolescence. Substance misuse: alcohol, tobacco, inhalants and other drugs. *British Medical Journal* **330**: 777–780.

Braunwald E, Antman E, Beasley J (2002) ACC/AHA 2002 guideline update for the management of patients with unstable angina and non ST segment elevation infarction – summary article. A report of the American College of Cardiology/American Heart Association Task Force on Practice Guidelines (Committee on the Management of Patients with Unstable Angina). *Journal of the American College of Cardiology* **40**: 1366–1374.

Carley S, Ali B, Mackway-Jones K (2003) Acute myocardial infarction in cocaine induced chest pain presenting as an emergency. *Emergency Medical Journal* **20**: 174–175.

Crea F (2003) Prevalence, pathogenesis, diagnosis and treatment of cardiac syndrome X. *E-Journal of Cardiology Practice.* **1**(15): 1–2 www.escardio.org/knowledge/cardiology_practice/ejournal_vol1/vol1_no15.htm.

Crea F, Lanza G (2004) Angina pectoris and normal coronary arteries: cardiac syndrome X. *Heart* **90**: 457–463.

Desideri G, Gaspardone A, Gentile M, Santucci A, Gioffre P, Ferri C (2000) Endothelial activation in patients with cardiac syndrome X. *Circulation* **102**: 2359–2364.

Dubinsky RM, Kabbani H, El-Chami Z, Boutwell C, Ali H (2004) Practice parameters: treatment of postherpetic neuralgia: an evidence-based report of the Quality Standards Subcommittee of the American Academy of Neurology. *Neurology* **63**(6): 959–965.

Egred M, Davis G (2005) Cocaine and the heart. *Postgraduate Medical Journal* **81**: 568–571.

Erwin M, Deliargyris E (2002) Cocaine associated chest pain. *The American Journal of Medical Sciences* **324**(1): 37–43.

Ewing J (1984) Detecting alcoholism. The CAGE questionnaire. *Journal of the American Medical Association* **252**(14): 1905–1907.

Fabian E, Varga A, Picano E, Vajo Z, Ronaszeki A, Csanady M (2004) Effect of simvastatin on endothelial function in cardiac syndrome X patients. *American Journal of Cardiology* **94**(5): 652–655.

Fallon E, Jaime R (1997) Acute chest pain. *AACN Clinical Issues* **8**(3): 383–397.

Gurjinder N, Weinman J, Bass C, Chambers J (2001) Chest pain in people with normal coronary arteries. *British Medical Journal* **323**: 1319–1320.

Harke H, Gretenkort P, Ulrich H, Koester P, Rahman S (2002) Spinal cord stimulation in post herpetic acute herpes zoster pain. *Anesthetic Analgesia* **94**: 694–700.

Herrington D, Reboussin D, Brosniham K, Sharp PC, Shumaker SA, Snyder TE, Furberg CD, Kowalchuk GJ, Stuckey TD, Rogers WJ, Givens DH, Waters D (2000) Effects of estrogen replacement on the progression of coronary artery atherosclerosis. *New England Journal of Medicine* **343**: 522–529.

Hollander JE (1995) The management of cocaine associated myocardial ischaemia. *New England Journal of Medicine* **333**(19): 1267–1271.

Hollander JE, Brooks DE, Valentine SM (1998) Assessment of cocaine use in patients with chest pain syndromes. *Archives of Internal Medicine* **158**: 62–66.

Hulley S, Grady D, Bush T, Furberg C, Herrington D, Riggs B, Vittinghoff E (1998) Randomisation trial of oestrogen plus progestin for secondary prevention of coronary artery disease in post-menopausal women: Heart and Estrogen/Progestin Replacement Study (HERS) Research Group. *Journal of the American Medical Association* **280**: 605–613.

Humphreys H, Irving W (2004) *Problem Orientated Clinical Microbiology and Infection.* Oxford, Oxford University Press.

Johnson R, Dworkin R (2003) Treatment of herpes zoster and post herpetic neuralgia. *British Medical Journal* **326**: 748–750.

Jones JH, Weir WB (2005) Cocaine-associated chest pain. *Medical Clinics of North America* **89**: 1323–1342.

Jung B, Johnson R, Griffin D, Dworkin R (2004) Risk factors for post herpetic neuralgia in patients with herpes zoster. *Neurology* **62**: 1545–1551.

Karch S (2005) Cocaine cardiovascular toxicity. *Southern Medical Association Journal* **98**(8): 794–799.

Kaski J (2002) Overview of gender aspects of cardiac syndrome X. *Cardiovascular Research* **53**(3): 620–626.

Kaski J (2004) Pathophysiology and management of patients with chest pain and normal coronary arteriograms (cardiac syndrome X). *Circulation* **109**: 568–572.

Kaski J, Aldma G, Cosin-Sales J (2004) Cardiac syndrome X: diagnosis, pathogenesis and management. *American Journal of Cardiovascular Drugs* **4**(3): 179–194.

Kaye D (2004) Office recognition and management of adolescent substance abuse. *Current Opinion in Paediatrics* **16**: 532–541.

Kayikcioglu M, Payzin S, Yavuzgil O, Kultursay H, Levent H, Inan Soydan C (2003) Benefits of statin treatment in cardiac syndrome X. *European Heart Journal* **24**: 1999–2005.

Kloner RA, Rezkalla S (2003) Cocaine and the heart. *New England Journal of Medicine* **348**(6): 487–488.

Lange R, Hillis D (2001) Cardiovascular complication of cocaine use. *New England Journal of Medicine* **345**(5): 351–363.

Lanza G, Crea F (2002) The complex link between brain and heart in cardiac syndrome X. *Heart* **88**: 328–330.

Lovitt S (2003) Treatment of post herpetic neuralgia. *Neurology* **60**(8): 6–7.

Maseri A (2004) Women's ischaemic syndrome evaluation. *Circulation* **109**: e62-e63.

McCann B, Hunter R, McCann J (2002) Cocaine/heroin induced rhabdomyolysis and ventricular fibrillation. *Emergency Medical Journal* **19**: 265–265.

McGrath A, Crome P, Crome IB (2005) Substance misuse in the older population. *Postgraduate Medical Journal* **81**: 228–231.

Melton C (2005) Herpes zoster. *E-Medicine Journal.* http://www.emedicine.com/EMERG/topic823.htm (accessed 28th February 2006).

Mirza M (2005) Angina like pain and normal coronary arteries: uncovering cardiac symptoms which mimic CAD. *Postgraduate Medicine Online* **117**(5): 41–46.

Mittleman M, Mintzer D, Maclure M, Tofler G, Sherwood J, Muller J (1999) Triggering of myocardial infarction by cocaine. *Circulation* **99**: 2737–2741.

Moon JE, Hospenthal DR (2006) Herpes zoster. *E-Medicine Journal.* http://www.emedicine.com/MED/topic1007.htm (accessed 16th May 2006).

Nallamothu B, Saint S, Kollas TJ, Eagle K (2001) Of nicks and time. *New England Journal of Medicine* **345**(5): 359–363.

On Y, Park R, Hyon M, Kim S, Kwon Y (2005) Are low total serum antioxidant status and elevated levels of C reactive protein and monocyte chemotactic protein-1 associated with cardiac syndrome X? *Circulation* **69**(10): 1212–1217.

Pasqui A, Puccetti L, Di Renzo M, Bruni F, Camarri A, Palazzuoli A, Biagi F, Servi M, Bischeri D, Auteri A, Pastorelli M (2005) Structural and functional abnormality of systemic microvessels in cardiac syndrome X. *Nutrition Metabolism and Cardiovascular Diseases* **15**(1): 56–64.

Qureshi A, Suri F, Guterman L, Hokins N (2001) Cocaine use and the likelihood of non fatal myocardial infarction and stroke. *Circulation* **103**: 502–506.

Reisz W, Gregory BS, Robinson D (1998) Evaluating non traumatic chest pain. *Lippincotts Primary Care Practice* **2**(5): 455–471.

Rosen S, Paulesu E, Wise R, Camici P (2002) Central neural contribution to the perception of chest pain in cardiac syndrome X. *Heart* **87**: 513–519.

Sadler C (2006) Snowed under. *Nursing Standard* **20**(35): 22–24.

Schwartz L, Bourassa MG (2001) Evaluation of patients with chest pain and normal coronary angiograms. *Archives of Internal Medicine* **161**(15): 1825–1833.

Valeriani M, Sestito A, La Pera D, De Armas L, Infusino F, Maiese T, Sgueglia GA, Tonali PA, Crea F, Restuccia D, Lanza GA (2005) Abnormal cortical pain processing in patients with cardiac syndrome X. *European Heart Journal* **26**(10): 975–982.

Vocci FJ, Elkashef A (2005) Pharmacotherapy and their treatments for cocaine abuse and dependence. *Current Opinion in Psychiatry* **18**: 265–270.

Wasilow-Mueller S, Erickson CE (2001) Drug abuse and dependency: understanding gender differences in aetiology and management. *Journal of the American Pharmaceutical Association* **4**(1): 78–90.

Weber JE, Shofer FS, Larkin GL, Kalaria AS, Hollander JF (2003) Cocaine-associated chest pain in the emergency department. *New England Journal of Medicine* **348**: 10–17.

Useful websites

Cardiac syndrome X

http://www.postgradmed.com/issues/2005/05_05/mirza.htm
http://www.texasheartinstitute.org/HIC/Topics/Cond/CardiacSyndromeX.cfm

Cocaine-related

www.crimestatistics.org.uk- Home Office
http://www.nta.nhs.uk/frameset.asp?u=http://www.nta.nhs.uk/publications/
  research_briefing1b.htm National Treatment Agency for substance misuse
http://whitehousedrugpolicy.org/publications/factsht/cocaine/index.html
http://store.health.org/catalog/facts.aspx?topic=41 (US Drug and Health information)

Herpes zoster

www.IHMF.org
www.vzvfoundation.org
http://www.emedicine.com/MED/topic1007.htm

Index

Page numbers in italic refer to tables or figures.